KU-733-376

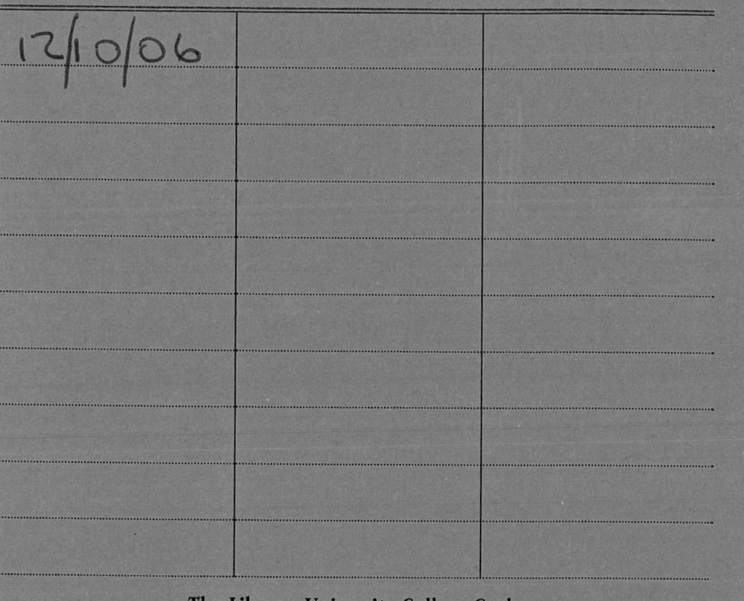
HEALTH SCIENCES LIBRARY, BROOKFIELD
COLÁISTE NA hOLLSCOILE CORCAIGH
Níl sé ceaduithe an leabhar seo a choimead thar an dáta is déanaí atá luaite thíos.
This book must be returned not later than the last date stamped below.
12/10/06
The Library, University College Cork
M.O. 21,204(a)

Global Inequalities at Work

Work's Impact on the Health of Individuals, Families, and Societies

Edited by

JODY HEYMANN, M.D., Ph.D.

OXFORD
UNIVERSITY PRESS
2003

OXFORD
UNIVERSITY PRESS

Oxford New York
Auckland Bangkok Buenos Aires Cape Town Chennai
Dar es Salaam Delhi Hong Kong Istanbul Karachi Kolkata
Kuala Lumpur Madrid Melbourne Mexico City Mumbai Nairobi
São Paulo Shanghai Taipei Tokyo Toronto

Published by Oxford University Press, Inc.
198 Madison Avenue, New York, New York 10016

http://www.oup-usa.org

Library of Congress Cataloging-in-Publication Data
Global inequalities at work :
work's impact on the health of individuals, families, and societies /
edited by Jody Heymann.
p. cm
Includes bibliographical references and index.
ISBN 0-19-515086-4
1. Industrial hygiene. I. Heymann, Jody, 1959–
RC967 .G56 2003 613.6'2—dc21 2002193005

2 4 6 8 9 7 5 3 1

Printed in the United States of America
on acid-free paper

The truth is that we are not yet free . . . We have not taken the final step of our journey, but the first step on a longer and even more difficult road. For to be free is not merely to cast off one's chains, but to live in a way that respects and enhances the freedom of others.

Nelson Mandela

To Tim and his global work

Acknowledgments

As I developed the ideas for, brought together expertise from around the world for, and edited *Global Inequalities at Work*, I was fortunate to have a number of people at my side. The book is far better for their contribution.

I decided from the start of this project that I didn't want to just bring together "the usual suspects." To ensure that individuals with new and fresh ideas had an opportunity to become part of this project, I cast the net wide. From the moment the net was cast through the 2 years of work that followed in carrying out this initiative, Patricia Carter of the Center for Society and Health served both as senior staff and logistical support. Her able help laid indispensable groundwork.

Soon after I conceived this project, I raised the idea of a book with Jeffrey House at Oxford University Press. His wisdom and guidance regarding the best way to develop a meaningful book out of this diverse and rich collaboration has both left an indelible mark on this book—and taught me a great deal for future ones.

It is true for all authors that their writing is strengthened by others turning a critical eye on it. In addition to my reviews and editorial comments, every chapter was carefully reviewed by Alison Earle. Her additional editorial eye was invaluable. Her critical insights improved countless aspects.

Authors faced the challenge of writing across linguistic and disciplinary bounds. Sharon Sharp helped edit the language so that the volume could speak with the more than a dozen different voices and perspectives it has but be accessible to readers. I am deeply grateful for her gifted work on this project.

The making of a book has craft to it as well as ideas, understanding, and writing. And part of the process of that craft is attending to the details from formatting manuscripts to checking references. I am particularly indebted to Stephanie Simmons, who patiently took on this task as her first job as a member of my team. The book you read reflects the care and quality of her work.

While they are thanked in the introduction to the text, particular thanks are due here to all the contributors to the volume. To the extent to which the book succeeds in being more than the sum of its parts, it owes a great debt to the individual authors who were willing to think beyond the boundaries of their own endeavors.

Neither last nor least, this initiative would not have been possible without the support of the Center for Society and Health at Harvard University, where I have served as Director of Policy. The support of the small faculty group that formed the Center with me at its start—Lisa Berkman, Ichiro Kawachi, and Nancy Krieger—as well as those who joined before the authors' conference—Norman Anderson and Laura Kubzansky—truly made the initiative both possible and far richer than it would have been without them.

As most people who have attempted this could tell you, pulling together a volume that spans regions and disciplines in a meaningful way turns out in the end to be far more work than you can ever imagine when undertaking the project. This project never would have been possible without the support and humor of close friends and family throughout.

Whatever nation you live in, if you read this book, you must already have decided that you care about people in parts of the world other than your own. Raised by parents whose commitments were both deep and wide-ranging—and who allowed mine to be—I had lived as a student in France, Iran, and Kenya, and worked in Tanzania and Mexico before Tim and I were married. He had been raised on a more local horizon but rapidly went global—from spending a honeymoon working together in a rural hospital in Gabon to leading programs to address infectious diseases worldwide. This book is dedicated to him and to everyone—no matter what their country of origin—who cares about the quality and dignity of life of *all* people.

Boston *J.H.*

Contents

About the Editor

JODY HEYMANN is Founder and Director of the *Project on Global Working Families* at Harvard University. This research program involves studies on the working conditions families face in five regions—North America, Europe, Latin America, Africa, and Asia. The project conducts in-depth studies of the impact of work and social conditions on the health and development of children, the care of the elderly and disabled, the ability of employed adults to obtain and retain work, and the ability of nations to decrease the number of families living in poverty. A member of the faculty at the Harvard School of Public Health and Harvard Medical School, Dr. Heymann is Director of Policy at the Harvard Center for Society and Health. Dr. Heymann has written extensively. Among dozens of other scholarly publications, her writing includes the recent book *The Widening Gap: Why America's Working Families Are in Jeopardy and What Can Be Done About It* (Basic Books 2000, 2002 paperback). Her articles have been published in the leading academic journals of many disciplines, including *Science, Pediatrics,* the *American Journal of Public Health,* the *Journal of the American Medical Association,* and the *American Economic Review.* She has served in an advisory capacity to the U.S. Senate Committee on Health, Education, Labor, and Pensions, the World Health Organization, and the U.S. Centers for Disease Control and Prevention, among other organizations. Dr. Heymann received her Ph.D. in public policy from Harvard University, where she was selected in a university-wide competition as a merit scholar, and her M.D. with honors from Harvard Medical School.

Contributors

PAVAN BAICHOO joined the International Labor Organization in 1997 to work on safety engineering, statistics, and ergonomics issues, and in 1999 drafted the ILO Guidelines on Occupational Safety and Health Management Systems (ILO-OSH 2001). He currently works in the ILO's program on Safety and Health at Work and the Environment, and serves as the chemical safety liaison with United Nations Environment Programme and as the officer concerned with issues surrounding the International Organization for Standardization (ISO).

MAYRA BUVINIC is Chief of the Social Development Division, Sustainable Development Department at the Inter-American Development Bank. Before joining the Bank in 1996, Ms. Buvinic was founding member and President of the International Center for Research on Women. Ms. Buvinic has published in the areas of poverty and gender, employment promotion, small enterprise development, reproductive health and, more recently, violence reduction.

LEONOR CEDILLO is currently leading the Risk Analysis program at the General Directorate of Environmental Health at the Federal Commission for the Protection of Sanitary Hazards of the Mexican Ministry of Health. She was founder of one of the first nongovernmental organizations in Mexico set up to collaborate with workers' organizations in evaluating and developing proposals for improving their occupational health conditions.

DAVID C. CHRISTIANI is Professor and Director of the Occupational Health Program in the Department of Environmental Health at the Harvard School of Public Health. His research interests are occupational, environmental, and molecular epidemiology. He has led major research projects in the respiratory field. Since the early 1980s, he has developed extensive cooperative ties with industrializing countries in Asia, Africa, and North America, and led and conducted many studies on environmental and occupational health in these countries.

MARINEL DALL'AGNOL is Associate Researcher in the Department of Social Medicine at the Federal University of Pelotas, Brazil. Her research is in the area of occupational epidemiology with an emphasis on child labor and health and the health of female workers. She has coordinated the Municipal Committee of the Child Labor Eradication Program.

CATALINA A. DENMAN is Senior Professor and Researcher at the Program on Health and Society at El Colegio de Sonora. Her research interests include women's health with an emphasis on working women, border health collaboration, and reproductive health. She was a founding member of the Red Fronteriza de Salud y Ambiente, a nongovermental organization initiated in 1992 to deal with improving environmental and health conditions in northern Mexico. She is Co-Coordinator of the Transborder Consortium for Research and Action on Women and Health at the United States–Mexico Border.

KIMBERLY ANN ELLIOTT is currently a Research Fellow at the Institute for International Economics and an adjunct professor at the Johns Hopkins School of Advanced International Studies. She has contributed to numerous books and articles on trade policy issues including international labor standards, the uses of economic leverage in international negotiations, and the causes and consequences of transnational corruption.

MICHAL ENGELMAN is a member of the Project on Global Working Families, led by Jody Heymann at the Harvard School of Public Health. She has analyzed data gathered by the Project from Mexico and Botswana, and launched the Project's most recent study in Russia. She has researched international comparative social policies and work and family issues including aging and eldercare, early childhood development in developing countries, and gender inequalities in education.

LUIZ A. FACCHINI is the Secretary of Health for the Municipality of Pelotas, State of Rio Grande do Sul, Brazil. Previously, he served as the Director of the Department of Social Medicine, Federal University of Pelotas. He has served as a consultant to the Pan American Health Organization (PAHO) and the Brazilian Council of Research among numerous other organizations. His research interests include occupational epidemiology, child labor and health, maternal work and child health, and women's work and health in agriculture and the food industry.

ANACLAUDIA FASSA is currently Chair of the Department of Social Medicine and Director of the Program of Occupational Epidemiology at the Federal University of Pelotas. Brazil. Her research interests include occupational epidemiology with an emphasis on child labor and health. She has served as consultant for the International Programme on the Elimination of Child Labour (ILO).

ARON FISCHER conducted research for the Project on Global Working Families. He analyzed qualitative and quantitative data from the Project's interviews in Mexico and Botswana and helped launch the Work, Family, and Democracy Initiative. He has researched global policy approaches to improving working conditions.

RICHARD B. FREEMAN currently holds the Ascherman Chair of Economics at Harvard University and is serving as Faculty Co-Chair of the Harvard University Trade Union Program. Professor Freeman is Program Director of the National Bureau of Economic Research Program in Labor Studies in the United States. He is also Co-Director of the Centre for Economic Performance at the London School of Economics. He has published extensively in labor economics and policy including the effects of immigration and trade on inequality, restructuring European states, and Chinese labor markets, among other areas.

ADEPEJU GBADEBO worked with the Project on Global Working Families to conduct interviews on the interactions between human immunodeficiency virus/acquired immunodeficiency syndrome and employment in Botswana. She has also researched health economics in the United States and co-authored "Economists on Academic Medicine" in the journal *Health Affairs.*

PARVIN GHORAYSHI is a Professor in the Department of Sociology at the University of Winnipeg, Canada. Her research interests include feminist theories and gender relations in developing countries, with a focus on the Middle East. She is the author of *Women and Work in Developing Countries* (1994) and coeditor of *Women, Work, and Gender Relations in Developing Countries: A Global Perspective* (1996). Her most recent publications appear in the *Canadian Journal of Development Studies, Women and Politics, Anthropologie et Sociétés,* and *Gender, Race and Nation: A Global Perspective.*

ANTONIO GIUFFRIDA is an Economist working at the Inter-American Development Bank on the design and implementation of health programs. He formerly worked at the Organisation for Economic Co-operation and Development (OECD), where he was responsible for an OECD Cross-National Study on Human Resources for Health Care. Prior to the OECD, he worked as a research fellow of the Centre for Health Economics at the University of York (UK).

AMANDA GLASSMAN is a Social Development Specialist at the Inter-American Development Bank providing technical assistance on projects and policies in the areas of health and social protection. Prior to working at the Bank, she was coordinator of the Latin America National Health Accounts Initiative at the Harvard School of Public Health and Population Reference Bureau Fellow at the U.S. Agency for International Development.

PETER GLICK is currently a Senior Research Associate with the Cornell University Food and Nutrition Policy Program. He has conducted research on such topics as the economics of health and schooling in developing countries, gender differences in employment earnings, health and employment interactions, and benefit incidence of public services in Africa.

SIOBÁN D. HARLOW serves as Associate Director of the International Institute and Associate Professor of Epidemiology at the University of Michigan. In collaboration with her Mexican colleagues, she has conducted research on the health status of female workers including projects focused on domestic workers, street vendors, and *maquiladora* workers. Her research focuses on understanding how life circumstances and biological processes unique to or more common among women influence their health status across the lifecourse.

ICHIRO KAWACHI is Professor of Health and Social Behavior and the Director of the Harvard Center for Society and Health at the Harvard School of Public Health. His research concerns the social and economic determinants of population health. He is the coeditor with Lisa Berkman of the first textbook on social epidemiology, published by Oxford University Press in 2000, as well as a forthcoming volume, *Neighborhoods and Health.* He is the Senior Editor of the journal *Social Science & Medicine.*

MARIA DE FÁTIMA MAIA is Associate Researcher in the Department of Social Medicine at the Federal University of Pelotas, Brazil. Her research in the area of occupational epidemiology focuses on child labor and health.

MARTHA MORROW is a Senior Lecturer at the Key Centre for Women's Health in Society, a multidisciplinary research and teaching center based within the School of Population Health at the University of Melbourne, Australia. Her research interests include social factors and health in developing countries and health promotion policy. Her teaching interests cover qualitative and rapid assessment research methods, social research for human immunodeficiency virus prevention, and health program evaluation methods.

STEPHEN PURSEY is Senior Advisor in the Office of the Director-General of the International Labor Organization. Before joining the Director-General's cabinet, he worked as chief economist for the International Confederation of Free Trade Unions (ICFTU) and in the International Labor Organization's International Policy Group, which services the Governing Body Working Party on the Social Dimension of Globalization. Among the issues he has worked on recently are the impact of globalization on poverty reduction and decent work, freedom of association and the right to bargain collectively, sustainable development, and trade and investment issues.

ALYSSA RAYMAN-READ is a member of the Project on Global Working Families. She has analyzed data from the Project's Botswana site. Previously, she wrote and edited pieces on a range of social and economic issues in both domestic and international contexts, including work and family policy, child and maternal health, reproductive rights, and the acquired immunodeficiency virus. She was formerly a Writing Fellow at *The American Prospect* magazine and a teacher at the American International School in Israel.

S. V. SUBRAMANIAN is Assistant Professor of Health and Social Behavior at the Harvard School of Public Health. His research includes refining the practical applications of multilevel methodologies to understand the macrodeterminants of health and social inequalities and developing comparative international perspectives in health and social behavior. He has published in international social science and health journals on the influence of income inequality, social capital, and, more broadly, geographic contexts on population health.

JUKKA TAKALA is the Director of the International Labor Organization's program on Safety and Health at Work and the Environment. Before holding this position, he served at the ILO as Chief Technical Advisor and Expert in Occupational Safety and Health in Nairobi and Bangkok, Chief of the International Occupational Safety and Health Information Centre (CIS), Chief of the Safety and Health Information Services Branch, and Chief of the Occupational Safety and Health Branch.

SUSANHA YIMYAM is an Associate Professor in the Faculty of Nursing, Chiang Mai University, Chiang Mai, Thailand. Her research interests and major areas of expertise are women's health, maternal and child health, human immunodeficiency virus prevention, and primary health care. Trained in maternal, children's, and women's health, she has published on breast-feeding and employed women in scholarly journals.

XIAO-RONG WANG is currently carrying out a 20-year longitudinal study of respiratory disease in cotton textile workers in Shanghai, China as a Senior Research Associate in the Occupational Health Program at the Harvard School of Public Health. Her research interest is in occupational and environmental epidemiology with a focus on respiratory diseases. Trained in occupational health medicine in China, she has worked on research projects involving China, Japan, and the United States.

Global Inequalities at Work

Introduction: The Global Spread of Risk

JODY HEYMANN

Leti, Humberto, and Laura each lived with their families in different corners of the hillside slums surrounding Tegulcigalpa. When the expression "pale as a ghost" is used, it is often employed in hyperbole. But the phrase hit the mark in describing Leti's infant daughter, Valentina. She was so malnourished that her skin was nearly translucent because there was none of the normal baby fat below the skin. Leti had had to return to work 42 days after giving birth or lose her job. She had no choice but to stop breast-feeding at that time—in spite of the fact that it was clear that she could not afford enough infant formula on her low wages to nourish Valentina adequately. Like the majority of children who are not breast-fed long enough in poor parts of the world where safe drinking water is unavailable, Valentina rapidly grew sick, first with intestinal and then with respiratory infections. When we met her, she was barely moving.

Humberto and his wife, Geralda, both worked in factories to make ends meet. If Geralda wanted to keep her job, she too had no choice but to return to work soon after giving birth and cease breast-feeding. Yet, not breast-feeding placed her son, like Valentina, at heightened risk of infections. Within a few months, Humbertocito was hospitalized with pneumonia. Like many overburdened hospitals in developing countries, the hospital relied on family members to provide essential care. Humberto asked for permission to take time off from work to care for his son. On the first day, permission was granted; on the second day, he received a warning. On the third day, he was fired and blacklisted from other factory jobs.

Laura was raising her 18-month-old daughter alone since the death of her husband. She worked in a foreign-owned factory 7 days a week. The shifts were inhumanely long—ranging from 15 to 22 hours a day. But it had been the only job she could find. It was summertime, and Laura's niece temporarily provided care for her daughter, but she was due to return to school in a month. Earning only $26 every 2 weeks and having to pay $14 to the factory for the one meal a day she received, Laura earned too little to afford child care. Soon she would have to choose between trying to get her 10-year-old niece to drop out of school to provide care—with the inevitable long-term consequences for the life options available to the girl—and leaving her own toddler home alone—as too many others in her neighborhood had been forced to do.

It was clear that the conditions Leti, Humberto, and Laura faced at work were having a dramatic impact on the health and welfare of their families.

A Focus on the Individual in the Field of Occupational Health

Throughout history, the field of occupational health has focused largely on the impact of exposures on the individual worker. In their extensive review of methods for the recognition and control of occupational disease, Landrigan and Baker (1991) focused on physical and chemical agents that affect individual workers. Similarly, guidelines on what to ask when taking an occupational health history suggest detailed questions about the exposure of individual workers to fumes and dust, elements and metals, solvents, and other chemicals, as well as a "miscellaneous" category to cover other individual exposures ranging from heavy lifting to radiation (Rosenstock and Cullen, 1986). These approaches have led to important reductions in toxic exposures at workplaces in North America and Europe.

The recent work examining how best to limit the primarily chemical and physical exposure of individuals to risks in the workplace has a long history that dates back more than two millennia. In ancient Greece, Hippocrates (est. 460–370 B.C.E.) observed and described the illnesses of metallurgists and clothmakers. In the first century C.E. in Rome, Pliny the Elder, and in the second century C.E. in Greece, Galen made new suggestions on how to address the risks faced by miners, those working with metals, and those exposed to dusts and vapors. Prevention has also long been prescribed. Pliny the Elder is known for being the first to describe bladder-derived respiratory masks for protection.

During the Renaissance, concern about the impact of dangerous jobs and trades on those who performed them reemerged. In 1473, Ulrich Ellenbog wrote *On the Poisonous Evil Vapours and Fumes*, a manuscript about the hazards to which those working with metals were exposed (Barnard, 1932). Georgius Agricola (1494–1555) underscored the effects on individual workers' health of mining and smelting gold and silver in *De Re Metallica*. Paracelsus (1493–1541), a physician who traveled throughout Europe, treated and wrote about those who fell ill while working at these occupations.

Perhaps not surprisingly it was the Enlightenment, with its many humanitarian reforms, that sparked the first detailed examination of how individual health was affected by a wide range of occupations. In 1713, the Italian physician and professor of medicine Bernardo Ramazzini wrote *De Morbis Artificum Diatriba*, an account of workers' diseases in approximately 100 professions. Ramazzini wrote about occupations that ranged from metalworking to sewer cleaning, from making glass to delivering infants as a midwife, from being an intellectual to being a potter.

Thus, a long and important history of both research and medicine has focused on the impact of working conditions on health. Originally dating back to ancient Greece, investigations into the risks of working in different occupations were first seriously revisited during the Renaissance. However, while both the breadth and the depth of our understanding of individual risks have expanded in important ways since the Enlightenment, the focus has remained largely on the individual.

Providing Individual Workers with Protection from and Compensation for Physical and Chemical Exposures

The focus on individual health effects has led to important policy developments as well as treatises. Beginning in the 1800s, a series of laws were passed to provide protection for individual workers. The British Factory Act of 1855 provided for the investigation of industrial accidents. In 1897, the Workmen's Compensation Act ensured that those injured on the job in Britain would receive remuneration from their employers. In 1906, compensation was expanded to include those who developed serious illnesses as a result of their work (Levenstein, Wooding, and Rosenburg, 2000). In theory, the combined legislation ensured that at least minimally safe conditions would exist, the factories would be inspected for compliance, and laborers who nonetheless became injured or ill as a result of their work would not be left destitute.

In the United States, as in Britain, tragedies often preceded public action. In 1869, a deadly fire in a Pennsylvania mine led to the passage of the first state legislation on mine safety. It took another two decades before federal legislation regarding mine safety was passed; in 1890 the Federal Bureau of Mines was created (Feitshans, 1999). It was concern for miners, whose occupation had the longest history of documented hazards, as well as for railway workers, that led to the first workers' compensation act in the United States. Maryland enacted compensation laws for miners and railway workers in 1902, and workers' compensation laws for railway workers followed in 16 states in 1906. In 1911, Wisconsin, and then seven other states, passed broader laws that compensated workers across occupations. By 1948, workers' compensation laws had been passed in all states (de la Hoz and Parker, 1998). In 1970, the U.S. Congress passed the Occupational Health and Safety Act—the first national mechanism for regulating hazards across a wide range of industries.

Often spurred by local crises, tragic accidents, or organized protests, many industrialized nations took steps on their own to address the hazards individuals faced in the workplace. While independent action by nations was common, countries also passed new policies to keep pace with the changes they saw occurring internationally.

Both the broader approach of factory inspections and the narrower one of banning specific toxins spread from one country to the next. The use of white phosphorus in making matches was first eliminated in Finland in 1872. The prohibition rapidly spread to Denmark in 1874, but it did not reach the Netherlands until 1901. The Bern Convention of 1906 eliminated the use of phosphorus in France, Italy, Luxembourg, Switzerland, and Germany. Factory inspections and medical examinations of workers began in Belgium in 1895 and in England in 1898, and then spread to the Netherlands in 1903, to Prussia in 1921, and to France in 1942 (Tepper, 1998). These examples describe only some of the policies passed and programs initiated to reduce the risks associated with work.

The efforts made by industrialized nations both independently and collectively, while not removing all hazardous exposures, have dramatically improved the safety of workplaces in these countries.

The Gaps Left by a Focus on Individuals

While the importance of the progress made in decreasing the risks faced by individual workers cannot be overstated, these advances have had two major limitations. First, while North American and European countries were addressing hazardous exposures, companies were moving factories to countries where regulations were less rigorously enforced or were nonexistent. Unskilled workers in poor countries were facing increasing hazards from both imported and home-grown industries as the speed of industrialization in their countries far outstripped the pace of new protections. Second, the protections, by and large, addressed only the health of individual workers. Working conditions were simultaneously having a dramatic effect on the health of families around the world, as they did for Leti, Humberto, and Laura. Yet, the broader effects of working conditions on the health and well-being of families and societies were not being addressed.

In effect, the field of occupational health has mapped one continent—that of individuals in industrialized countries—extremely well, but much territory has been left uncharted. A map of the relationship between work and health that is truly global—both geographically and in its coverage of the impact of work on the health of individuals, families, and societies—has not been drawn.

The relative paucity of attention paid to the impact of working conditions on the health of families, societies, and the global community is evident from an examination of published research on occupational health and a review of what is being taught. In a review of 30 occupational and environmental health programs from the United States, Canada, Australia, the United Kingdom, South Africa, Finland, Sweden, Thailand, Singapore, and Hong Kong, only two listed courses that examined the impact of working conditions on levels beyond the individual.[1]

Examining How Work Affects the Health of Individuals, Families, and Society

This is the first book to look in detail at how working conditions globally are affecting the health of families and societies as well as individuals. The need to understand the impact of work on families is particularly acute as we enter the twenty-first century. Over a billion adults now work away from home and family members for whom they provide care. This is the result of several major demographic changes that have taken place over the past two centuries, including marked urbanization; declines in agricultural labor; rapid rises in manufacturing, trade, and service work; and the worldwide entry of the majority of men and then of women into the industrial and postindustrial labor forces. In the slums of Tegulcigalpa, when parents have to work over 70-hour weeks just to survive, and no child care is available, toddlers die of injuries and accidents when left alone or in the care of their preschool siblings. In poor U.S. neighborhoods, elementary and high school children are at the greatest risk of being victims of crime when they are home alone after school while their parents are working and no other adult supervision is available. In Botswana, too many working adults have to make the untenable choice between caring for a husband, wife, brother, or sister who is dying of acquired immunodeficiency syndrome (AIDS) and losing a job—often the sole source of family income—if they take unapproved leave. In Vietnam, working conditions determine whether adults can check on their sick and ailing elderly parents to ensure that they have had food or needed medicine during the day. In short, poor working and social conditions can undermine the health of dependent family members of all ages.

This volume critically examines the impact of work on the health of societies as well as families. Work-related factors play an enormous role in determining the extent of gender, social class, racial and ethnic, and other inequalities in societies. These inequalities, in turn, have an enormous effect on health. Previously, these two facts were considered only in isolation. The field of social epidemiology has laid an important foundation for understanding how social inequalities affect health. But to date, little attention has been paid by those concerned with health to the role of wages, working conditions, occupational structure, and segregation in exacerbating and perpetuating economic and gender inequalities. This book explores their interconnections, and does so at a particularly important time in history. In recent decades, global disparities in income have risen dramatically—so much so that by the 1990s, the assets of the world's 358 billionaires were greater than the combined income of 45% of the world's population (Faux and Mishel, 2000).

Though this book emphasizes the impact of working conditions on families, societies, and the global community, the ongoing effects on individuals' health are not ignored, particularly since knowledge of these effects can lead to dramatic improvements in workers' health and safety conditions. That knowledge, however, has not yet mitigated the marked risks that the most marginalized workers in the world face. Well-known and well-understood chemical and physical hazards that have been dramatically reduced in wealthy industrialized countries persist in poor countries. Moreover, while the dangers presented by working with some compounds—from phosphorus to asbestos—are well understood, rapid progress in the biological, physical, chemical, and material sciences means that workers are constantly being exposed to new agents whose risks are unknown. In the United States alone, a thousand new chemicals—most of which have unknown consequences for health—are introduced into the workplace each year (Levenstein, Wooding, and Rosenburg, 2000).

Current Context of Rapid Globalization: Pitfalls and Possibilities

This book addresses these issues at a time when globalization is both markedly changing the impact of work on the health of individuals, families, and societies and radically revising what can be done about it.

For most of the twentieth century, nations throughout the industrial world responded to the risks and opportunities that the changes in work were presenting to individuals by adopting new policies in their own countries. While safety and health inspections often spread from one nation to another, there was no economic imperative to try to achieve an international consensus. Fifty years ago, individual nations could still improve the conditions their own citizens experienced at work with little risk that jobs would be lost to other countries. Over the past 50 years, however, economic globalization has undermined the extent to which countries can respond unilaterally to problems.

The end of the nineteenth and the beginning of the twentieth century experienced what has been referred to as *early globalization*, and countries saw the growth of a more integrated international economy. However, barriers to communication, transportation, and the flow of capital and goods across national borders remained large. As we enter the twenty-first century, the old obstacles are largely gone. Each nation-state makes its own choices, but capital, goods, and jobs now flow readily across borders, placing pressure on individual nations not to provide far better health or safety protection to their own workers than other countries do. As Robert Kuttner (2000) wrote in The Role of Governments in the Global Economy, "With globalism, areas of the world that insist on retaining [good] standards find themselves priced out of the market, in a general race-to-the-bottom." (p. 154) Countries are now aware that if they alone set high standards for working conditions—high enough to ensure good health for their citizens—it is likely that capital will flee to countries with worse conditions.

While industrialized countries continue to have better wages and working conditions than most developing nations, the argument is being made with increasing frequency in North America and Europe that working conditions cannot be improved if nations in these regions are to remain competitive with other countries and keep jobs. One of the ways that poor countries have competed for jobs is to create export processing zones that offer far lower rates of taxation and far less regulation than are typical in the companies' home countries. Export processing zones and nations that compete by offering companies few regulations and workers few assurances of decent working conditions have argued that their need to compete for jobs has prevented them from insisting on decent working conditions.

But while globalization of the economy has made it more difficult for individual countries to lead the way in improving working conditions, it has also created a unique opportunity to work toward improving conditions around the world simultaneously through new global agreements and global governance institutions. When it comes to improving the effect of work on the health of individuals, families, and societies, it may be possible for the first time to make truly global policy changes as part of international trade agreements and to provide essential supports to individuals and families worldwide through institutions designed to provide assistance globally. Examples of recent improvements in global working conditions include those resulting from initiatives over the past decade to end forced labor and eliminate the most abusive forms of child labor.

In summary, at the same time that rapid globalization is changing the risks of work in different parts of the world, it is reconfiguring the possible avenues for improving labor conditions. *Global Inequalities at Work* describes how globalization has put the health of new groups at risk, as well as how it has simultaneously undermined old solutions and provided opportunities for new approaches.

Overview of *Global Inequalities at Work*

To help map out this new environment and to broaden our ability to address the impact of work on the health of individuals, families, and societies, I brought together experts from around the world in public health, economics, epidemiology, sociology, medicine, public policy, and anthropology. They included specialists from leading universities, international organizations, nongovernmental organizations, and research institutions who brought to this project experience from a wide range of countries around the world, including Thailand, Brazil, China, Iran, Switzerland, Canada, Vietnam, Botswana, Australia, Mexico, and the United States, among others. *Global Inequalities at Work* is an outgrowth of this initiative.

To bring together these divergent voices, approaches, and experiences in one volume requires a great deal of effort on the part of all who contribute. While such wide nets are rarely cast because the work involved is great, the harvest is richer still; nothing less than a global effort that spans disciplinary bounds would be sufficient to address the complex and vital relationship between work and health.

Part I of *Global Inequalities at Work* (Chapters 1–3) focuses on the effect of labor conditions on the health of individual workers. It opens with a chapter on chemical and physical exposures. Chapter 1 addresses these risks in the new context of a global economy. As noted in the chapter, the use of some chemicals, such as benzene, has long been restricted in industrialized countries, yet in developing countries their use continues to rise. Likewise, physical hazards that have been banned in the United States and Europe continue to grow in developing countries. Hazardous production is being transferred from wealthier to poorer countries globally. Still, the chemical and physical hazards are not only a problem that developing nations face since the consequences of chronic exposure, those resulting from the rapid introduction of new substances, and the rise of an unprotected informal sector continue to occur in industrialized countries.

Chapter 2 provides an important example of biological and social risks in the workplace by examining the case of human immunodeficiency virus (HIV) in Africa. Social and biological experiences at work can both increase and decrease an individual's risk of contracting HIV. Sexual harassment or coercion at work, low wages that lead to increased economic vulnerability to exposure, and occupational exposure to infected blood products can all increase the risk of a laborer becoming infected with HIV. Social conditions at work can influence not only the likelihood that employees will become infected but also the perils they face if they develop AIDS. The workplace response to the condition will influence whether HIV infection results in stigma, discrimination, income or job loss, and thus more rapid health deterioration—or conversely, whether infected individuals will be able to keep their jobs, sustain an adequate income, and access health care.

How workplace risks affect individuals' health depends both on who is exposed and on what they are exposed to. Chapter 3 examines child labor and describes how the characteristics of those working can influence the health consequences of work. Children are more susceptible than adults to a wide range of occupational hazards. This chapter assesses occupational health risks that range from injuries to illnesses. It both examines risks that all workers face—while examining how the risks and their impact are greater for child workers—and discusses hazards that affect only children. For example, the chapter describes how young children who work full-time and fail to attend school face potentially devastating consequences for their long-term opportunities, income, and health. The case of child labor in Brazil is examined in detail.

Part II (Chapters 4–6) of the book provides a detailed analysis of several ways in which working conditions can dramatically influence the health and welfare of the families of those working. Chapter 4 focuses on the ways in which working conditions shape the nature, quality, and amount of time adults can spend caring for children, elderly parents, and disabled family members as well as other family members in need. This chapter details new research findings on how working conditions affect adults' ability to provide essential care for family members in North America, Latin America, Africa, and Asia. The analysis is global in scope as well as in geography.

The impact of working conditions on the health of family members is felt as profoundly in the developing world as in industrialized countries. Chapter 5 discusses a subject that is particularly important in poor countries and poor regions of middle-income countries—the relationship between work, breast-feeding, and health. Breast-feeding provides important benefits for both infant and maternal health, including lower rates of diarrheal disease, pneumonia, malnutrition, and death among infants and lower risks of certain cancers among women. This chapter both reviews the literature and describes a detailed case study from Thailand examining the challenges at home and at work faced by women who seek to combine work and breast-feeding in this industrializing nation. Working conditions that significantly increase the ability of working mothers to breast-feed—ranging from adequate paid parental leave to the availability of breast-feeding breaks and child care near workplaces—are explored.

Chapter 6 looks at the relationship between parents' working conditions and children's nutrition beyond infancy. This chapter reviews the relevant literature and demonstrates that the nature of parents' working conditions, rather than the mere fact of parents' employment, is what determines whether the effects of parental work on children's nutrition will be beneficial or detrimental. As noted in the chapter, characteristics of the parent's job, such as the wage earned, and the nature of available social supports, such as the quality of alternative child care, all make a critical difference in children's nutritional status.

Part III (Chapters 7–9) examines the relationships between work and health at the societal level. This part focuses on two examples: the ways in which working conditions affect income inequalities and health, and the ways in which working conditions influence gender inequalities and health. Chapter 7 examines the effect of work and wage structures on societal levels of poverty and income inequality. It assesses how the poverty and income inequality that result from wage disparities, in turn, significantly undermine social health. Inequalities both across and within countries have been increasing, with deeply damaging consequences for health.

Conditions of work have had as profound an effect on societies' gender inequalities as they have had on income inequalities. Chapter 8 examines the relationship between gender inequality at work and health. Trends in Latin American and Caribbean women's labor force participation over the past two decades are explored in detail, and the positive and negative effects of the associated working conditions are assessed. As noted in the chapter, work itself has been shown to provide many positive health effects, but the lower wages that women receive, the occupational segregation that exists, and the overall worse working conditions that prevail have all led to detrimental health consequences.

Chapter 9 examines the health impacts of gender inequality at work in the context of a single country. It examines how state policies in Iran institutionalize gender inequality by restricting women's work, education, and movement. The chapter details the result: women are often limited in the type of work they can perform and in their ability to seek better work conditions. These limitations result in dire health and welfare consequences.

Part IV (Chapters 10–12) investigates the new challenges to and opportunities for improving the relationship between work and health that are presented by a rapidly globalizing economy. Chapter 10 appraises what is known about the extent to which border industries, the *maquilas*, bring with them better or worse working conditions than those in the nations from which the companies originated, as well as better or worse working conditions than those in other local industries. The case of Mexico is examined in detail.

Chapter 11 begins with the premise that increased competition in the context of a global economy currently creates incentives for businesses to locate in countries with the worst labor standards. However, the chapter moves rapidly from the recognition of that current economic condition to a discussion of what can be done to ensure decent working conditions and healthy economic development globally. The policy efforts of the International Labor Organization are detailed.

Central to improving working conditions globally is addressing the question of whether it is possible to create global labor standards, as well as whether it is possible to ensure that healthy labor standards will eventually provide the foundation for free trade in the global economy. These issues are the focus of Chapter 12. The case is compellingly made that economic strength, free trade, and global labor standards are strongly complementary.

Work and Health

The centrality of work in human life cuts across cultures and national boundaries, though each culture has different words to express it—from the Chinese proverb "You must judge a man by the work of his hands" to the Talmudic commentary "No labor, however humble, is dishonoring" to the Buddhist saying "Your work is to discover your work and then with all your heart to give yourself to it." The Irish dramatist Sean O'Casey (1952) wrote, "Work . . . the one great sacrament of humanity from which all other things flow—security, leisure, joy, art, literature, even divinity itself." But for as long and as widely as there has been an awareness of the riches that work lives can bring, there has been a growing knowledge of the hazards that can accompany them.

The quality of work strongly influences human health, just as the quality of one's health dramatically affects one's ability to work. Recent World Bank studies of nations around the world documented that people dreaded having any family member in ill health, not only because of illness's direct effects but also because that person consequently could not work, thus often pulling the family into poverty (Narayan et al., 2000).

While the relationship between work and health has long been important because of how deeply both are valued and how tightly the two are intertwined, a new urgency about understanding the subject has arisen from rapid globalization and rising socioeconomic inequalities. The contributors to *Global Inequalities at Work* provide a probing and insightful beginning to understanding how the inequalities at work in the global economy are affecting the health of individuals, families, and societies.

Note

1. These universities were chosen from an online directory of public health graduate programs around the world. Programs with information online in English, French, Russian, and Spanish were examined. Of those programs, 29 offered comprehensive course information on their websites. Lists of courses offered and required for occupational health concentrations were examined, as well as course descriptions and syllabi when available.

References

Barnard, C. 1932. A translation of Ulrich Ellenbog's "On the Poisonous Evil Vapours and Fumes." *The Lancet* 1: 270–71.

de la Hoz, R., and J. E. Parker. 1998. Occupational and environmental medicine in the United States. *International Archives of Occupational and Environmental Health* 71(3): 155–61.

Faux, J., and L. Mishel. 2000. Inequality and the global economy. In *Global capitalism*, edited by W. Hutton and A. Giddens. New York: New Press.

Feitshans, I. 1999. Lessons learned: Three centuries of occupational health laws. In *Contributions to the history of occupational and environmental prevention*: First International Conference on the History of Occupational and Environmental Prevention, Rome; 4–6 October 1998, edited by A. Grieco, S. Iavicoli, and G. Berlinguer. New York: Elsevier.

Kuttner, R. 2000. The role of governments in the global economy. In *Global capitalism*, edited by W. Hutton and A. Giddens. New York: New Press.

Landrigan, P. J., and D. Baker. 1991. The recognition and control of occupational disease. *Journal of the American Medical Association* 266(5): 676–80.

Levenstein, C., J. Wooding, and B. Rosenberg. 2000. Occupational health: A social perspective. In *Occupational health: Recognizing and preventing work-related disease and injury*, edited by B. S. Levy and D. H. Wegman. Philadelphia: Lippincott, Williams & Wilkins.

Narayan, D., R. Patel, K. Schafft, A. Rademacher, and S. Koch-Schulte. 2000. *Voices of the poor: Can anyone hear us?* New York: Oxford University Press (published for the World Bank).

O'Casey, S. 1952. In New York now. In *Rose and crown*. London: Macmillan.

Rosenstock, L., and M. R. Cullen. 1986. *Clinical occupational medicine*. Philadelphia: W. B. Saunders.

Tepper, L. B. 1998. History of international occupational medicine. In *International occupational and environmental medicine*, edited by J. A. Herzstein, W. B. Bunn III, L. E. Fleming, J. M. Harrington, J. Jeyaratnam, and I. R. Gardner. St. Louis, MO: Mosby.

Part I

Global Health Risks in the Workplace: The Impact on Individuals

1

Impact of Chemical and Physical Exposures on Workers' Health

DAVID C. CHRISTIANI AND XIAO-RONG WANG

Work is a central part of human life, and it has both positive and negative impacts on workers' health. Exposure to chemical and physical hazards in the workplace, resulting in a variety of occupational illnesses, is a common negative impact. Historically, industrialized countries have witnessed numerous industrial disasters (Raffle et al., 1987). Today more challenges in occupational health are faced by industrializing countries, which not only account for more than 70% of the world's population (World Bank, 1993), but also have undergone rapid increases in population, industrial transformation, and economic growth over the past three decades. That process is accompanied, however, by grave health problems related to people's exposure to various industrial hazards. Changes in the patterns and intensities of industrial exposures have created a great challenge for occupational health. Along with rapid expansion of the formal sector of industry and commerce, a large informal sector has developed, including workers in agriculture, small industry, construction, and casual work (Chen and Huang, 1997; Christiani, Durvasula, and Myers, 1990; Loewenson, 1998). The informal sector is less regulated for occupational hazards than the formal sector, which encompasses large manufacturers and business enterprises.

Conservative estimates indicate that there are 160 million cases of occupational disease worldwide. It is generally agreed that if the industrializing countries continue their current rate of industrial growth, that figure will double by the year 2025 (Murray and Lopez, 1996). The majority of occupational diseases are occurring almost exclusively in developing countries. Although industrialized and industrializing countries share many similarities in the impact of chemical and physical exposure on workers' health, differences exist, particularly in the patterns which are influenced by the sociopolitical and economic structures of each country. In general, occupational health activities have not kept pace with rapid industrialization and economic changes in industrializing countries, but rather have matched these countries' patterns of uneven economic and social development. This chapter provides an overview of several major health problems related to chemical and physical agent exposures in workplaces, highlights occupational problems faced by industrializing countries where the relevant data are available, and compares the exposures that occur in industrialized countries with those that occur in industrializing ones.

Exposure to Industrial Chemicals and Metals

Many chemical substances encountered in the workplace are toxic and have harmful effects on the human body. Workers absorb chemicals by three main routes: the respiratory system, the skin, and the gastrointestinal tract. Exposure to hazardous industrial chemicals may lead to serious immediate or delayed damage to workers' health and environment. According to the 1995 *World Disaster Report* covering 1969 to 1993, accidents (including industrial disasters) are second only to floods in frequency; chemical disasters of industrial origin, with serious human and environmental consequences, rank tenth, just after infectious epidemics and followed by landslides (Walker, 1995). Until the 1970s, major chemical accidents occurred predominantly in industrialized countries, where there was a much higher concentration of industries. Since the 1970s, however, the number of accidents in developing countries has increased steadily. The worst chemical accidents with the most fatalities in the twentieth century happened in India, Brazil, and Mexico (Firpo de Souza Porto and de Freitas, 1996). In Brazil, for instance, the official number of accidents at work between 1980 and 1989 was 10,500,000, resulting in 260,000 permanent injuries and 46,000 fatalities. The total number of accidents may be greater, however, since accidents at work are not always reported in Brazil (Bertazzi, 1989). Currently, the most extensively expanding exposure to industrial chemicals is in the newly industrializing countries, such as China, India, and Thailand.

Heavy metal poisoning induced by exposure to lead, mercury, cadmium, manganese, arsenic, and other metals is a traditional problem in occupational health. While work-related chemical poisoning has been well controlled in industrialized countries, both acute and chronic poisonings have been increasing dramatically in industrializing countries. In some of these countries, such as China (He, 1998), Korea (Lee, 1999), and Croatia (Šarić, 1999), lead is reported to be the most prevalent etiologic agent in industrial poisoning.

Organic solvents are another class of chemicals that are important to industry today and can be found in many consumer products. Among the solvents, benzene is the most dangerous because of its hematotoxic and leukemogenic properties. Acute benzene poisoning usually occurs in workplaces with poor ventilation. Chronic exposure to benzene has been associated with leukemia and other cancers (Parmeggiani, 1983). In industrialized countries, the use of benzene has been restricted or the permissible exposure limit has been reduced (Stellman, 1997). In Italy, for instance, after two epidemics of aplastic anemia caused by benzene, this solvent was banned in 1965 by law (Chen and Chan, 1999). In the United States, the time weighted average permissible exposure limit was reduced from 10 parts per million to 1 in 1987, and the National Institute of Occupational Safety and Health recommended a further reduction to 0.1 part per million (Graham, Green, and Roberts, 1988). But in many industrializing countries, benzene is still used widely in manufacturing (as in the chemical, plastics, and shoe manufacturing industries) as a solvent, often with poor protective measures. Although solvent poisoning is an occupational health issue in other countries, including Zimbabwe in Africa (Loewenson, 1998), the worst situation may be in some Asian countries—such as China, Korea, India, Indonesia, and Malaysia—where labor-intensive industries, including especially shoe making and rapidly developing high-technology microelectronics, are gathered (Chen and Chan, 1999; LaDou and Rohm, 1998; Lee, 1999).

China officially reported 5943 cases of chronic benzene poisoning between 1984 and 1993 (Chen and Chan, 1999). This figure is likely to be underestimated considerably, however, because the nonstate industrial sector, such as collective, rural, and private enterprises, was not included in the statistics. The industries in this sector have worse occupational safety and health problems and now dominate the Chinese economy. One study revealed a marked increase in hematologic abnormalities due to benzene exposure among workers in rural small-scale industries (Christiani 1988). A retrospective cohort study, conducted from 1987 to 1991, of 75,000 benzene-exposed state workers in 12 Chinese cities reported the effects of benzene in relation to leukemia and hematolymphoproliferative disorders. There were excess deaths caused by leukemia, malignant lymphoma, and neoplastic diseases of the blood among benzene-exposed workers (Yin, 1996).

The problems resulting from exposure to organic solvents are also conspicuous in Vietnam, Indonesia, and other Asian countries. One of the worst cases reported in Asia involved a Korean-owned Nike subcontractor in Vietnam. Built in 1995, the plant is one of the most technologically advanced of all Nike plants and employs 10,000 workers. According to Nike's own internal investigation conduced in 1996, workers wore no protective equipment in a work environment where the lax Vietnamese permissible exposure limit standard for toluene (26.6 parts per million or 100 milligrams per cubic meter) was exceeded by over six times in different sections of the plant (Chen and Chan, 1999). Medical checkups of 165 workers in three of the factory's sections revealed that 77.5% of them had respiratory diseases, and "an increasing number of employees" suffered from skin, heart, and throat diseases (Greenhouse, 1997).

Pesticide Poisoning

Pesticides occupy a special position among the chemicals to which workers can be exposed because of widespread global use and the remarkably extensive populations involved. People exposed to pesticides include industrial workers (producers) and agricultural workers (applicators), as well as the general population (consumers). The occupational exposures differ remarkably: for instance, skin exposure is prevalent among applicators in agriculture, while inhalation exposure is more common among producers during the formulation and manufacturing of pesticides (Maroni et al., 2000).

At present, pesticides are highly valued in industrializing countries. Most countries use large quantities of insecticides, since insects create the most serious problems. Many older, nonpatented, extremely toxic, environmentally persistent, and inexpensive chemicals (such as DDT and some organophosphorus mixtures) are used extensively in the industrializing nations. Due to the lack of appropriate regulations, equipment, and training, acute pesticide poisoning is a major health problem in the industrializing countries, while the industrialized ones have virtually eliminated this problem (Jeyaratnam, 1992).

The World Health Organization (1990) estimated an annual worldwide total of some 3 million cases of acute, severe poisoning (including suicides)—matched by a possibly greater number of unreported cases of mild to moderate intoxication—with 220,000 deaths. Around 99% of all deaths due to acute pesticide poisoning occur in the industrializing countries, where only 20% of the world's agrochemicals are used (Kogevinas, Boffetta, and Pearce, 1994). The reliance on pesticides is also related to personnel availability. Most developing nations use greater quantities of insecticides than developed nations. For example, in Vietnam, 80% of the product volume used is insecticides, weeding still being done by hand (Tennenbaum, 1996). According to incomplete statistics from China, the annually reported cases of acute pesticide poisoning have numbered about 50,000. Among the total cases reported from 1992 to 1994, occupational pesticide poisoning accounted for 23.6% (He, 1998). In a report from a national survey of hospital cases in Sri Lanka, investigators reported an incidence of 100,000 persons admitted to hospitals for acute intoxications annually, with almost 1000 deaths, out of a population of twelve million (Jeyaratnam, 1982). In Thailand in 1983, an estimated 8268 pesticide-related intoxications occurred in an agricultural community of 100,000 workers (Boon-Long et al., 1986). Few attempts have been made to estimate the extent to which agrichemicals are used in Africa. One survey in South Africa's Western Cape Province estimated that 8.5% of the 120,000 workers employed in deciduous fruit production may be exposed directly to agrichemicals (London, 1994).

Exposure to Dusts, Fibers, and Occupational Respiratory Diseases

Many kinds of dust in industrial and agricultural activities can cause occupational respiratory diseases such as pneumoconioses and asthma. For centuries, the most frequently and widely used minerals in manufacturing activities have been silica, coal, and asbestos, which cause pneumoconiosis. In addition to causing pneumoconioses, silica and asbestos are known as carcinogens, inducing lung cancer and mesothelioma. Asbestos use has declined in North America and Europe since the International Agency for Research on Cancer classified asbestos as being carcinogenic to humans, based on sufficient toxicologic and epidemiologic evidence (IARC, 1987). Some countries have completely banned asbestos use. However, production and sales in other countries (such as those in parts of Southeast Asia, South America, and Eastern Europe) have increased, primarily due to the use of asbestos-based construction materials (Lemen and Bingham, 1994).

Since the 1980s, the incidence of pneumoconioses in the industrialized countries has decreased dramatically, although pneumoconioses remain a major occupational problem. In the 1980s, an estimated 1.7 million workers were exposed to crystalline silica outside of the mining industry, and approximately 700,000 workers exposed to asbestos in the United States (Steenland and Stayner, 1997). By 1997, dust-related lung diseases, including silicosis, asbestosis, and coal workers' pneumoconiosis, accounted for only 2900 cases (NIOSH, 2000).

The profile in the industrializing countries, however, is very different. On the basis of a nationwide 1986 Chinese epidemiologic survey, there were about 400,000 patients with verified pneumoconioses throughout China since 1949. Subsequently, 10,000 to 15,000 new cases were reported each year. The cumulative number of cases reached 600,000 by 2000 (He, 1998). An additional 520,000 workers were suspected of having pneumoconioses. Silicosis and coal workers' pneumoconiosis are the major forms of the disease, accounting for 48% and 39% of the cases, respectively. Again, this estimate included only state-owned enterprises. Township, village, and private industries have been creating a large number of acute and chronic cases. Therefore, the actual number of pneumoconiosis cases could be much higher.

China does not stand alone in having dust-related health problems. In the late 1980s, the prevalence of coal workers' pneumoconiosis reportedly ranged from 5.6% in Brazil to 20% in Zimbabwe (Van, 1990). In some countries, such as India, respiratory quartz dust levels may exceed 10 milligrams per cubic meter, causing the majority of the workforce to suffer from silicosis (including acute silicosis) and silicotuberculosis (Jindal and Whigg, 1998).

Organic dusts are probably the most ubiquitous respiratory insults in the agricultural setting. Plants such as tea, coffee, tobacco, cotton, cereal, grains, sisal, and jute are major products of the formal sector in many industrializing countries. Respiratory diseases including asthma and asthma-like syndromes are important clinical problems among agricultural workers. Unfortunately, the investigation of agricultural respiratory hazards has lagged behind that of hazards in industrial settings. The diseases induced by occupational exposure to agricultural hazards have not been recognized as legitimate occupational diseases even in the industrialized countries, and even less attention has been paid to these diseases in the industrializing countries. In fact, diseases resulting from exposure to organic dusts afflict a much larger number of persons worldwide, because more than 70% of the workforce may be involved in agriculture in many industrializing countries (Christiani, Durvasula, and Myers, 1990).

Noise-Related Hearing Loss

Noise is a major occupational health risk. The connection between noise exposure and decline in hearing ability has been known for centuries. Noise hazards are present in a variety of environments, especially in manufacturing, construction, agriculture, mining, transportation, and the military (Dunn, 2000). Work-related noise presents three fundamental risks to workers' health: (*1*) acute hearing deficits, which are secondary to loud noises such as blasts and explosions; (*2*) chronic hearing impairment, which is due to continuous or long-term exposure to hazardous noise levels; and (*3*) extra-auditory effects, including alterations of blood pressure and adverse influences on existing illnesses such as hyperlipoproteinemia and diabetes (McCunney and Meyer, 1998). Studies conducted in the United States have shown that, given the same level of noise exposure, men are more susceptible to noise-induced hearing loss than women, and Caucasians are more susceptible than African Americans. Also, the left ear tends to be more susceptible than the right ear to the effects of noise (Dunn, 2000). The discrepancy in gender and ethnicity may be partly explained by inadequate control of many confounding factors such as age, type of noise exposure, intensity of noise exposure, use of protective equipment, cigarette smoking, and the environmental milieu. However, some studies support the belief that white men are more vulnerable to the harmful effects of noise than nonwhite men, even when these confounding factors are taken into account (Cooper, 1994; Ishii and Talbott, 1998). Studies also have shown that individuals with blue eyes are more susceptible to noise-induced cochlear ear damage than green- or brown-eyed individuals (Carter, 1980; Cunningham and Norris, 1982).

Noise-induced hearing loss at the workplace is a major problem in both industrialized and industrializing countries. Recent estimates have indicated that 30 million U.S. workers are exposed to hazardous noise on the job, and an additional 9 million are at risk of hearing loss from other agents such as solvents and metals (NIOSH 1996). The National Institute of Occupational Safety and Health has rated noise-induced hearing loss as one of the top 10 work-related problems, involving at least 11 million workers in the United States (Ishii and Talbott, 1998). Yet, the situation is much worse in industrializing countries because of poorer protection. Noise-induced hearing loss is the leading occupational disease in some countries, such as Singapore (Tay, 1996), South Korea (Lee, 1999), the Philippines (Department of Labor and Employment, 1999), and Croatia (Šarić, 1999). A study investigating workers in the Lesotho Highlands Dam and Tunnel Construction Program in Africa showed that 92% of the 258 subjects experienced noise-induced hearing loss (Colvin et al., 1998). Despite such serious situations, however, no systematic data are available on the incidence or prevalence of noise-induced hearing loss in many industrializing countries, and occupational noise-induced hearing loss is not compensated in some countries.

In the workplace, workers rarely are exposed to a single industrial hazard. Noise and chemicals often coexist in many industries. Interactions between noise and chemicals may pose challenges to occupational health research. Animal studies have suggested that exposure to both noise and some industrial chemicals may result in enhanced ototoxicity—for example, single simultaneous exposure to noise and carbon monoxide or exposure to noise and toluene (Cary, Clark, and Delic, 1997). Combined exposure to noise and lead or cadmium resulted in histopathological heart lesions of undefined severity, a finding that was not observed for either of these agents in isolation. A number of studies have investigated human populations exposed to both noise and industrial chemicals. Due to confounding factors, however, conclusions about interactions have been difficult to reach.

Work-Related Musculoskeletal Disorders

Work-related musculoskeletal disorders primarily affect soft tissues and commonly involve the back, cervical spine, and upper extremities. These disorders are also known as *cumulative trauma disorders*, *repetitive motion disorders*, *repetitive strain injury*, *occupational overuse syndromes*, and *occupational cervicobrachial disorders*. The environment and performance of work contribute significantly to the development, exacerbation, or acceleration of these multifactorial disorders. In spite of the fact that work-related musculoskeletal disorders are the oldest occupational health problems in history, epidemiologic research remains in its infancy compared to research on other diseases. The currently available data have been reported chiefly by industrialized countries rather than industrializing countries, where such information is scarce.

Low back pain is one of the most common work–related musculoskeletal disorders. It involves acute or chronic pain of the lumbosacral, buttock, or upper leg areas. Millions of workers around the world are afflicted by an occupational lower back illness. In the United States, the incidence of disabling low back pain increased 26% from 1974 to 1978, while the population increased only 7% (Pope, 1989). The lifetime prevalence of at least one major episode of low back pain is 60% to 90% (Borenstein, Wiesel, and Boden, 1995). The U.S. Department of Labor has estimated that 100 million workdays are lost annually because of low back pain (Johanning, 2000). Low back pain is also the most costly occupational health problem: this problem is responsible for 34% to 40% of the total costs, although 16% to 20% of all workers' compensation cases involve low back pain. More than $16 billion (in direct costs) is spent each year on the treatment and compensation of low back pain in the United States alone (Levy and Wegman, 2000).

Most of the epidemiological studies on low back pain have been restricted to industrialized countries, which comprise less than 15% of the world's population

(Volinn, 1997). Little is known about the epidemiology of low back pain in industrializing countries, but it is believed that such problems are more serious in these countries because harder physical labor is more prevalent and is often unavoidable even for older workers. A limited number of studies conducted in Nigeria, China, Indonesia, and the Philippines have shown that low back pain rates are higher among urban workers than among rural ones. This suggests that the prevalence of this problem may be on the rise with urbanization and rapid industrialization. In addition, high rates prevail among workers in particular industries, such as sewing machine operators, as well as among those with tedious work or close supervision (Volinn, 1997). In most industrializing countries, however, low back pain has not yet been defined as a compensable occupational disease. A recent study identifying research priorities in occupational health in Malaysia (Sadhra et al., 2001) showed that chemical poisoning and injuries from accidents at work remained the main areas of concern for both industry and the government. By contrast with findings from Western countries, workplace psychosocial problems and musculoskeletal injuries were deemed less important. Workforces and occupational health professionals are often not well equipped to cope with these new demands.

Occupational Cancer

Cancer was one of the major public health problems of the twentieth century, and it will continue to be so in the twenty-first. Workplace exposures to carcinogens are important contributors to the total burden of cancer in both industrialized and industrializing countries. Carcinogens can be chemicals such as aniline dyes, physical agents such as ionizing radiation, or biological agents such as viruses or aflatoxin. By 1999, the International Agency for Research on Cancer (IARC, 1972–1999) had classified more than 35 chemical agents used in industries or industrial processes as carcinogenic to humans. The cancers most closely associated with workplace exposure (chiefly industrial) are lung cancer and skin cancer, followed by bladder cancer, leukemia, and brain cancer (Frumkin, 1997).

How much cancer is occupational? This has been a matter of debate. In the United States, occupational exposure, environmental pollution, and ionizing radiation have been estimated to cause about 10% of all cancers in humans (Colditz et al., 1996; Doll and Peto, 1981a). Doll and Peto (1981b) attributed between 2% and 8% of all cancers to workplace exposures, representing between 25,000 and 100,000 new cases of cancer each year in the United States alone. The burden of lung and bladder cancers attributable to occupations in Western countries has been estimated to range between 5% and 20% (Vineis et al., 1995). In high-risk groups such as chemical workers, the proportion of cancers related to work may be substantially higher. Vineis and Simonato (1991) reviewed several population-based and hospital-based studies from Western countries (the United States, Italy, Sweden, the United Kingdom, and Norway) and found that in specific populations located in industrial areas, the proportions of lung cancer ranged between 1% and 5% (when only exposure to asbestos was considered) and might be as high as 40% (in a high proportion of subjects exposed to ionizing radiation). The proportions of bladder cancers attributable to occupational exposures have ranged between 16% and 24% in several investigations (Vineis and Simonato, 1991). The variation in the proportions observed in different studies very likely has depended on the different levels of exposure for particular types of occupations, in different countries, or in different factories within the same country. It is believed that in industrialized countries, occupational cancers likely account for less than 10% of all cancers (Frumkin, 1997), and the risk from occupational exposures has been greatly reduced over the past several decades.

By contrast, in many industrializing countries cancer is becoming a major cause of death. However, epidemiological research on occupational cancer conducted in these countries is scanty, making it difficult to estimate accurately the burden of occupational cancer. The decentralized nature of many industries and the limited control of exposure to known and suspected carcinogens suggest that the workplace plays a great relative role in cancer causation. Workers in industrializing countries are more likely to have much higher levels of exposure than those in industrialized countries. Due to the weaker economic structure in industrializing countries, the permissible exposure levels are higher than elsewhere. For example, for 1,3-butadiene, the limit set by the American Conference of Governmental Industrial Hygienists is 10 parts per million, while it is 780 parts per million in Brazil and 1000 parts per million in Mexico and Taiwan (Vineis et al., 1995).

Since the 1970s, many hazardous production activities have been transferred to the industrializing countries (Pearce et al., 1994). Chemicals previously banned in the United States or Europe are now produced and used in the industrializing countries. For example, asbestos milling has been transferred from the United States to Mexico, and benzidine production has been shifted from European countries to the former Yugoslavia and to Korea (La Dou, 1991; Pearce, et al., 1994; Simonato, 1986). The massive transfer of manufacturing and agricultural chemical use to the industrializing nations of Asia, Africa, and Latin America has resulted in exposure of large working populations to known and suspected workplace carcinogens (Christiani and Monson, 1997). Hence, we believe that cancers associated with occupational exposure in industrializing countries will increase dramatically in the next few decades.

Limited Current Knowledge

Although great progress was made during the twentieth century in understanding the health effects of human exposure to chemicals and physical agents, our current knowledge still is very limited. More than 104,000 chemical and physical agents in the working environment have been identified, but the effects of most of them on workers' health have not been assessed (Gold, Lasley, and Schenker, 1994). For example, only approximately 732 agents have been evaluated for evidence linking occupational exposures to human cancer (Patellos and Garabrant, 1994).

Compounds used in the growing plastics and synthetic fiber industries have not been fully examined for their potential toxicity. Soon after the compound polytetrafluoroethylene (PTFE) was introduced, pyrolysis products–induced "polymer fume fever" and pneumonitis were discovered in the polymer industry. Most of the information documenting adverse human health effects from environmental and occupational contaminants has come from animal studies focused on exposure to single chemicals, and there is little information on how two or more contaminants affect humans. Occupational exposure levels are generally set for single compounds. Unlike laboratory animals, however, workers are usually exposed to a wide variety of hazardous chemicals and physical agents. Two or more compounds and agents may show additive, antagonistic, or synergistic interactions or may act on totally different systems (Carpenter et al., 1998). Solvents form the most frequently used multicomponent mixtures in industry today, and they have the ability to inhibit the metabolism of other chemicals. Interactive effects of exposure to noise and other chemicals on hearing loss are another example of coexposure. Furthermore, the effects of coexposure of chemicals can occur at different stages of metabolism, including uptake, elimination, biotransformation, and binding (McCauley, 1998).

In the United States, research programs on the toxicology of chemical mixtures have existed for several decades. Until the 1990s, however, this problem did not receive a great deal of attention or research outside the United States (Feron, Cassee, and Groten, 1998). A positive development is that in the past decade there has been growing attention and research in other countries, with an increasing awareness of simultaneous exposure to several compounds (though largely confined to the industrialized countries).

Control of Work-Related Diseases

Work has a special place in human life in most cultures and political systems. But the negative aspects of work, such as work-related diseases and injuries, bring tremendous losses both in economic terms and in the quality of workers' lives. Occupational exposures to harmful agents are of greater intensity and longer duration than those in other environments, but the occupational ones can often be more readily identified, measured, and prevented.

In Chinese, the word *crisis* (*wei ji*) has two meanings: "danger" and "opportunity," both of which can be used to describe the situation of occupational health today. There are many dangers and opportunities that face workers, employers, occupational health and safety researchers, and other professionals. Most occupational diseases such as pneumoconioses and occupational cancers are *incurable*, but they are *preventable*, so there is a crucial opportunity for preventive interventions by governmental agencies, scientific researchers, and businesses.

Control of workplace exposures is a big challenge in both industrialized and industrializing countries. Safety standards for chemical and physical hazards in the workplace are not yet high enough in industrialized countries, and a major task for these countries is to determine or evaluate the potential effects of various chemical and physical agents on workers' health at low exposure levels. However, greater challenges are faced by industrializing countries in which industrial hazardous exposures are at significantly higher levels (India, the Philippines, Mexico) or notably on the rise (China). An effective preventive strategy based on interactions among social, political, economic, scientific, and legal sectors is necessary to achieve the ultimate goal of preventing work-related diseases in each country. Specific occupational health profiles are significantly determined by the sociopolitical and economic structures of each country. In general, occupational health systems in industrializing countries are weakly and unevenly developed. Establishing stronger legal systems to develop necessary national polices and regulations may be another crucial step for industrializing countries to control and reduce high levels of primary hazardous exposures in the workplace. The legislation regulating the decision-making process for new installations is very precarious in many industrializing countries (ILO, 1994). For instance, hardly any country in Latin America has legislation equivalent to the European "Seveso Directive" or the North American "Emergency Planning and Right-to-Know." Where legislation exists, the technical and financial deficiencies of the regulatory institutions, added to the lack of effective pressure groups in political systems that are not fully democratic, strongly limit enforcement of the law (Firpo de Souza Porto and de Freitas, 1996). In addition to forcible compliance with national standards for industrial hazards by legislation, the awareness of employers and workers should be enhanced through education campaigns. Employers need to realize that providing safe working conditions is essential to having healthy, productive workers with minimal workers' compensation costs.

In the past, industrial hazards and related health problems were considered concerns restricted to hazardous industries. But now it is increasingly recognized that these are problems of global concern and global activity. As noted earlier, the transfer of hazardous industries to the developing world is a problem of growing concern (Jeyaratnam, 1993). Divergent conditions in the industrialized and industrializing nations often gives rise to the problem of double standards in the control of industrial hazards. Double standards arise when one country bans or restricts a product or process and another country does not. A uniform set of international standards based on health considerations and international control mechanisms must be formulated to ensure that exporting nations will inform importing nations of the health risks associated with the industries in question. Such efforts require cooperation between international organizations, and between industrialized and industrializing countries.

The rapid expansion of labor forces, including women and children, and rapid industrial transformations have created complex and broad occupational health problems particularly in industrializing countries. These include both classic problems experienced by the industrialized countries decades ago, such as chemical intoxication from lead, mercury, and other metals, as well as pneumoconioses, and new hazards due to introduction of modern technology, such as those discussed thus far—and all of these problems have been compounded by poor socioeconomic and often unstable political conditions (Xu and Christiani, 1995). However, only 5% of all health research projects are conducted in industrializing countries (Jeyaratnam, 1992). There is a great need for epidemiological studies in each country to determine the prevalence and distribution of occupational diseases and to identify other major health problems that are arising because of chemical and physical hazards in the workplace.

As discussed earlier, research capabilities and research programs in industrializing countries need to be strengthened to identify and resolve relevant problems. The selection of research priorities and the translation of results into effective policy are paramount but difficult. There is little uniformity between industrializing countries with respect to sociopolitical structure. Researchers need to find ways to balance disparate sociopolitical interests, taking scientific value, social impact, and feasibility into account to set priorities. However, up to the present, much research in industrializing countries has not focused on priority health problems because priorities are not well established, because funding may not be forthcoming for the priority problems, and because researchers and government may not collaborate sufficiently to create an effective response (Barker, 1995). In southern African countries, for example, relevant health research has had disappointingly little impact on policy changes (Joint Project on Health Systems Research, 1994). In summary, much remains to be done for research to be regarded as integral to the process of policy formulation and informed decision making in the occupational health of industrializing countries.

Greater cooperation between industrialized and industrializing countries is also an important step toward the reduction of prevailing differences in occupational health problems and work-related diseases. As they face new problems associated with industrialization, developing countries should take advantage of existing information about occupational health available from countries with relevant experience. The active industrial transformations in industrializing countries offer an exceptional opportunity for improving conditions and conducting natural experiment studies that are of global relevance. In addition, the highly centralized social and administrative structures of many industrializing countries, such as China, make it possible to achieve high response rates and to minimize loss to follow-up in occupational health studies (Xu and Christiani, 1995). Routinely collected data and unpublished material residing in various government departments and corporations may be rich sources of information that is generally unavailable. International cooperative research efforts and training programs should be encouraged and expanded to enhance the chances of success by identifying priorities, selecting important and feasible topics, taking advantage of a country's unique features, and improving quality control.

ACKNOWLEDGMENTS
Supported by the National Institute of Occupational Safety and Health Grant OH2421 and the National Institutes of Health Grants ES00002 and ES69780.

References

Barker, C. 1995. Research and the health services manager in the developing world. *Social Science & Medicine* 41: 1655–65.

Bertazzi, P. A. 1989. Industrial disasters and epidemiology: A review of recent experiences. *Scandinavian Journal of Work and Environmental Health* 15: 85–100.

Boon-Long, J., T. Glinsukon, P. Pothisiri, S. Srianujata, V. Suphakarn, and M. Wongphanich. 1986. Toxicological problems in Thailand. In *Environmental toxicity and carcinogenesis. Proceedings of a regional workshop*, edited by M. Ruchirawat and R. C. Shank. Bangkok: Text and Journal Corporation.

Borenstein, D. G., S. W. Wiesel, and S. D. Boden. 1995. *Low back pain. Medical diagnosis and comprehensive management.* Philadelphia: Saunders.

Carpenter, D. O., K. F. Arcaro, B. Bush, W. D. Niemi, S. Peng, and D. D. Vakharia. 1998. Human health and chemical mixtures: An overview. *Environmental Health Perspectives* 106: 1263–70.

Carter, N. L. 1980. Eye colour and susceptibility to noise-induced permanent threshold shift. *Audiology* 19: 86–93.

Cary, R., S. Clarke, and J. Delic. 1997. Effects of combined exposure to noise and toxic substances: Critical review of the literature. *Annals of Occupational Hygiene* 41: 455–65.

Chen, M. S., and A. Chan. 1999. China's "Market economic in command": Footwear workers' health in jeopardy. *International Journal of Health Services* 29: 793–811.

Chen, M. S., and C. L. Huang. 1997. Industrial workers' health and environmental pollution under the new international division of labor: The Taiwan experience. *American Journal of Public Health* 87: 1223–31.

Christiani, D. C. 1988. Modernization and occupational cancer (editorial). *Journal of Occupational Medicine* 30: 975–76.

Christiani, D. C., R. Durvasula, and J. Myers. 1990. Occupational health in developing countries: Review of research needs. *American Journal of Industrial Medicine* 17: 393–401.

Christiani, D. C., and R. R. Monson. 1997. Introduction: Cancer in relation to occupational and environmental exposures. *Cancer Causes and Control* 8: 269–70.

Colditz, G., W. Dejong, D. Hunter, D. Trichopoulos, and W. Willett, eds. 1996. Harvard Report on Cancer Prevention. *Cancer Causes and Control* 7(suppl.): S55.

Colvin, M., A. Dalvie, J. E. Myers, I. A. Macun, and B. Sharp. 1998. Health and safety in the Lesotho Highlands Dam and Tunnel Construction Program. *International Journal of Occupational and Environmental Health* 4(4): 231–35.

Cooper, J. C. 1994. Health and nutrition examination survey 1997–1975: I. Ear and race effects in hearing. *Journal of American Academic Audiology* 5: 30–36.

Cunningham, D. R., and M. L. Norris. 1982. Eye color and noise induced hearing loss: a population study. *Ear Hear* 3: 211–214.

Department of Labor and Employment (DLE). 1999. *Annual medical report of the Bureau of Working Conditions.* Manila: DLE.

Doll, R., and R. Peto. 1981a. *The causes of cancer.* New York: Oxford University Press.

Doll, R., and R. Peto. 1981b. The causes of cancer: Quantitative estimates of avoidable risks of cancer in the United States today. *Journal of the National Cancer Institute* 66: 1191–308.

Dunn, D. E. 2000. Noise. In *Occupational health: Recognizing and preventing work-related disease and injury*, 4th ed., edited by B. S. Levy and D. H. Wegman. Philadelphia: Lippincott Williams & Wilkins.

Feron, V. J., F. R. Cassee, and J. P. Groten. 1998. Toxicology of chemical mixtures: International perspective. *Environmental Health Perspectives* 106: 1281–89.

Firpo de Souza Porto, M., and C. M. de Freitas. 1996. Major chemical accidents in industrializing countries: The socio-political amplification of risk. *Risk Analysis* 16: 19–29.

Frumkin, H. 1997. Cancer epidemiology and the workplace. *Salud Pública de Mexico* 39: 356–69.

Gold, E. B., B. L. Lasley, and M. B. Schenker. 1994. Introduction: Rationale for an update. Reproductive hazards. *Occupational Medicine* 9: 363–72.

Graham, J. D., L. C. Green, and M. J. Roberts. 1988. *In search of safety: Chemical and cancer risk.* Cambridge, MA: Harvard University Press.

Greenhouse, S. 1997. Nike shoe plant in Vietnam is called unsafe for workers. *New York Times*, November 8, p. 1.

He, F. 1998. Occupational medicine in China. *International Archives of Occupational and Environmental Health* 71: 79–84.

International Agency for Research on Cancer (IARC). 1972–99. *IARC monographs on the evaluation of carcinogenic risks of chemicals to humans.* 71 vols. Lyon, France: IARC.

International Agency for Research on Cancer (IARC). 1987. *Overall evaluations of carcinogenicity: An updating of IARC monographs 1–42*, supplement 7. Lyon, France: IARC.

International Labor Office (ILO). 1994. *Seminário Latino-Americano Sobre Accidentes Mayores.* São Paulo, Brazil: ILO.

Ishii, E. K., and E. O. Talbott. 1998. Race/ethnicity differences in the prevalence of noise-induced hearing loss in a group of metal fabricating workers. *Journal of Occupational and Environmental Medicine* 41: 661–66.

Jeyaratnam, J. 1982. Survey of pesticide poisoning in Sri Lanka. *Bulletin of the World Health Organization* 60: 615–19.

Jeyaratnam, J., ed. 1992. *Occupational health in developing countries.* Oxford: Oxford University Press.

Jeyaratnam, J. 1993. Occupational health issues in developing countries. *Environmental Research* 61: 207–12.

Jindal, S., and J. Whig. 1998. Silicosis in developing countries. In *Occupational lung disease: An international perspective*, edited by D. E. Banks and J. E. Parker. London: Chapman & Hall.

Johanning, E. 2000. Evaluation and management of occupational low back disorders. *American Journal of Industrial Medicine* 37: 94–111.

Joint Project on Health Systems Research. 1994. Peer review of the joint project on health systems research for southern African countries, June 1993. *Health System Research Newsletter.* Feb., No. 12, 6.

Kogevinas, M., P. Boffetta, and N. Pearce. 1994. Occupational exposure to carcinogens in developing countries. In *Occupational cancer in developing countries*, edited by N. Pearce,

E. Matos, H. Vainio, P. Boffetta, and M. Kogevinas. IARC Scientific Publication 129. Lyon, France: IARC.

LaDou, J. 1991. Deadly migration. *Technological Review* 7: 47–53.

LaDou, J., and T. Rohm. 1998. The international electronics industry. *International Journal of Occupational and Environmental Health* 4: 1–18.

Lee, S. H. 1999. Occupational medicine in Korea. *International Archives of Occupational and Environmental Health* 72: 1–6.

Lemen, R., and E. Bingham. 1994. A case study in avoiding a deadly legacy in developing countries. *Toxicology and Industrial Health* 10: 59–78.

Levy, B. S., and D. H. Wegman. 2000. Occupational health: An overview. In *Occupational health: Recognizing and preventing work-related disease and injury*, 4th ed., edited by B. S. Levy and D. H. Wegman. Philadelphia: Lippincott Williams & Wilkins.

Loewenson, R. H. 1998. Health impact of occupational risks in the informal sector in Zimbabwe. *International Journal of Occupational Environmental Health* 4: 264–74.

London, L. 1994. Agrichemical safety practices on farms in the Western Cape. *South African Medical Journal* 84: 273–78.

Maroni, M., C. Colosio, A. Ferioli, and A. Fait. 2000. Introduction. In: Biological monitoring of pesticide exposure (review). *Toxicology* 143: 5–8.

McCauley, L. A. 1998. Chemical mixtures in the workplace. Research and practice. *American Association of Occupational Health Nurses Journal* 46: 29–40.

McCunney, R. J., and J. D. Meyer. 1998. Occupational exposure to noise. In *Environmental and Occupational Medicine*, 3rd ed., edited by W. N. Rom. Philadelphia: Lippincott-Raven.

Murray, C. J. L., A. D. Lopez. 1996. *The global burden of disease*, Vol. I. World Health Organization, World Bank. Cambridge, MA: Harvard School of Public Health.

National Institute for Occupational Safety and Health (NIOSH). 1996. *Criteria for a recommended standard. Occupational noise exposure. Revised criteria 1996.* Washington, D.C.: U.S. Department of Health and Human Services.

National Institute for Occupational Safety and Health (NIOSH). 2000. Worker Health Chartbook. U.S. Department of Health and Human Services; CDC and NIOSH. DHHS (NIOSH). Publication Number 2000-127.

Parmeggiani, L. 1983. *Encyclopaedia of occupational health and safety*, 3rd ed. Geneva: International Labor Organization.

Patellos, M. C., and D. H. Garabrant. 1994. Occupational cancer. *Primary Care* 21: 329–47.

Pearce, N., E. Matos, H. Vainio, P. Boffetta, and M. Kogevinas, eds. 1994. *Occupational cancer in developing countries.* IARC Scientific Publication 129. Lyon, France: IARC.

Pope, M. H. 1989. Risk indicators in low back pain. *Annals of Medicine* 21: 387–92.

Raffle, P. A. B., W. R. Lee, R. I. McCallum, and R. Murray. 1987. *Hunter's diseases of occupations*, 7th ed. Boston: Little, Brown.

Sadhra, S., J. R. Beach, T. C. Aw, and K. Sheikh-Ahmed. 2001. Occupational health research priorities in Malaysia: A Delphi study. *Occupational and Environmental Medicine* 58: 426–31.

Šarić, M. 1999. Occupational health services in Croatia. *International Archives of Occupational Environmental Health* 72: 481–95.

Simonato, L. 1986. Occupational cancer risk in developing countries and priorities for epidemiological research. In *Proceedings of the international symposium on health and environment in developing countries.* Haikko, Finland.

Steenland, K., and L. Stayner. 1997. Silica, asbestos, man-made mineral fibers, and cancer. *Cancer Causes and Control* 8: 491–503.

Stellman, J. M., ed. 1997. *Encyclopaedia of occupational health and safety*, 4th ed. Geneva: International Labor Organization.

Tay, P. 1996. Severe noise-induced deafness—a 10-year review of cases. *Singapore Medical Journal* 37(4): 362–64.

Tennenbaum, D. 1996. The value of Vietnam. *Environmental Health of Perspectives* 104: 1280–5.

Van, S. 1990. Pneumoconiosis: The situation in developing countries. *Experimental Lung Research* 16: 5–13.

Vineis, P., K. Cantor, C. Gonzales, E. Lynge, and V. Vallyathan. 1995. Occupational cancer in developed and developing countries. *International Journal of Cancer* 62: 655–60.

Vineis, P., and L. Simonato. 1991. Proportion of cancers in males due to occupation: A systematic approach. *Archives of Environmental Health* 46: 6–15.

Volinn, E. 1997. The epidemiology of low back pain in the rest of the world. A review of surveys in low- and middle-income countries. *Spine* 22: 1747–54.

Walker, P. 1995. *World disaster report.* Geneva: International Federation of Red Cross and Red Crescent Societies.

World Bank. 1993. *World Development Report, 1993: Investing in Health.* Oxford: Oxford University Press.

World Health Organization (WHO). 1990. *Public health impact of pesticides used in agriculture.* Geneva: WHO.

Xu, X., and D. C. Christiani. 1995. Occupational health research in developing countries: Focus on U.S.–China collaboration. *International Journal of Occupational and Environmental Health* 1: 136–41.

Yin, S. 1996. A cohort study of cancer among benzene-exposed workers in China: Overall results. *American Journal of Industrial Medicine* 29: 227–35.

2

Biological and Social Risks Intertwined: The Case of AIDS

ADEPEJU GBADEBO, ALYSSA RAYMAN-READ, AND JODY HEYMANN

Biological and social exposures at work can play as strong a role in determining individual health as physical and chemical ones. AIDS provides a prime example of the relationship among social and biological conditions at work and health. No greater threat to health has arisen in centuries than the human immunodeficiency virus/acquired immunodeficiency syndrome (HIV/AIDS) epidemic. The World Health Organization (WHO) has estimated that by the end of 2001, 40 million people were infected with HIV/AIDS worldwide. That year, there were approximately 14,000 new infections per day. Although the incidence of HIV is rising fastest in Eastern Europe and Southeast and Central Asia, the AIDS epidemic is now most dire in sub-Saharan Africa, where 3.4 million new infections in 2001 alone resulted in more than 28.1 million people living with HIV/AIDS (UNAIDS/WHO, 2001). Moreover, HIV/AIDS is overwhelmingly concentrated among working-age adults. Social and biological conditions are critical determinants of both HIV infection and how those who become infected with HIV fare.

We begin this chapter by exploring the bidirectional relationship between HIV/AIDS and the workplace. In the second section, we outline what has already been done to address the relationship between HIV/AIDS and the workplace. This international review of existing social policy and research regarding HIV/AIDS and the workplace reveals that most current efforts to address the relationship between work and health do not respond adequately to the HIV/AIDS epidemic in nations and regions of the world with very high disease prevalence rates. In the third section, we present the findings of our research team's study of the impact of social conditions on the relationship between work and health in Botswana, where HIV prevalence rates approach 40% of working age adults. In the final section, we offer program and policy recommendations.

The Relationship between HIV/AIDS and the Workplace

Impact of HIV/AIDS on the Workplace

As a result of the epidemic, workplaces in hard-hit regions are suffering losses with the potential to cripple both the public and private sectors. These losses have profound long-term implications. HIV/AIDS affects the workplace for five main reasons.

First, workplaces—from public schools to private firms—face a shrinking labor pool. Although the number of people infected varies by region and nation, the overwhelming majority of those suffering from HIV/AIDS in both industrialized and developing nations are in their working prime. At least 25 million workers aged 15 to 49 are infected with the HIV virus (ILO, 2001). High HIV prevalence rates correspond to high morbidity and mortality, lowered life expectancy rates, and diminished work spans of healthy workers—all of which negatively affect the labor force. In the year 2000, 85% of the 300 deaths among the Central African Republic's teachers were caused by AIDS. In Zambia, the number of AIDS-related teacher deaths equaled approximately 50% of the number of teachers Zambia trains each year. In countries facing the worst of the epidemic, life expectancy has dropped precipitously. Those born in the sub-Saharan African nations of Botswana, Malawi, Mozambique, and Swaziland can expect to live for only four decades. Life expectancy in sub-Saharan Africa is currently about 47 years. Were it not for the HIV/AIDS virus, the average life expectancy would be 62 years (UNAIDS/WHO, 2001).

Second, the workplace suffers increased absenteeism and turnover due to the high prevalence of HIV. These problems are particularly severe in the developing world, where the majority of workers do not have access to antiretroviral therapies that extend periods of relative health. In fact, fewer than 4% of those residing in the most seriously affected nations have access to these therapies (UNAIDS, 2002a). A study of 15 firms in Ethiopia showed that during a 5-year period more than 53% of employee-reported illnesses were due to AIDS (UNAIDS/WHO, 2001). According to a report on sub-Saharan Africa from the UNAIDS program, "illness and death" had moved from last place (UNAIDS, 2000c, 2) to first place on the list of reasons people gave for leaving a company. While old-age retirement accounted for the majority of employee attrition as recently as the 1980s, it accounted for a small minority of all employee attrition as of 1997 (UNAIDS, 2000c).

Third, there are new burdens for healthy workers, since remaining workers often must compensate for lost productivity by shifting their job duties or taking on residual workloads. Fourth, HIV/AIDS affects workplaces by increasing the costs, sometimes dramatically, of work benefits and subsidies such as health insurance and disability payments. Work benefits and policies are typically sustainable because most workers are well. In countries where a large percentages of workers are ill, health-care and disability benefits, among others, cost much more than many workplaces originally projected and ultimately may be able to sustain. Finally, HIV/AIDS hurts the workplace because social stigmatization and discrimination, along with the problems they precipitate, have not yet been adequately addressed.

In summary, the influences of HIV/AIDS on workplaces range from profound humanitarian losses to marked economic threats, from individual employee losses to workplace-wide losses to national losses. Shrinking labor pools, increased absenteeism and turnover, increased burdens on healthy workers, rising costs of benefits, and the loss of job security and earning capacity for infected workers and their colleagues all add enormous burdens to individuals and to the workplace.

Impacts of the Workplace on HIV/AIDS

Not only does HIV/AIDS significantly affect workplaces, but the workplace significantly influences the transmission and consequences of HIV/AIDS in various ways. The primary structural and environmental factors affecting HIV transmission that have been demonstrated include mobility, economic vulnerability, and inequalities related to such issues as gender-based discrimination and disease-based stigmatization. All of these transmission factors are relevant to the workplace (UNAIDS, 2000a).

Likewise, a limited number of employment opportunities and heightened fears of job loss influence how HIV-infected workers respond to their illness. If workers believe a positive HIV status will result in negative outcomes at work, such as loss of employment or advancement opportunities, they often are less likely to get tested for HIV and to seek appropriate treatment and counseling. Workplaces that create fearful or discriminatory environments for those suffering from HIV/AIDS may therefore contribute to the disease's spread and impede medical treatment.

The Consequences of Inaction

The relationship between HIV/AIDS and the workplace is already influencing every economic sector in countries with high prevalence rates. Calculations from WHO indicate that some of the highest-prevalence countries will lose as much as 20% of their gross domestic product (GDP) by 2020 (UNAIDS/WHO, 2001). South Africa has estimated that it has lost and will lose 1% of GDP each year between 1998 and 2005 if current trends continue. Likewise, the World Bank has projected that in Tanzania, GDP growth for the period 1985 to 2010 will be reduced 15% to 25% due to AIDS. In India, recent analyses found that 90% of the 3 to 5 million people living with HIV/AIDS were under 45 years of age, and as of the year 2000, the cost to Asian economies of HIV/AIDS was between $38 billion and $52 billion (UNAIDS, 1998). Finally, the annual per capita growth rate in half of the nations of sub-Saharan Africa has been reduced 0.5% to 1.2% as a consequence of the AIDS crisis, according to WHO estimates (UNAIDS/WHO, 2001).

Workplace Prevention, Research, and Policy Efforts to Date

Although interest in the relationship between the work world and HIV/AIDS among leaders in the global campaign against AIDS is clear, program and policy action remains inadequate. Many of the private and public initiatives addressing HIV/AIDS in the workplace today are limited in scope to specific target populations and do not address the range of factors underlying disease transmission. This section explains why the workplace deserves greater focus as a site for HIV/AIDS prevention and treatment programs and why the scope of such programs must account for the factors of disease transmission in high prevalence regions.

Inadequate Attention to High-Prevalence Areas

Although workplace efforts to date have not effectively addressed the general at-risk population in the high-prevalence countries, some workplace intervention programs implemented thus far in sub-Saharan Africa have succeeded in reducing high-risk sexual activity in defined subpopulations. For instance, a behavioral intervention in Kenya among male truckers—which involved HIV counseling and testing, condom promotion, and diagnosis and management of sexually transmitted diseases during a 1-year follow-up period—revealed a significant decline in self-reported contact with female sex workers and in sexually transmitted disease rates (Jackson et al., 1997). Similarly, an intervention in Tanzania among barmaids and restaurant workers decreased self-reported high-risk sexual behavior, including commercial sex work (Mhalu et al., 1991).

As validated public health approaches, programs targeting high-risk individuals remain valuable in preventing HIV transmission in many regions of the world, especially where the epidemic's impact is highly concentrated in definable at-risk groups. However, this narrowly targeted approach is inadequate in regions where HIV/AIDS is affecting populations in which virtually every working-age adult, regardless of job title or grade, can be identified as at significant risk for infection.

Initial Focus on Legal Measures

In addition to prevention efforts targeted at subpopulations, early approaches focused on legal protections whose goal was to secure for people with HIV/AIDS the right to "full, freely chosen and productive employment," (N'Daba and Hodges-Aeberhard, 1998, 7), the right to confidentiality regarding disease status, specific rights such as the right to certain employee benefits (social security, pensions, medical coverage, and so on), and the right to such accommodations to failing health as flexibility in work duties or schedules. For example, in Australia, Canada, and the United States, having HIV/AIDS was defined as a protected disability under civil rights and labor laws, which prohibit employment discrimination on the basis of disability (Hodges-Aeberhard, 1999).

Although legal approaches can offer important protections for HIV-infected workers and establish grievance procedures regarding infringed rights, these approaches have limitations in terms of their effectiveness at preventing discrimination. First, legal measures may subject workers to breaches of medical confidentiality, which may lead to further stigmatization and discrimination (Hodges-Aeberhard, 1999). Second, current legislation is often incomplete in its application because infected workers do not merely face discrimination in relation to hiring, promotion, and dismissal; they also confront challenges regarding their access to employment benefits, including medical coverage and pensions. Third, the legislation does not address the practices and beliefs underlying stigmatization and discrimination. (Gostin, Feldblum, and Webber, 1999). Moreover, the legal approach to antidiscrimination generally does not address the social and economic conditions that affect the spread of HIV in the workplace and how those who are infected fare.

Recent Attention to Treatment

In world regions where the HIV/AIDS epidemic is most severe, employers are finding it necessary to attend more to the health of their workforce. The case of Debswana provides an important example of this more recent response.

Debswana Diamond Company is 50% owned by DeBeers and 50% owned by the government of Botswana, and employs more than 5300 people in the areas of diamond mining, refining, and sales via its urban-based corporate headquarters and its rural mining facilities.[1] After the first AIDS deaths were observed in the hospitals located at the Jwaneng and Orapa mines in 1987 and 1989 (Botswana and UNDP, 2000), Debswana initiated education and awareness programs in 1988 and 1989. In response to a knowledge, attitude, and practice survey conducted by a physician at the Jwaneng mine in 1990, full-time AIDS coordinators were hired for the mines at Jwaneng and Orapa in 1991 and 1992, respectively, to educate and counsel Debswana's workforce (Botswana and UNDP, 2000).

In the late 1990s, the company began to experience more intensely the impact of increased HIV/AIDS-related morbidity and mortality on its workforce. Ill-health retirements increased from 40% in 1996 to 75% in 1999—and a high percentage were due to AIDS-related conditions (Debswana Diamond Co., 2001). Moreover, the percentage of AIDS-related deaths increased rapidly throughout this period: in 1996, it was 37.5%; in 1997, 48.3%; and in 1999, 59.1% (Debswana Diamond Co., 2001). The threat to workers' health was rising, as was the threat to the company's viability. Increased morbidity and mortality led not only to increased absenteeism (due to sickness and funeral attendance), retraining costs, and payout of medical and retirement benefits, but also to lowered employee morale and productivity.

In 2000, an AIDS Impact Assessment estimated the costs and benefits (as measured by units of productivity, sick leave allowances, and employee benefits) of providing life-prolonging antiretroviral therapies. The findings suggested that antiretroviral therapy would prolong the active lives of employees living with HIV/AIDS and would be affordable because the benefits would offset the costs. As a result, in 2001 Debswana's board of directors decided to become the first company on the African continent to subsidize the cost of prophylactics and antiretroviral drugs, as well as the related costs of monitoring viral loads and CD4 counts (Actuarial Solutions, 2000; Debswana Diamond Co., 2001). The company pays 90% of these costs for the employee and one family member who is HIV positive for as long as the employee remains in the employ of Debswana (Debswana Diamond Co., 2001).

While Debswana has taken remarkable steps to combat HIV/AIDS-related illnesses in the company by offering workers voluntary testing and by subsidizing antiretroviral drug costs for all workers, to date only 12% of the workers known to have the disease have taken advantage of the program. According to Debswana officials, the discrepancy occurs because of persistent, deep-seated stigmatization and discrimination in the community, which create fears of retributive responses to a positive disease status among workers who may worry that their privacy will be lost by testing and treatment (PLUSnews, 2001).

Since Debswana's 2001 decision, other companies including Anglo American and DeBeers in South Africa have decided to develop antiretroviral therapy programs. The importance of these programs in beginning to address the suffering of those already infected cannot be overstated. Yet, it is equally clear that these programs cannot stand alone. It remains the case that any worker would prefer not to become infected rather than to become ill and receive treatment. Treatment programs on their own do not begin to address prevention. The social conditions that raise the risk of infection need to be addressed. Moreover, it is essential to address discrimination for treatment to be accepted.

Work, HIV/AIDS, and Health in Botswana: A Case Study

The HIV epidemic is dramatically more severe in sub-Saharan Africa than in much of the rest of the world: approximately 70% of people living with HIV/AIDS in 1999 resided in that region. Furthermore, sub-Saharan African nations account for all of the world's 16 countries in which more than 10% of the adults aged 15 to 49 are infected with HIV; and in 7 southern African countries, 20% or more of adults in that age range are infected with HIV (UNAIDS, 2000a). Botswana, with a population of 1.6 million, faces a particularly grim HIV/AIDS epidemic, making it an important site for AIDS research and prevention work. Yet, Botswana has several advantages when it comes to addressing HIV/AIDS because it has a stable democracy, a decent health infrastructure, and a relatively strong economy. Even with these strengths, however, the relationship between work and HIV/AIDS in Botswana illustrates the problems that workers in high-prevalence regions experience.

The Botswana Epidemic and the Project on Global Working Families

Botswana currently has the highest HIV prevalence rate in the world. In 1999, sentinel surveillance statistics from Botswana showed an adult seroprevalence rate of 36% among sexually active adults (UNAIDS, 2000a), with the highest rate occurring among 20- to 30-year-olds (Government of Botswana, Ministry of Health, 2000). Furthermore, mathematical modeling has shown that if the HIV incidence rate remains unchanged, more than 85% of Botswanan males currently aged 15 will eventually die of AIDS (and more than 65% will die of AIDS even if the current HIV incidence rate is halved) (UNAIDS, 2000a). This means that without proper medical care, one-third of Botswana's adult population could die by 2010. Such grim trends will have extensive economic repercussions as well. Before the HIV epidemic, Botswana had one of the most rapidly growing economies in sub-Saharan Africa (UNDP, 2000), but HIV/AIDS now completely threatens the economy. A government study on the macroeconomic impacts of HIV/AIDS has estimated that Botswana's GDP will be 24% to 38% less by 2021 than it would have been without the disease (Botswana and UNDP, 2000).

The Botswana case study presented below includes both existing information from the research literature and new findings from the Project on Global Working Families, led by Heymann. Heymann's multicountry study, examining the relationship between work and health, has investigated the impact of HIV/AIDS on work and caregiving by adults in Botswana.

The study involved both closed-ended and semistructured, open-ended interviews. Since June 2000, the project team has conducted more than 200 in-depth and over 1000 closed-ended interviews for this study. Participants were recruited at government health clinics in one city (Gabarone), one town (Lobatse), and one urban village (Molepolole). People were eligible if they were working or had been working during the previous 6 months in either the informal or formal sector and if they were the primary caregiver for at least one other person. Results of the in-depth interview study are reported here; the large follow-up survey is currently underway. The response rate for the in-depth study was 96%. Of those interviewed, 8% had had no formal education, 33% had attended primary school, 37% had attended junior secondary school, 13% had attended senior secondary school, and 9% had attended a tertiary education program or university. Seventy-six percent of respondents work in the formal sector and 24% in the informal sector. Fifty-seven percent of respondents both work and care for a family member or friend with HIV/AIDS at least once per week. In addition, more than 50 professionals were interviewed, including physicians, teachers, child-care providers, and employers. The professional interviews were conducted in a range of locations, including urban, town, and village areas in 2001. Professional respondents were chosen based on the advice of people knowledgeable about the given area.

In the following sections, we examine the evidence relevant to the key socioeconomic and environmental factors discussed at the beginning of the chapter, including stigmatization and discrimination at work, economic inequalities at work, gender disparities at work, and workers' mobility. Each subsection begins with a presentation of current understandings from previous research and then expands this discussion by presenting insights from Botswanan participants in the Project on Global Working Families. In addition, we provide new research findings on the relationship between HIV/AIDS caregiving and work.

Stigmatization and Discrimination

Addressing the social, institutional, and legal discrimination related to an HIV-positive status is a universal and widely recognized challenge. For those countries with high prevalence rates, this challenge is particularly pressing, as a higher percentage of the population is exposed to the effects of stigmatization and discrimination. According to a report issued as part of the World AIDS Campaign 2002–2003, "stigma and discrimination associated with HIV and AIDS are the greatest barriers to preventing further infections, providing adequate care, support and treatment and alleviating impact" (UNAIDS, 2002b, 5).

Even in countries like the United States, which currently has strong public policies to protect workers from discrimination, the U.S. Equal Employment Opportunity Commission reported in 2000 that, since 1992, 2400 HIV-related cases had been filed (U.S. Equal Employment Opportunity Commission, 2000). In countries where labor codes are not well developed or enforced, HIV stigmatization can be even more damaging.

While the prevalence and consequences of HIV discrimination in the workplace have not been carefully studied in sub-Saharan Africa, trade unions and nongovernmental organizations have documented discrimination through mandatory testing of job applicants, dismissal of workers with AIDS, employment of only those who are thought to be at low risk for HIV, and exclusion of HIV coverage from medical benefits schemes (UNDP, 1998). Silence, prejudicial attitudes, myths, and misinformation bred by stigmas have acted as fuel for the HIV epidemic, since many people have been reluctant to be tested for HIV and to seek medical treatment in countries such as Uganda and Kenya (Moss et al., 1999; Muyinda et al., 1997). This reluctance to be tested may prevent individuals from taking appropriate preventive measures if they are HIV negative or, if they are HIV positive, may affect whether they expose others to the disease.

Individuals interviewed in the Project on Global Working Families in Botswana reported that they deeply feared social stigmas in the workplace. Some reported that they were unwilling to be tested for HIV in part because they feared repercussions—perceived or real—that their HIV information-seeking would have on their jobs and, therefore, their ability to earn a living.

According to the clinic patients and the professionals interviewed in the Botswana study, the medical community often encouraged patients to keep their medical records confidential, especially from their employers. Some respondents noted that doctors were sometimes so concerned about the social stigmas their patients might face that they were guarded even in their written comments about their patients' medical conditions.

One 32-year-old man, Phadi,[2] described the locally common practice of doctors writing coded symptom observations on medical cards (which each Botswanan carries to and from clinic visits) to limit the likelihood of public knowledge of HIV status.

Physicians may be particularly inclined to write ambiguous diagnoses when they perceive that a patient's job security might be at risk. Dr. Leatile Ayo explained what she did when such cases arose:

> We only say their symptoms, but we don't mention that they're HIV positive. We know that once we mention that, maybe that patient will lose their job. We just discuss the objectives [with the] employers and what we are doing with the patient and what we expect, but we don't say anything more.

Another physician, Dr. Tiego Jacobs, explained:

> The attitude of the shrewd employers has been to fire them, actually. They lose their jobs. Because if you are a food handler who is found to be positive, that's the end of you. Even if you tell them that it's treatable—all you have to do is lay off somebody for a couple of weeks, then their job—that is why we never, never write their diagnosis. They always write to us, "Doctors, send me this patient—furnish us with the diagnosis." We never [do that].

Dr. Jacobs also explained that employers sometimes went to great lengths to uncover their employees' health status. He said that employers usually try to convince their employees to relinquish their hospital record cards, which patients keep in their possession between health care visits. Dr. Jacobs said that employers call sick workers into their office and demand to see their hospital card—the one with a diagnosis. If workers do not share their cards voluntarily, he said, some employers physically "grab" their medical cards. According to Dr. Jacobs, employers read these medical cards and say "'Aha, no wonder you always come to the hospital so frequently.'" Because of the likelihood of this violation of privacy regarding disease status, Dr. Jacobs explains, "That's why we always say [that] what's written on the card is always confidential. It should not be shown to the employer." In cases in which employers try to access their employees' medical records, either voluntarily or forcibly, Dr. Jacobs says he tells his patients not to comply.

Clearly, both doctors and workers feared the repercussions to employment that a loss of privacy could precipitate.

Poverty and Economic Inequalities

Poverty is a critical factor in HIV/AIDS transmission. As the *Botswana Human Development Report* of 2000 states, "Poverty is both a cause and a consequence of ill health. . . . Thus poverty and HIV and AIDS tend to be mutually reinforcing realities" (Botswana and UNDP, 2000, 17). Although poverty statistics in Botswana are limited, the most recent widely used study (the BIDPA *Study on Poverty and Poverty Alleviation in Botswana*), conducted in 1997, found that 47% of the population fell below the national poverty line in 1994 (UNCTAD and UNDP, 2000) and 21% were unemployed in 1997.

Economic factors underlie the decisions that individuals make about their work and health behaviors when confronting the impact of the AIDS epidemic on their personal and professional lives. Gakale, an HIV-positive 36-year-old separated mother of three children (aged 13 to 17 years), "had to work," even though her physical pain was amplified by her work duties and demanding schedule. Gakale said that quitting was not an affordable option for her and her family. The financial losses she already had incurred for medical leaves had made it difficult to provide for even her family's basic needs:

> If I quit I won't have anything to live on. I go to work as much as possible. I only come to the hospital if I feel the pain is too great or if the doctor has asked me to come back for review. . . . This problem has caused me some financial problems. I don't get as much money as I used to when I was healthy and working all the time. Because of that, I find myself running into shortages that I didn't used to have. . . . Food is also a problem these days. We run short of food before the end of the month.

The overall reduction of productivity due to illness impoverished individual workers and businesses as they struggled to compensate for lost human capital, but medical treatment sometimes ended up being pitted against job security. Phadi, a 32-year-old father of a 4-year-old daughter, explained that taking frequent medical leaves had increased the pressures at his workplace, intensifying his relationship with managers every time he sought medical care:

> Whenever I have something that needs medical attention, my supervisors allow me to go to the hospital, but they always ask me to return as soon as possible. They want me to finish my work. The problem is that I have a lump of work remaining. . . . When I come back, I find I have piles of work to do. I also have new inquiries coming in. That means the work gets harder when I come to the hospital.

Phadi believed his position was insecure and as a result often felt compelled to work even when ill to avoid losing his position. He had been fired from a previous job because of his disease:

> The way [companies] operate is this: when you get seriously sick, they dismiss you. I was admitted [to the hospital], so they dismissed me. What they do is pay you for the month you've worked and then for the next month and your leave days. That's it.

HIV/AIDS also takes a particularly devastating toll on poor workers by further restricting their choices about work. Workers become locked into jobs and into limited financial futures.

Socioeconomic conditions are inextricably linked to the relationship between HIV/AIDS and the workplace. The influence of working conditions on health outcomes is magnified when poor people become sick and face losing needed income. Furthermore, our interviews with workers in Botswana show that income and economic status affect a range of work-related choices. Those without access to economic resources clearly report a diminished ability to select protective working conditions, to seek job advancement, to obtain job security, and to meet their health needs.

Gender Disparities

Crucial risks related to HIV, work, and health are dictated by gender disparities. Although more research is needed on work-related sexual harassment and coercion, there is already compelling evidence that sexual harassment in the workplace is common globally and is overwhelmingly experienced by women rather than men. A review of 18 studies estimated that 44% of women have experienced sexual harassment at work at some point (Gruber, 1990). Women may be coerced into having sexual relations with employers as a condition of employment or promotion (Schoepf, 1988, 1992, 1993a, 1993b; Walu, 1991). In fact, a study in Tanzania found that women who work in the formal sector (such as the manual labor, office, and business jobs that employ most women in Botswana's formal sector) are significantly more likely to be HIV infected than women who work independently on their farms (Quigley et al., 1997). Another study—involving women in Botswana—revealed that the first sexual experience for 20% of the respondents interviewed had been coerced under physical duress (MacDonald, 1996). When societywide gender discrimination creates workplaces prone to sexual harassment and exploitation, workplace environments can crucially affect modes of transmission of HIV infection. As in other countries, examining these issues is an essential first step toward meeting Botswana's national goal of designing comprehensive prevention programs addressing women's health hazards in the workplace (MacDonald, 1996).

In addition, studies in several sub-Saharan African countries have demonstrated the degree to which sexual relationships are characterized by male attitudes and societal norms that sanction sexual relationships between young girls and older men. Girls in these studies were found to be at higher risk of HIV infection than boys; in fact, 14-year-old girls in Ndola, Zambia, were four times more likely than their male counterparts to be HIV positive (Botswana and UNDP, 2000). In Botswana, there are two HIV-positive girls under the age of 14 for each HIV-positive boy in this age group. Among 15- to 29-year-olds, the ratio rises to three HIV-positive women for every HIV-positive man. Experts believe these data are explained by the Botswanan tendency for young girls to engage in sexual relationships with older men (Botswana and UNDP, 2000).

Poor women throughout the developing world who are unable to support themselves financially are more dependent on partners—either temporarily or long-term—for their subsistence, and this dependence may be associated with the exchange of sex for money or material gifts (deBruyn, 1992; Schoepf, 1988, 1993b; Schoepf et al., 1988; Stoller and Schneider, 1993; Susser and Stein, 2000). In creating development goals, Botswanan officials cited anecdotal evidence that the feminization of poverty in Botswana was one of the causes of female prostitution (Meekers and Calves, 1997). It may also be associated with the need for women to remain sexually active with partners even when they fear their partners are at high risk for HIV infection or are already infected (Botswana and UNDP, 2000). At a meeting outside Durban, women stated that the best method for preventing HIV would be to provide work for women, and that the exchange of sex for money was not restricted to sex workers but was a last option for women whose families desperately needed food or money (Susser and Stein, 2000). Nongovernmental organizations have identified women's education, job training, and economic independence as potential means of reducing women's HIV infection risks (Smith and Cohen, 2000).

The Project on Global Working Families interviews indicated that even when women were employed, they could not protect themselves from HIV infection when economic hardship was paired with gender inequality. In one such interview, a 27-year-old mother of one child, who opened her own *tuck shop* (a type of convenience cart, from which she sold food, beverages, and small household items), said she could not insist on safe sex with her abusive boyfriend because she was financially dependent on him to help support her.

Workers' Mobility

The workforce in Botswana, like the workforces in many other sub-Saharan African countries, is highly mobile. In a 1995–1996 government survey, 35.6% of employed individuals said that they had migrated for the purposes of a job (20.1% had been seeking jobs, and 15.5% had been transferred in their jobs) (Government of Botswana, 1998). Botswana's relatively strong transportation infrastructure, recently improved further with the completion of the Kalahari Highway linking Botswana to both Namibia and South Africa, has only increased the frequency of work-related migration, travel, and mobility (Botswana and UNDP, 2000).

Current public and private practices include transferring employees across Botswana in order to staff remote outposts. The government often sends teachers, police personnel, health-care workers, and other government employees—usually separated from their families—to remote locations to work for several years at a time in underserved areas. Until 1999, when the practice eased because of concerns regarding HIV exposure, the government also had a youth Year of Service program (Tirilo Sechaba), in which girls and boys graduating from senior secondary (high) school were sent away from home to work as government employees for 1 year, often in remote areas (Eberly, 1992).

Other forms of work-related migration in Botswana are also common. Workers travel both to obtain work and to keep it (such as construction jobs that require workers to move from site to site), and they travel both within Botswana and to neighboring countries. Mining, in particular, has created many job opportunities for which workers travel. Almost half of the laborers in South Africa's gold mines, for example, come from the neighboring countries of Botswana, Lesotho, and Mozambique (UNAIDS, 2000b). Furthermore, partners often separate and travel for weeks or months to tend to their fields and cattle herds during certain times of the year; even 50% of relatively poor urban dwellers still have land in the villages in which they grew up (Kruger, 1998). Frequent traveling means that workers are frequently separated from their families and communities and are exposed to the stresses of social and cultural transitions (UNAIDS, 2000a).

In terms of health risks, employees required to work in remote locations or to travel frequently tend to engage in high-risk sex more frequently than do their less mobile counterparts (UNESCO and UNAIDS 2000). Along with gender and income inequalities, mobility factors play a large role in the spread of AIDS. One 44-year-old teacher who had lived apart from his wife for several years because of his job described in an interview for the Project on Global Working Families how risks increased when employment separated partners:

> One serious risk is the risk of HIV/AIDS. If you are not with your spouse, there is this tendency for people to lose their self-control and they sleep around. . . . Promiscuity is a problem. I think relationships tend to suffer if you are apart.

Especially for new and younger workers, as well as workers whose circumstances (such as poverty) limit their choice of jobs, separation from family as a result of job-related travel may be unavoidable. As one 25-year-old man we interviewed explained, this placed both the workers and the communities they migrated to at risk:

> At my home village, during the time the police college was being built, construction people came from South Africa to work for the company and build the school. These girls in the village fell for these guys. These guys use no protection and they go sleeping around with people. When the company leaves, it leaves disaster. It leaves AIDS.

Although it has been established that mobile work populations are at greater risk for HIV infection than the population at large, a study conducted in Botswana in 1999 found that only half of the mobile workers interviewed consistently used a condom during sex (Botswana and UNDP, 2000).

Impact Beyond Individual Workers: Caregiving and the Workplace

In addition to the workplace factors discussed thus far affecting the outcomes of HIV-infected individuals, the Project on Global Working Families interviews with Botswanan workers indicated that there were other important ways workplace conditions affect workers. Particularly striking was the relationship among caregiving for ill family members and friends, caring for children orphaned by HIV, and adults' work.

Caregivers often had to make impossible choices between caring for their loved ones and keeping their jobs, because many workplaces did not have policies that enabled workers to take leaves without threatening their employment status. These untenable choices were often manifested in loss of job security, unpaid leaves of absence, lost income, inadequate care and supervision of sick family members, including children, as well as the necessity to work difficult hours or in low-quality employment conditions.

Phuduhudu, for example, was a 63-year-old mother of eight children, three of whom had died—one of AIDS in 1999—leaving three grandchildren in her care. These grandchildren were registered with the government as orphans of an AIDS victim and were receiving *destitute support*, which was being shared among all of the family members. Phuduhudu was also caring for another grandchild. For the previous 9 years, Phuduhudu had been working as a maize meal grinder in a local primary school. Like many others we interviewed, she, as one of her family's primary sources of economic support, had worked odd and long hours to care for her child with AIDS.

Some respondents in our interviews noted that workers had to negotiate ways to meet their caregiving demands—bringing a sick child to work, taking half a day off from work to get a child to the hospital, or even taking an extended leave from work—on a case-by-case basis because their workplaces offered no guaranteed protection of their employment. Ultimately, in many of these cases, the extended and progressive nature of the AIDS-related illnesses forced many working caregivers to leave or lose their jobs. Some respondents found themselves in situations that required them either to quit a job entirely or take a lower-quality position.

Seetasewa, a 45-year-old mother of five children aged 5 to 24, found herself in such a situation. Her youngest child, Kesego, had a moderately severe form of cerebral palsy but was able to attend school. Her 24-year-old daughter, Banyana, had recently returned home after having been away for 5 years; she was suffering from advanced AIDS and had been rejected everywhere else. While supporting her older children and providing extensive care for her younger ones, including managing Kesego's special needs, Seetasewa had been working. However, she explained that working had become impossible while she was caring for both Kesego and her AIDS-infected daughter:

> When I took her [the daughter with AIDS] to stay with me, I was working then. I would wake up, prepare something for her, and then ask the younger ones to fetch water for her and give her the food so that she could eat. When I saw that her health was always going down, I took her to the hospital. As soon as I was sure that she was HIV positive, I found it very difficult to keep working. . . . I was not working back then because I couldn't. I had to look after Kesego and others. I had no time to work and there was no job that could allow me to do all that I needed to do.

Kapinga, a 52-year-old mother of five children (one who died soon after childbirth), also described a situation in which caring for her HIV-positive child disrupted and then ended her work life. Kapinga explained that she was not well educated and therefore had to settle for poorly paid work for long hours as a maid or cleaner in order to provide for her family. When Dorcas, Kapinga's oldest daughter, grew more and more ill from advanced AIDS, Kapinga decided to take some time off from her job as a maid. Yet she found that caring for Dorcas demanded full-time attention, and Kapinga could not return to work:

> The thing that prompted me to leave work was that Dorcas could not do anything for herself or for the household. She wasn't able to do anything anymore. She became seriously ill in late November and early December, which is when I realized that I must leave work to take care of her. For the past four years she has been sick, during that time . . . she was able to do some work in the house and do things for herself. In December is when I realized that she couldn't do anything for herself at home. . . . It was kind of a leave when I decided to go and take care of my child, but I was supposed to go back to work on the first of January. I haven't been able to go.

While caring for ill family members often made it difficult to fulfill employment responsibilities, several of the workers interviewed also said that, conversely, their work requirements made it difficult to care adequately for sick family members, including young children. Phuduhudu, whose situation was described earlier, reported that she had taken sick children to work with her or left them at home while she worked for lack of a better child-care option:

> When my kids or my grandchildren are sick, or if it's the one who doesn't attend school, I'll boil some water, put the water in a flask, and take the kid to work with me. They can sleep somewhere while I'm busy doing my job. That day, I won't do a home visit. But if a kid who attends school has been brought back because they are sick, I'll make sure that I get some herbs, mix them and boil them, give them to the kid, and ask the kid to sleep while I go to work.

Tragically, we found that many of the respondents struggling to provide care and work while dealing with HIV/AIDS found themselves trapped in a downward spiral. When income or benefits were lost because work was disrupted, job security threatened, or productivity diminished as a result of HIV/AIDS caregiving, workers often found that their ability to care for themselves and their families was compromised. Income loss as a result of HIV/AIDS strained already limited household budgets. Breadwinners too often did not have enough savings to cover the essential costs of living, such as those for medical care, food, housing, schooling, and other costs associated with caregiving.

Ndebele described the new financial burdens she carried because she was left to raise her orphaned grandchildren after her daughter, Marie, died of AIDS. Ndebele and Marie were the only earners for their family, and Ndebele losing the ability to work would have made providing for basic needs such as food, medication, and housing virtually impossible:

> It's very difficult to work and take care of my family at the same time. . . . I have to take care of Marie's kids since she passed away, but I can't do that and go to work at the same time, so I had no choice but to take [my granddaughter] to a day-care center, which also requires fees. Most of the time, this kid is sick. I once took her to a private practitioner, but I've since stopped . . . every consultation or every visit that she made cost money. I can't afford that because I am not getting enough.

As communities in high-prevalence regions are dismantled by the AIDS epidemic, it becomes clear that what happens at the workplace must be understood as fundamental to the health of all. The workplace provides a crucial environment in which the design and implementation of effective interventions can reduce HIV spread and limit the negative impacts of the disease on families, communities, and the economy.

Recommendations

The relationship between HIV/AIDS and the workplace makes it clear that to address the HIV/AIDS epidemic in the world's highest-prevalence regions, a broader approach—one that would address more fully the factors that place people at risk and that enhance the most effective means to prevent and contain the impact of HIV/AIDS—is critically needed. Since the majority of infections in high-prevalence areas such as sub-Saharan Africa strike working-age populations, it is clear that the workplace is an important locus of education, prevention, and treatment programming. The workplace provides an important site for intervention because it matches the incentives of employers (to keep their employees healthy and productive) with those of employees (to remain healthy and wage earning). Moreover, workplaces affect risk because they determine the social conditions that can significantly affect infection rates, including the extent of income stability, sexual harassment and coercion, and itinerant and mobile working patterns. Social ecological frameworks provide a model for worksite interventions, since such frameworks recognize that individual behavior, the environment, and social factors all influence health and health practices (Green, Richard, and Potvin, 1996). Successful social ecological models must take into account a range of settings and circumstances when investigating the cumulative effect of conditions faced by targeted individuals (Stokols, 1996). Table 2–1 provides an example of how these models might be adapted to address HIV/AIDS, work, and health.

In programs targeting individual behavioral change, a workplace intervention may counsel an individual truck driver about his need to use condoms and to avoid sex with commercial sex workers. The more comprehensive approach we advocate would, in addition, address the social factors affecting high-risk sexual practices, such as the accessibility and cost of condoms or the frequency and duration of time the worker spent away from his home and primary sexual partner. Addressing the social environment in which individuals live and work is critical to preventing further transmission of the AIDS virus. Even in Botswana, where the epidemic is most severe, where there are impressive efforts by many governmental leaders and a few groundbreaking companies, many workplaces have not yet made the substantial changes in response to the epidemic that policy makers would recommend (Botswana Business Coalition on AIDS, 2000).

Table 2–1. Adaptation of the Social Ecological Model to HIV/AIDS, Work and Health

Theoretical framework for approaching change	Examples of determinants of health-related behaviors	Implications for policy
Behavioral change	Individual behavior choices regarding initiation and frequency of sexual contact, number of sexual partners, extent of safe sexual practices	Interventions targeted at individual behavior, such as partner reduction and condom promotion
Environmental enhancement	Availability of condoms, confidential HIV testing, diagnosis and treatment clinics for sexually transmitted diseases (STDs)	Interventions targeted at STD treatment, availability of condoms and other barrier methods, and testing
Social ecological approach	Itinerant work Mandated transfers Exposure to sexual harassment or coercion Workplace stigmas or discrimination	Interventions targeted at all three levels: • Individual • Health environment • Work environment

Source: Model adapted from Stokols (1996).

Increasingly, leaders in the global anti-AIDS campaign have agreed not only that AIDS efforts must focus on the relationship between work and HIV/AIDS but also that a more comprehensive approach is necessary. We argue that such an approach needs to include elements such as the following:

- Prevention and education programs in high-prevalence countries need to target all working-age adults in those countries, not just adults in so-called high-risk jobs. When the HIV prevalence rate is over 20%, as it is in many countries in the southern cone of Africa, *all* working-age adults are at high risk.
- Policy makers should address the impact of itinerant work and mobility on family disruption and the destabilization of monogamous relations. These work-related practices need to be reexamined particularly in relation to staffing patterns and issues such as hiring practices, promotions, and expected daily activities. Policies that support workers' ability to live with their families should be developed, including policy actions that reduce the number of days employees must spend away from family members and those that increase the possibility for a spouse or significant other to stay with or visit the mobile worker.
- Researchers and policy makers should collaborate to better understand why, when, and how sexual harassment and coercion occur at work and how to eliminate them. Extensive policies and programs to address such abuses need to be developed by employers and governmental policy makers.
- Poverty and economic inequalities place individuals at markedly increased risk. Employers can play an essential role by ensuring that all workers earn a living wage for their family.
- Because gender inequalities influence HIV transmission, efforts to combat gender inequalities in the workplace must be undertaken jointly by employers, businesses leaders, and policy makers. There is also a pressing need for better research on both the factors predicting and the effects of gender inequity and discrimination in the workplace on HIV/AIDS. Region-specific recommendations for comprehensive workplace prevention and education programs as well as protective legal provisions should grow out of this research.
- Employers need to develop policies to address workplace stigmatization and discrimination in both high- and low-prevalence countries. Addressing these problems is critical in encouraging those individuals whose HIV status is unknown to get tested, decreasing the probability of spread to uninfected people, increasing the likelihood of treatment for infected people, and improving the quality of life for those infected.
- Clearly, routine infection-prevention measures should not be ignored. All workers should have access to condoms. Health-care workers and other workers subject to infection through job responsibilities should have access to such materials as safe syringes and latex gloves, as well as education about their proper use.

- Workplaces should provide employees with the flexibility and leave they require to meet the caregiving needs of sick family members. Both the challenges and importance of work and caregiving have been greatly magnified by the AIDS pandemic. Policies and programs need to be developed to support adults' ability to care for sick partners, siblings, children, and others while earning enough to sustain their families.

The work–HIV/AIDS relationship demands the attention and collective action of researchers and policy makers across geographical, national, and cultural divides if we are to overcome the threat HIV/AIDS poses to human development. Moreover, it is a deadly reminder of how critical a role social conditions can play in the health of working-age adults.

Notes

1. In addition to written documents, details on Debswana are based on interviews with Tsetsele Fantan, HIV/AIDS Coordinator at the Debswana Diamond Company, 2001.
2. All names have been changed to respect respondents' privacy.

References

Actuarial Solutions. 2000. *AIDS impact assessment for Debswana Diamond Company (PTY) Ltd.* November. Debswana Private Document.

Botswana Business Coalition on AIDS. 2000. AIDS at the workplace. In *Conference on HIV/AIDS for chief executives.* Gaborone, Botswana: Botswana Ministry of Health, Occupational Health Unit.

deBruyn, M. 1992. Women and AIDS in developing countries. *Social Science & Medicine* 34: 249–62.

Debswana Diamond Company (PTY) Ltd. 2001. *Summary of Debswana's response to HIV/AIDS to date.* May 16.

Eberly, D. J. 1992. *National youth service: A global perspective.* Based on the advanced papers and discussions held at the National Youth Service conference, held at the Wingspread Conference Center, Wisconsin, 18–21 June. Washington, D.C.: National Service Secretariat. Available from http://www.utas.edu.au/docs/ahugo/NCYS/first/1-Botswana.html

Gostin, L. O., C. Feldblum, and D. W. Webber. 1999. Disability discrimination in America: HIV/AIDS and other health conditions. *Journal of the American Medical Association* 281: 745–52.

Government of Botswana, Central Statistics Unit (CSU), Labor Statistics Unit. 1998. *1995/96 Labour force survey.* Gaborone, Botswana: CSU.

Government of Botswana, Ministry of Health, AIDS/STD Unit. 2000. *Sentinel surveillance report 1999.* Gaborone, Botswana: Botswana Ministry of Health.

Government of Botswana and United Nations Development Programme (UNDP). 2000. *Botswana human development report 2000: Towards an AIDS-free generation.* Gaborone, Botswana: UNDP.

Green L., L. Richard, and L. Potvin. 1996. Ecological foundations of health promotion. *American Journal of Health Promotion* 10(4): 270–81.

Gruber J. E. 1990. Methodological problems and policy implications in sexual harassment research. *Population Research and Policy Review* 9: 235–54.

Hodges-Aeberhard, J. 1999. Policy and legal issues relating to HIV/AIDS and the world of work. November. Geneva: International Labor Organization. Available from http://www.ilo.org/public/english/protection/trav/aids/policy.htm

International Labor Organization. 2001. Why AIDS is a workplace issue. Available from http://www.ilo.org/public/english/protection/trav/aids/about/pages_whyissue.htm

Jackson, D. J., J. P. Rakwar, B. A. Richardson, K. Mandaliya, B. H. Chohan, J. J. Bwayo, J. O. Ndinya-Achola, H. L. Martin, Jr., S. Moses, and J. K. Kreiss. 1997. Decreased incidence of sexually transmitted diseases among trucking company workers in Kenya: Results of a behavioural risk-reduction programme. *AIDS* 11: 903–9.

Kruger, F. 1998. Taking advantage of rural assets as a coping strategy for the urban poor: The case of rural–urban interrelations in Botswana. *Environment and Urbanization* 10(1): 119–34.

MacDonald, D. S. 1996. Notes on the socio-economic and cultural factors influencing the transmission of HIV in Botswana. *Social Science and Medicine* 42(9): 1325–33.

Meekers, D., and A. E. Calves. 1997. Main girlfriends, girlfriends, marriage, and money: The social context of HIV risk behaviour in sub-Saharan Africa. *Health Transition Review* 7(Suppl): 361–75.

Mhalu, F., K. Hirji, P. Ijumba, J. Shao, E. Mbena, D. Mwakagile, C. Akim, P. Senge, H. Mponezya, U. Bredberg-Raden, and G. Biberfeld. 1991. A cross-sectional study of a program for HIV infection control among public house workers. *Journal of Acquired Immune Deficiency Syndromes* 4: 290–96.

Moss, W., M. Bentley, S. Maman, D. Ayuko, O. Egessah, M. Sweat, P. Nyarang'o, J. Zenilman, A. Chemtai, and N. Halsey. 1999. Foundations for effective strategies to control sexually transmitted infections: Voices from rural Kenya. *AIDS Care* 11(1): 95–113.

Muyinda, H., J. Seeley, H. Pickering, and T. Barton. 1997. Social aspects of AIDS-related stigma in rural Uganda. *Health Place* 3(3): 143–47.

N'Daba, L., and J. Hodges-Aeberhard. 1998. *HIV/AIDS and employment.* Geneva: International Labor Organization.

PLUSnews. 2001. Botswana: Diamond giant leads the fight against HIV/AIDS. UN Office for the Coordination of Humanitarian Affairs, 14 November. Available from http://www.irinnews.org/AIDSreport.asp?ReportID=1119&SelectRegion=Southern_Africa

Quigley, M., K. Munguti, H. Grosskurth, J. Todd, F. Mosha, K. Senkoro, J. Newell, P. Mayaud, G. ka-Gina, A. Klokke, D. Mabey, A. Gavyole, and R. Hayes. 1997. Sexual behaviour patterns and other risk factors for HIV infection in rural Tanzania: A case-control study. *AIDS* 11: 237–48.

Schoepf, B. G. 1988. Women, AIDS and economic crisis in central Africa. *Canadian Journal of African Studies* 22: 625–44.

Schoepf, B. G. 1992. Women at risk: Case studies from Zaire. In *The time of AIDS: Social analysis, theory and method,* edited by G. Herdt and S. Lindenaum. Newbury Park, CA.: Sage.

Schoepf, B. G. 1993a. AIDS action-research with women in Kinshasa, Zaire. *Social Science and Medicine* 37(11): 1401–13.

Schoepf, B. G. 1993b. Gender, development and AIDS: Political-economy and culture framework. In *Women and international development,* edited by R. Gallin, A. Ferguson, and J. Harper. Boulder, CO.: Westview Press.

Schoepf, B. G., N. Payanzo, N. Rukarangira, E. Walue, and C. Schoepf. 1988. Women and society in central Africa. In *AIDS 1988: Proceedings of the AAAS symposium*, Washington, D.C., edited by R. Kulstad. Philadelphia: Current Science.

Smith, S., and D. Cohen. 2000. *Gender, development and the HIV epidemic.* UNDP. Available from http://www.undp.org/hiv/publications/gender/gendere.htm

Stokols, D. 1996. Translating social ecological theory into guidelines for community health promotion. *American Journal of Health Promotion* 10(4): 282–98.

Stoller, N., and B. E. Schneider, eds. 1993. *Women as the key: Leadership in the HIV epidemic.* Philadelphia: Temple University Press.

Susser, I., and Z. Stein. 2000. Culture, sexuality, and women's agency in the prevention of HIV/AIDS in southern Africa. *American Journal of Public Health* 90(7): 1042–48.

United Nations Conference on Trade and Development (UNCTAD) and United Nations Development Programme (UNDP). 2000. Botswana globalisation, liberalisation and sustainable human development: Country assessment study. June. Available from http://www.bw.undp.org/docs/Globalisation-Liberalisation-Human%20Development%20in%20Botswana.pdf

United Nations Development Programme (UNDP). 1998. *HIV/AIDS and human development, South Africa.* Pretoria, South Africa: UNDP.

United Nations Development Programme (UNDP). 2000. *Human development report 2000.* New York: Oxford University Press.

United Nations Programme on HIV/AIDS (UNAIDS). 1998. HIV/AIDS and the workplace: UNAIDS technical update. July. Geneva: UNAIDS.

United Nations Programme on HIV/AIDS (UNAIDS). 2000a. *Report on the global HIV/AIDS epidemic* June 2000. Geneva: UN.

United Nations Programme on HIV/AIDS (UNAIDS). 2000b. A human rights approach to AIDS prevention at work: The southern African development community's code on HIV/AIDS and employment. June. Available from http://www.unaids.org/publications/documents/human/law/Brochure_SADC.pdf

United Nations Programme on HIV/AIDS (UNAIDS). 2000c. Fact sheet. July. Available from http://www.unaids.org/fact_sheets/files/Dev_Eng.doc

United Nations Programme on HIV/AIDS (UNAIDS). 2002a. New UNAIDS report warns AIDS epidemic still in early phase and not leveling off in worst affected countries. Press release, July 2. New York.

United Nations Programme on HIV/AIDS (UNAIDS). 2002b. *World AIDS Campaign 2002–2003. A conceptual framework and basis for action: HIV/AIDS stigma and discrimination.* Available from http://www.unaids.org/publications/documents/human/JC781-WAC-ConceptFramework_en.pdf

United Nations Programme on HIV/AIDS (UNAIDS) and the World Health Organization (WHO). 2001. *AIDS epidemic update.* English original. Geneva: UNAIDS and WHO.

U.S. Equal Employment Opportunity Commission. 2000. La Cruz Azul (Blue Cross) of Puerto Rico to pay $200,000 in disability discrimination lawsuit. Press release, December 6. Available from http://www.eeoc.gov/press/12-6-00.html

Walu, E. 1991. Women's work in the informal sector: Some lessons from Kinshasa, Zaire. The Hague: Institute for Social Studies.

3

Individuals at Risk: The Case of Child Labor

LUIZ A. FACCHINI, ANACLAUDIA FASSA,
MARINEL DALL'AGNOL,
MARIA DE FÁTIMA MAIA,
AND DAVID C. CHRISTIANI

In 1919, the International Labor Organization (ILO) developed the first Minimum Age Convention establishing the age at which children could legally work. The present Minimum Age Convention, No. 138, was adopted in 1973, and it remains the fundamental standard (International Labor Conference, 1999; International Labor Organization, 1973). Yet children around the globe are toiling as domestic servants in homes, laboring behind the walls of workshops, and working hidden from view on plantations (UNICEF, 2001).

It is estimated that there are 352 million children younger than 18 years old in the world who are economically active, that is, who perform productive activities, including unpaid and illegal work, as well as work in the informal sector. Estimates suggest that nearly half, 48%, are girls and that children between 5 and 14 years old comprise 211 million of the total number of economically active children, while 141 million are 15 to 17 years old. Among the economically active children, 88% of the 5- to 14-year-olds and 42% of the 15- to 17-year-olds work in activities that are inappropriate for children of their age, that is, in forms of child labor that need to be eliminated according to the ILO Minimum Age Convention, 1973 (No. 138), and the ILO Worst Forms of Child Labour Convention, 1999 (No. 182), standards (ILO, 2002; International Labor Conference, 1999; International Labor Organization, 1973).

The ILO (2002) estimates that more than 96% of all child workers live in developing countries. Whereas in developed countries 18% of the economically active children are younger than 14, in developing countries 62% are younger than 14. Still, child labor continues to be a problem in many industrialized as well as developing nations. According to the U.S. Department of Labor, for example, there are approximately 6 million children employed in the United States, and 30% of them are working illegally based on laws regarding the minimum age for employment, permitted tasks, and number of hours worked (Landrigan and McCammon, 1997).

As the world's most populous region, Asia accounts for more than 50% of child laborers (Fig. 3–1). Furthermore, Asia has the largest number of child workers in the 5 to 14 age category, with 127.3 million in total. Sub-Saharan Africa has 48 million children working, while Latin America and the Caribbean has 17.4 million. However, Africa has the highest percentage of working children: roughly one in three below the age of 15. In Asia, the Middle East, and Latin America and the Caribbean, it has been estimated that 15% to 20% of all children work. Developed economies and transition economies have the lowest proportion of child workers. It is estimated that about 2% of all children below 15 years of age are economically active in developed countries (Forastieri, 1997; ILO, 1998b, 2002).

Poverty and economic disparities are closely linked with the prevalence of child labor, but the nature and causes of child labor have now become increasingly complex, with new forms arising as global realities and relations have changed (UNICEF, 2001). The connection between globalization and child labor could be seen as a threat as well as an opportunity. Although there is general agreement that globalization itself is not the cause of child labor, it can have a negative influence on child labor. Structural policies of adjustment have resulted in many developing countries spending less on social programs, social security, and basic services such as education and health. This may lead to an increase in the number of families needing to turn to child labor to meet basic needs. The growing competition among developing and developed countries may lead to the deregulation of labor laws and thus to a lower level of employment protection of both adults and children.

On the positive side, globalization has increased awareness of child labor throughout the world and can provide an opportunity to resolve the problems surrounding child labor, especially in the longer term. The international community can ensure the use of globalization as a positive instrument in the fight against child labor. Actions must focus on education, health, and the standardization of fundamental labor

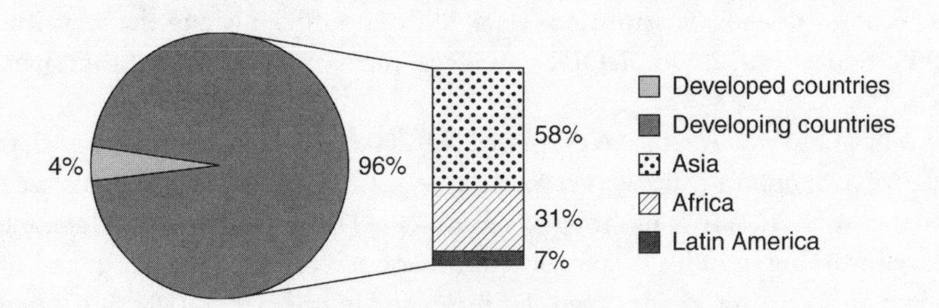

Figure 3–1. World distribution of child labor.

standards, and must involve both the private and public sectors as well as workers (ILO, 1997a).

Despite the troubling issues regarding child labor raised above, the extent and nature of work's impact on children's health and development have been investigated relatively little (Scanlon et al., 2002). In this chapter, we examine child labor worldwide and review the evidence on the major problems associated with and potential benefits of child labor in general, as well as the associations between work and children's health. We also discuss the limitations of the currently available data on all of these topics. To provide a more specific context within which to examine child labor issues, we then focus on employment laws, child labor rates, and problems associated with child labor in Brazil as a whole. Our own study in Pelotas, Brazil, in which the focus was on health risks related to child labor, is then examined in detail. We conclude by discussing alternatives to the existing policies designed to reduce child labor and exploitation and closely examine the principal aspects of a child labor eradication policy developed in Brazil. The relevance of this approach for other areas is considered, and we discuss broad methodological and policy-related issues that need further attention with regard to child labor and health.

Effects of Work on Children's Health

A 1998 Institute of Medicine Report noted that work can positively affect children by helping them develop discipline, responsibility, self-confidence, and independence; teaching them how to manage money; and providing them with valuable role models for work skills (Committee on the Health and Safety Implications of Child Labor, 1998). However, it is the nature and type of work children perform that determine whether work will harm their health and development (Parker, 1997a, 1997b). Child labor is likely to be more harmful if it occurs at younger ages; interferes with school, recreation, and rest; involves an erratic work schedule, long hours, or frequent nocturnal work; or includes hazardous occupations and low wages (Fig. 3–2) (Fassa, 2000). The effects of child labor may be neutral or even positive in only a minority of activities, such as helping out in a family-run shop during school holidays. On the other hand, it is very easy to identify hazardous and exploitive work such as bonded labor, prostitution, work in drug trafficking, and the recruitment of child soldiers. All are intolerable and illegal forms of child labor (Scanlon et al., 2002).

In central and west Africa, it is estimated that 200,000 children are traded each year. Landlords can bond a child worker for as little as US$1.50, and family debts are manipulated so that there is no hope of repayment. The growth and development of children working in industry and agriculture are severely compromised, and these children are at risk for a wide range of diseases and injuries (ILO, 1998b). Numerous reports describe poisoning, serious skin and other infections, chronic lung disease,

BENEFICIAL	None	**Interference with school, recreation, or rest**	Very much	HARMFUL
	Teen	**Age**	Very young	
	Few hours	**Number of hours per day**	Long hours	
	Day	**Work schedule**	Night	
	Not hazardous	**Nature of work**	Hazardous	
	High	**Wage**	Low	

Figure 3–2. Balance between beneficial and harmful conditions related to child labor.

cancers, burns, amputations, skeletal deformities, and impairments to hearing, vision, and immune function (Scanlon et al., 2002).

The commercial sexual exploitation of children is increasing, and organized networks can be found in Latin America, Asia, Africa, and, most recently, Eastern Europe. An estimated 1 million children in Asia alone are victims of the sex trade, much of it focused on sex tourism. Child prostitutes risk pregnancy and sexually transmitted diseases including human immunodeficiency virus (HIV) infection. Paradoxically, as prostitutes, the children often fall victim to the same legal system that should be protecting them (United Nations High Commisioner for Human Rights, 1996). Children in domestic service are often victims of physical, psychological, and sexual abuse.

The recruitment of children as combat soldiers is a growing problem. Children in combat risk disease, disability, and violent death. Former child combatants suffer from aggression, alienation, and an inability to interact socially (Amnesty International, 2000; Somasundaram, 2002).

While most child workers are not in these—the most harmful and exploitive—situations, significant health hazards occur for children laboring in adult workplaces. Children and teens differ from adults in their anatomical, physiological, and psychological characteristics, and thus frequently are more susceptible to occupational hazards in their workplaces than adult workers exposed to the same hazards might be (Committee on the Health and Safety Implications of Child Labor, 1998; Fassa, 2000; Forastieri, 1997; ILO, 1998a; UNICEF, 1997).

There is epidemiological evidence that children are more susceptible than adults to lead, silica, benzene, noise, heat, ionizing radiation, and the risk of accidents. Moreover, there is theoretical concern that children are more susceptible to carcinogenic, chemical, and ergonomic exposures (Fassa et al., 2000b). Moreover, because children's anatomical and physiological characteristics are different from those of adults, children doing heavy work, carrying heavy loads, or maintaining awkward body positions for long hours can become deformed as a result of excessive stress placed on the bones before the epiphysis has fused. This may lead to skeletal damage or impaired growth. In addition, children suffer more than adults from exposure to dangerous chemical substances and to radiation. The level of concentration of these substances needed to cause damage is lower than that of adults. They are not physically suited to long hours of strenuous and monotonous work, and they suffer the effects of fatigue more quickly than adults (Fassa et al., 2000b). This is particularly true if the children suffer from malnutrition, which is very often the case. The children are often not aware of dangers, nor do they have any knowledge of the precautions to be taken (ILO, 1997c).

Most studies of child labor's role in injuries have been conducted in the United States, and these studies have shown that children have a higher risk of injuries than adults. The National Center for Health Statistics in the United States reported an occupational injury rate in 1997 for 15- to 17-year-olds of 4.9 per 100 full-time equivalent (FTE) workers, while for all workers aged 16 and older, it is 2.8 (Committee on the Health and Safety Implications of Child Labor, 1998). Surveys of young workers have further highlighted the extent of the problem. Layne and associates (1994), in a study of 679 injuries that occurred in the United States from July to December 1992, found a yearly nonfatal injury rate among 15- to 17-year-olds of 5.8 per 100 FTE. A 1998 Institute of Medicine Report has noted that 7% to 16% of working teens reported experiencing a serious injury at work that required them to seek medical care (Committee on the Health and Safety Implications of Child Labor, 1998). Clearly, additional data are needed on the injuries experienced by child and adolescent workers.

A Case Study: Brazilian Child Workers

To examine the experience of child workers in greater depth, we will now discuss findings from our study of working children in the Brazilian city of Pelotas. Under Brazilian law, no one younger than 16 can be hired to do paid work, and schooling until this age is mandatory (Ministério do trabalho e emprego, 2000). (Before 2000, the minimum age was 14 years). Employees are required by law to have a work registration card, which is provided at no cost and with very little bureaucracy, and employers are required to register each person's employment. Since children are not allowed to work before the age of 16, they cannot have a work card before that age. Furthermore, the Brazilian Federal Constitution and the Statute on Children and Adolescents forbid children younger than 18 to work at night (10 P.M. to 5 A.M.) or in dangerous, arduous, or unhealthy jobs. The work activities of 16- and 17-year-olds should still permit them to attend school, and their employers are obliged to allow them the necessary time to attend school (Ministério do trabalho e emprego, 2000).

However, the regulations are frequently flouted. For instance, when the study on the national legislation of 1998 was performed, 30% of the working children in Pelotas were younger than 14, and 51% of all child workers there had had their first job when they were younger than 14. The Brazilian employment laws are not strictly enforced on the whole, and the problem is even worse for working children. It is estimated that Brazil has 9.3 million children between 10 and 17 years old doing paid and nonpaid work, and 1998 data (the latest available) showed that 25% of the children in this age group were active in the labor force (Cruz Neto and Moreira, 1998; Fausto and Cervini, 1996). Data from the 1999 National Household Sample Study, the last one carried out in Brazil, reveal that approximately 9% of children 5 to 14 years old in the country were working. From 1995 to 1999, child labor in this age group fell from 14.5% to 11.8% among boys and from 7.8% to 6% among girls. In this period, the same trend was seen among children 5 to 9 years old (Instituto Brasileiro de Geografia e Estatística, 2001).

The country's situation regarding child labor is very heterogeneous, and its enforcement of the legal restrictions on child labor is lax. In the less developed regions of the country (north and northeast), where approximately 36% of the total population lives, and in the big cities throughout the country, it is easy to find some types of outlawed bonded labor, the sale and trafficking of children, debt bondage, use or procurement of children for prostitution or pornographic purposes, use of children in illicit activities such as trafficking of drugs, and work that is likely to harm the health, safety, or morals of children (UNICEF, 2001). Even in the more developed regions of the country (southeast and south), where approximately 57% of the total population lives, very poor children do not have the minimum skills to get a better job, often doing primarily menial labor such as domestic work and garbage recycling (Fassa et al., 2000a).

In Brazil, as in many other countries, street children are a big problem, particularly in cities with 500,000 or more inhabitants. There children pick through trash dumps, sell goods, and beg, but are also involved in prostitution, drug trafficking, and other criminal activities. The national figure is imprecise and depends on the concept's definition, which can include children without a family who use the street as their home, as well as children who stay predominantly on the street and are exploited as street sellers, as beggars, or in illegal activities even when they have a family or a relative at home. In Rio de Janeiro there are an estimated 30,000 street children and, in São Paulo, around 12,000 (ECACL, 2002).

Despite some progress, in Brazil as in most of the developing world, official data on child labor are generally fragmentary, underestimate informal sector work and family work, and frequently exclude unpaid work. In Brazil the official data are collected and compiled by IBGE (the Brazilian Institute of Geography and Statistics) from such sources as the National Census, the National Household Sample Studies, and the Monthly Employment Study, each with its own methodology. The National Census and the Monthly Employment Study gather a limited amount of data on employment and work activities, with no focus on child labor. The National Household Sample Studies gather data on selected social issues such as work, health, and education in order to obtain a more detailed focus on a representative sample of households in the country and its regions and states. Although this approach ensures that more data relevant to child labor in Brazil are available, the last official survey containing detailed information on child labor was carried out in 1999 (Instituto Brasileiro de Geografia e Estatística, 2001).

The collection and availability of primary data on child labor are increasing, but population-based studies on child labor and health are rare in Brazil, as in many developing countries (Cruz Neto and Moreira, 1998; Fausto and Cervini, 1996; Forastieri, 1997).

The Pelotas Child Labor and Health Study

Lacking an adequate system for obtaining accurate data on child labor and health in Brazil, we developed a detailed cross-sectional population-based study in the low-income neighborhoods of Pelotas, which is located in one of the most developed regions of Brazil. Pelotas has 300,000 urban inhabitants, 23% of whom are between 6 and 17 years old (Instituto Brasileiro de Geografica e Estatística, 1992).

In the past two decades, Pelotas has experienced economic stagnation and deindustrialization with the closing of several food industries, mainly due to the opening of the Brazilian market to the global economy and the technological gaps in the local industries. These changes have, in turn, led to high rates of unemployment of around 10% to 15% (Fausto and Cervini, 1996) and an increase in the informal sector. Currently, 50% of the adult workers are in the informal sector (Wunsch Filho, 1995). This social context has affected the city's entire labor force, especially the adults and children living in the low-income urban neighborhoods, where the living conditions, educational levels, and occupational skills are worse.

In Pelotas, as other places in Latin America, access to good living conditions, education, job skills, social security, and health is not evenly distributed but strongly concentrated. Social inequity is huge in Latin America, both in mid-sized and large cities, even in southern Brazil, where Pelotas is located and social conditions are better. The Pelotas study is one of the few investigations involving a detailed examination of child labor in Latin America, and although the frequency of child labor and its profile vary from one setting to another, the working conditions in each type of occupation are likely to be similar. Moreover, this study provides information about some previously unstudied occupations such as domestic service work.

Data Collection

In 1998, we interviewed 4924 children aged 6 to 17 living in 3171 households in 22 randomly selected low-income neighborhoods of Pelotas. Based on the Brazilian National Census of 1991, we estimated a population of 5298 children in this age group living in the selected neighborhoods. We were not able to interview about 374 children in the target age group, that is, 7.6% of the subjects in the estimated sample. The children and their mothers or other guardians gave their informed consent to participate in the study. In the few cases in which children were not living with their mothers, the adults most commonly asked to provide consent and be interviewed were grandmothers, aunts, and stepmothers. Each adult was interviewed about general characteristics of the family such as parents' age, schooling, employment, and the availability of household goods, while each child answered questions about his or her work, health, and education. As we interviewed all children at home, abandoned children and those living on the street were not included in the sample. However, the sample included children working on the streets who return home each night and provide critical financial support for their families.

We defined the *work of children and teens* as activities performed by 6- to 17-year olds that contributed to the production of a marketable product, good, or service. In that definition, we included activities done without pay—for example home-based work such as helping in a small business at home. It also includes household chores performed at home when these require children's full-time work and are essential to enabling the parents to work outside of the home (such as cleaning the home or caring for younger siblings). Our broad definition incorporated aspects traditionally excluded from the official statistics, such as unpaid work, informal work, and work by the very young. Although household chores performed at home could be considered an economic activity in some circumstances, this particular type of work is not analyzed in this chapter due to its particularities and the difficulty of determining the circumstances in which this work was an economic activity.

These unique population-based data allowed us to examine the work profiles in relation to age, gender, socioeconomic level, and other variables of interest, and to evaluate the children's workloads and the effects on their health.

Findings Regarding Child Labor in Pelotas

Of the 4924 children surveyed, 51% were boys and 49% were girls, 76% were white and 24% were nonwhite. Fifty percent were from families with a monthly income lower than the equivalent of US$375. Among the 8- to 13-year-olds ($n = 2526$), 98% were attending school and 6% were combining work and school, while among the 14- to 17-year-olds ($n = 1608$), 89% were attending school and 17% were combining work and school. Among the study children, 9.7% were working at that time, 20.6% had ever worked, 3.4% were unemployed at the time of the study, and 66.3% had never worked. Children who reported that they were looking for a job and were not working at the time of the study were classified as unemployed.

The prevalence of workers increased with age and was higher for boys than for girls. Among the boys, the prevalence of workers aged 6 to 9 was 2.4%; for those aged 10 to 13, 10%; and for those aged 14 to 17, 28.8%. Among the girls, the prevalence of workers aged 6 to 9 was 0.5%; for those aged 10 to 13, 4%; and for those aged 14 to 17, 12.6%.

In the group of children working at the time of the study ($n = 476$), 71% were boys and 29% were girls. Seventy percent were 14 to 17 years of age; 24.8%, were 10 to 13; and 5.3%, were 6 to 9. Of the workers older than 7, 87.7% were also attending school. Among the workers, 16.4% had worked for the first time when they were between 5 and 9 years old; 40.5% were between 10 and 13 years old; and 40.3% were between 14 and 17 years old. Whereas 19.3% of the boys had first worked between the ages of 5 and 9, only 10.6% of the girls had done so while in that age range.

Type of employer and informal or formal sector work. Among the employees and subjects who performed home-based work ($n = 396$), 47.6% worked for an employer who was not a family member, 36.9% worked for a parent, and 15.4% worked for some other family member. *Home-based work* included both work done to support the child's own family's business as well as the child's efforts to help a family member get his or her own work done when that family member was working "for a boss" (a non-family member). More than half of the child workers in the manufacturing, construction, and retail sectors worked for their parents (55.6%, 52%, and 54.6%, respectively). The highest prevalence of children working for a family member other than a parent was found in domestic services (32.4%), followed by construction (18%). More than 60% of the child workers in nondomestic services (e.g., auto repair, receptionist, telephonist, messenger) and domestic services worked for a nonrelated employer, while 30% of those working in retail, manufacturing, and construction had this type of employer.

In low-income areas in Brazil, almost all self-employed workers did not register themselves. Therefore, the study did not investigate the working conditions for this group of workers. Of the employees aged 14 to 17, 83.2% were nonregistered workers. Construction, manufacturing, and retail were the types of work with the highest prevalence of nonregistered workers in this age group (94.3%, 86.7%, and 86.4%, respectively); in domestic services the prevalence was 80.4%, and in nondomestic services it was 75.7%. Among the subjects aged 14 to 17 who worked for their parents, 97% were not registered; for those who worked for a family member other than the parent, the rate was 92.9%, and for those with a nonrelated employer it was 73.8%. In addition, none of the unpaid workers were legally registered.

Types of compensation. Most of the child workers (71%) received money, and only money, as compensation for their work. More boys received money exclusively (75.6%) than did girls (59.7%). However, more girls received money and other things (such as food, clothes, and toys) or things except money (35.9%) than did boys (19.8%). Of those receiving money as at least part of their compensation, the average wage was $61 a month. The mean wage was $84 for manufacturing, $77 for nondomestic services, $72 for construction, $55 for retail, and $50 for domestic services. Among child workers, 16.2%

did not receive any money for their work, and 4.5% did not receive compensation of any sort.

Type of work and common jobs. Almost half (44.5%) of the Pelotas child workers we interviewed were laboring in services; among those, just over half (54.4%) were performing domestic services and just under half (45.6%) nondomestic services. The second most frequent type of work was retail (34.1%). In addition, 12.7% of the children worked in construction, 4.7% in manufacturing (primarily home-based food industries), and 2.5% in marginal activities (such as gardening, guarding and washing cars, and delivering things). As shown in Table 3–1, girls were three times more prevalent in domestic services and 37% more prevalent in retail than boys, whereas boys were 77% more prevalent in nondomestic services than girls. Construction and manufacturing were almost exclusively male activities.

The most frequent jobs children held were stonemason assistant (10.1%), restaurant and grocery assistant (9.5%), seller (9.2%), yard cleaner (6.5%), nanny (6.1%), and maid (5.3%). The majority of the workers were employees (74.4%), 9.3% helped regularly with family work, 9.3% were self-employed, and 7.0% had temporary jobs.

Work schedule. While 31.8% of the child workers worked for 40 hours or more a week (a full-time schedule), 51.7% worked for more than 20 hours a week (more than part-time). Data on the number of hours worked were missing for 18.4% of the sample. Among the 6- to 9-year old workers, 20% were working full-time. Construction, domestic services, and manufacturing had the highest prevalence of children working for 40 or more hours per week (approximately 36% in each sector). The highest prevalence of part-time work was among those engaged in marginal activities (41.7%), followed by nondomestic services (36.8%).

In our study, *night work* was defined as work done from 6 P.M. to 6 A.M. Although Brazilian law considers work done between 10 P.M. to 5 A.M. as night work, the law also requires a minimum of 11 hours of rest between two periods of work, and Rec-

Table 3–1. Prevalence of Child Labor in Each Type of Work, by Gender, in Pelotas, Brazil, 1998 ($n = 4924$)

Type of work	Boys ($n = 339$)	Girls ($n = 137$)	Total ($n = 476$)	RR (95% CI)*
Nondomestic services	27.6	15.6	24.2	1.77 (1.1–2.7)
Domestic services	13.1	38.5	20.3	.35 (.24–.48)
Retail	30.9	42.2	34.1	.73 (.56–.91)
Construction	17.2	1.5	12.7	11.62 (2.9–46.9)
Industry	6.2	0.7	4.7	8.41 (1.1–61.9)
Marginal activities	3.0	1.5	2.5	2.0 (0.4–9.0)
Agriculture	2.1	—	1.5	—
Total	100	100	100	

*RR = Relative risk for boys with reference to the female prevalence. CI = confidence interval.

ommendation 146 of ILO Convention 138 requires a minimum of 12 hours of rest between two periods of work (Ministério do trabalho e emprego, 2000). Among those who responded, 12.9% labored more than 10 hours per week in the evening or at night. Child workers engaged in marginal activities and in retail had the highest prevalence of work involving 10 or more hours per week in the evening or at night (25% and 19.9%, respectively). For those in nondomestic services, domestic services, and construction, the respective rates were 11.4%, 9.4%, and 6.7%.

Child workers engaged in nondomestic services, manufacturing, and retail had the highest prevalence of attendance in school (more than 90% for each), compared with 80% of those in domestic services and construction and 54.5% of those in marginal activities.

Workloads and type of work in relation to health. For the 88% of respondents on whom data were available, extreme temperatures, chemical products, repetitive movements, the need to work fast, and monotonous work were among the more frequently reported workload issues. Table 3–2 contains data on the prevalence of the workloads by the types of activities. As noted there, construction, manufacturing, and marginal activities entailed some of the worst working conditions, as perceived by the children. The ergonomic risks were highest in the work conditions perceived to be the worst, especially in nondomestic work.

Musculoskeletal disorders. More than 60% of the children in our study reported musculoskeletal pain in at least one site during the year before the interview, and 41.5% of them said the pain had made it difficult to perform some activity. The association with age and gender varied widely, according to the sites of pain. The workers in manufacturing, domestic services, and construction had the highest prevalence of musculoskeletal pain experienced in any site during the year before the interview: 90.9%, 79.2%, and 73.3%, respectively. In the same groups, reports of musculoskeletal pain during the week before the interview were made by 36.4%, 27.4%, and 30%, respectively. The sites of pain reported by manufacturing workers were the neck (42.9%), shoulders (19.0%), wrists or hands (42.9%), upper back (23.8%), and thighs (19.0%). Construction workers had the highest prevalence of pain in the elbows (6.9%) and the lower back (17.2%). The workers in domestic services had the highest prevalence of pain in the legs (18.9%) and the knees (25.6%), and those in nondomestic services had the highest prevalence of pain in the ankles and feet (13.6%).

Injuries. In our study, 65% of the children aged 6 to 17 reported having experienced a minor injury (a hurt, a cut, a wound that that did not require them to seek a doctor) in the year before the interview, and 15.7% reported a serious injury (that produced at least 1 day of disability and required them to seek medical care). In addition, 4.8% reported having had frequent (more than one episode of the same kind) injuries, either minor or serious, in the year before the interview. (To reduce the prob-

Table 3–2. Prevalence of Occupational Risks by Type of Activity in Pelotas, Brazil, 1998

	Type of activity						
Occupational risk	Nondomestic services (%)	Domestic services (%)	Retail (%)	Construction (%)	Manufacturing (%)	Marginal activities (%)	Average (%)
Extreme temperatures	21.5	20.5	20.0	28.8	28.6	50.0	24.2
Outdoor work	43.0	34.2	34.0	71.2	22.7	70.0	45.9
Inadequate ventilation	18.7	13.7	22.7	25.0	18.2	20.0	19.7
Exposure to harmful gases or steams	14.0	2.7	6.0	3.8	13.6	0	6.7
Exposure to harmful dusts or fumes	29.0	32.9	34.0	67.3	36.4	30.0	38.3
Noise	10.3	6.8	9.3	3.9	27.3	20.0	12.9
High humidity	18.7	16.4	10.0	19.2	13.6	40.0	19.7
Chemical exposures	23.4	6.8	4.0	32.7	45.5	30.0	23.7
Risk of accidents	8.4	5.5	4.0	25.0	18.2	10.0	11.8
Risk of falling down	7.5	8.2	1.3	34.6	9.1	0	10.1
Need to work fast	22.4	6.8	22.7	17.3	36.4	0	17.6
Awkward work posture	24.3	16.4	20.7	28.8	31.8	10.0	22.0
Lifting or carrying heavy loads	20.6	15.1	17.3	30.8	22.7	0	17.7
Repetitive movements	44.9	21.9	36.0	53.8	63.6	30.0	41.7
Monotonous work	15.0	13.7	18.7	11.5	36.4	0	15.9
Work with wet clothes	16.8	11.0	8.0	38.5	13.6	40.0	21.3
Work with broken tools	2.8	6.8	0.7	5.8	4.5	10.0	5.1
Boss pressure	2.8	4.1	5.3	0	9.1	0	2.2

Note: Data are missing for 11.6% of the sample.

ability of overlap between categories, musculoskeletal problems were defined as a pain not related to an accident.)

The occurrence of minor and serious injuries was higher among 10- to 13-year-olds and boys. The prevalence of frequent injury was also higher among boys and child workers.

The rate of frequent injuries was higher among workers (8.1%) than among non-workers (4.5%). The type of work was not associated with the different kinds of injuries, but working children reported being exposed to greater risks of serious injuries than did nonworking ones: risk of falling down (26.3% versus 14.8%), risk of accidents (20.5% versus 15.4%), exposure to noise (20% versus 15.2%), and hazardous outdoor work (18.8% versus 13.8%).

Smoking. In our study, the prevalence of smoking was 5.1% for the whole sample, with no differences between boys (5.2%) and girls (4.9%). We found that smoking rates were significantly higher among the older children ($p < .0001$) and among workers than nonworkers for all age groups ($p < .05$), as shown in Table 3–3. The prevalence did not vary significantly by type of work (average rate of 14.9%, in industry and retail, 13.6%, and nondomestic services and construction, 15%), with the exception of marginal activities. Among the marginal workers, almost 42% ($n = 12$) smoked.

Comparisons of Children's Work and Health Effects in Pelotas and Other Locales

Our study of child labor in Pelotas contributes to a broader understanding of where children work and under what conditions. However, further analyses are needed to place the Pelotas experience in context and detail the impact of child labor on health elsewhere.

While placing our findings in a global context is very challenging due to the lack of similar data and differences among the groups studied in terms of age, economic ac-

Table 3–3. Childhood Smoking Rates, by Work Status and Age, in Pelotas, Brazil, 1998

Age group	Percentage of workers who smoke	Percentage of nonworkers who smoke	Percentage of sample that smokes
6–9	—	—	0.2
10–11	—	—	0.5
12–13	5.9	1.8	2.2
14–15	16.0	9.5	10.4
16–17	21.7	16.5	17.9
Total	14.9	4.0	5.1

Note: $p < .05$ for the comparison of smoking rates between workers and nonworkers across all age groups; $p < .0001$ for the comparison of smoking rates across age groups.

tivities, and social context, a tentative analysis can be made. The overall 9.7% prevalence rate of child labor among 6- to 17-year-olds found in Pelotas was lower than that found among children in urban Brazil (25% among children 10 to 17 years old) (Fausto and Cervini, 1996), in Latin America countries (15% to 20% among children 5 to 17 years old), and in the world (23% among 5- to 17-year-olds) (Forastieri, 1997; ILO, 1998b, 2002).

Among very young workers, the prevalence of child labor in Pelotas (1.5% among 6- to 9-year-olds) was similar to the prevalence in developed economies (1.4% among 5- to 9-year-olds) and lower than that found in Asian and Pacific countries (3.1% among 5- to 9-year-olds), in Latin America countries (12% among 5- to 9-year-olds), in sub-Saharan Africa (23.6% among 5- to 9-year-olds), and in the world (12.2% among 5- to 9-year-olds) (Forastieri, 1997; ILO, 1998b, 2002).

The 8% prevalence rate of child labor among 10- to 14-year-olds found in Brazilian urban populations was similar to that found in our study. However, in Pelotas the prevalence among 15- to 17-year-olds (23.3%) was lower than that in developed countries (31.3%), Brazil (46.6%), Latin America (35%), and globally (42.4%) (Fausto and Cervini, 1996; Forastieri, 1997; ILO, 1998b, 2002).

In Pelotas, the prevalence of workers was higher for boys (13.4%) than for girls (5.7%) in all age groups. Previous estimates for Brazil (Fausto and Cervini, 1996) and for the world (ILO, 1998b) have also shown that more boys than girls work. However, the last ILO estimate (2002) showed that in both the 5- to 9-year-old and 10- to 14-year-old age brackets, boys and girls are equally likely to be engaged in economic activities. Only as boys and girls grow older do we observe a widening gap, with more boys working than girls (ILO, 2002). The difference is probably explained, at least partially, by the fact that the number of girls who work is often underestimated by statistical surveys, which usually do not take into account unpaid economic activity carried out in and around the home (ILO, 1998b).

Almost half (44.5%) of the Pelotas child workers were laboring in services. This finding is similar to estimates among Brazilian urban child workers (45.9%) (Fausto and Cervini, 1996) but higher than global estimates (around 10%) (ILO, 1998b) that include children working in agriculture (around 70% of child workers). In Pelotas, retail was the second most frequent type of work. Thirty-four percent of the sample were employed in retail, a rate higher than that estimated among urban child workers in Brazil (17.4%) (Fausto and Cervini, 1996) and globally (approximately 8.3%) (ILO, 1998b). The study in Pelotas showed a lower prevalence of child labor, lower rates of female participation in the labor force, a lower intensity of work, and a higher prevalence of nonregistered workers than in other urban population in Brazil (Fausto and Cervini, 1996).

Given the fact that Pelotas had a lower prevalence of child labor and a lower intensity of work than urban Brazil and many regions globally, the economic exploitation of children may be significantly worse elsewhere. In Pelotas, as elsewhere in Brazil, employment practices frequently deviate from those established by law. The serious problems associated with child labor include the following: work by very young children, work in hazardous activities, work under conditions that could be harmful to health or development, work under conditions that could disturb school attendance or school performance, and work in illegal situations.

As noted earlier, we found that in Pelotas, rates of school attendance were lower for children who worked than for those who did not. Most of the workers combined work and school, and 30% worked full-time. Research has shown that for children, such time overloads can negatively affect both their health and their school performance (Committee on the Health and Safety Implications of Child Labor, 1998). These findings, along with others discussed in this chapter, suggest that the negative effects on children's health, school attendance, and school performance will, in turn, be associated with long-term negative effects on their economic opportunities and, therefore, their health as adults. Up to now, however, longitudinal research on such issues has been very limited.

As for domestic work, its informal and hidden nature increases the difficulty of estimating the number of domestic workers around the world, but it is recognized as one of the most common forms of urban child labor in developing countries. In addition, it involves a large number of girls as employees (ILO, 1997b). Despite these facts, very little is known about the impact of domestic services on health and education. Researchers have noted, however, that the hazards associated with domestic work by children vary widely, according to cultures and places, but that it is a typical job in developing countries, particularly in Latin America, where girls often work as servants without access to education or payment (ILO, 1997b).

The occupational hazards associated with domestic services are largely related to the long hours and to the potential for physical, mental, and sexual abuse by an employer (ILO, 1997b). The attitude of the employer (such as beating or castigating children or giving them heavy workloads) has been shown to largely determine the child's level of exploitation. Domestic services also include hazards related to cooking, boiling water, chopping vegetables, using chemical fluids, and carrying heavy items (Black, 1997; Bureau of International Labor Affairs, 1994; Fassa et al., 2000a; UNICEF, 1997). Such issues are of particular concern for the youngest workers.

Construction and manufacturing, two activities typically engaged in predominantly by boys (ILO, 2002; Instituto Brasileiro de Geografia e Estatística, 2001) are often very hazardous. Construction often involves a high risk of accidents—particularly fatal ones—and workers' exposure to silica, asbestos, harmful dusts, and heavy loads. Manufacturing has hazards that are specific to the production process, as well as hazards resulting from the lack of safety protections and procedures (Bequele and Meyers, 1995; Committee on the Health and Safety Implications of Child Labor, 1998).

The prevalence of child workers engaged in marginal jobs that involve work on the street is a worldwide problem occurring in countries in Africa, Asia, and the European countries in transition to a market economy, such as Georgia, Poland, Romania, Russia, and Ukraine. The problem is particularly acute in Latin America and the Caribbean countries. Despite its general relevance, child labor in marginal activities is a relatively smaller problem in Pelotas than in Brazil as a whole and in other Latin American countries. The global number of street children is not known, but national figures are available for several countries. For instance, there are approximately 20,000 street children in Angola (Luanda and Catchiungo), 100,000 in Bangladesh (Dhaka), 8000 in Bolivia; 50,000 in Brazil; 30,000 in Colombia; and 20,000 in Ecuador (ECACL, 2002).

Among the common activities performed by children in the streets are shining shoes; washing cars; carrying water; begging; scavenging and collecting garbage; selling fruits, flowers, newspapers, cigarettes and other goods; loading and unloading goods; and pushing handcarts. However, many children are being exploited and abused in the streets, particularly in the developing countries, where they can be involved in petty crime, stealing, prostitution, and drug trafficking or are being bonded as soldiers and members of criminal gangs. The risks faced by children engaged in street work in Pelotas are the same as those that have been noted among street-based child workers in other countries: exposure to alcohol, tobacco, and drug use, especially glue and paint sniffing or crack smoking; traffic accidents; and injury in street violence.

Policies to Address Problems Associated with Child Labor

The efforts to end child labor require political will. Law enforcement can be an important strategy to combat harmful child labor practices. However, various initiatives to combat child labor in other parts of the world have led to a migration of workers from one group of hazardous jobs, such as sport and carpet industries in South Asian countries, to others even more hazardous, poorly paying, and informal (such as forced and bonded labor in agriculture, armed conflicts, prostitution and pornography, and drug trafficking).

A coherent multidisciplinary program needs to be developed by governments, employers' organizations, trade unions, nongovernment organizations, the representatives of working children and their families, and other members of the civil society. This program should focus on key areas such as education and enactment and enforcement of child labor legislation, as well as poverty alleviation. The program should involve the development and implementation of policies targeted at the immediate removal of children from the most intolerable forms of child labor, as well as their rehabilitation and the provision of adequate alternatives to the children and their families; the prevention of child labor through the universal provision of access to quality education, and to an adequate social infrastructure including systems for the provision of health care, social protection for families, and enhanced opportunities for adult employment; and the creation of better awareness and understanding of the rights of children and the need to end child labor (ILO, 1997a).

When considering policies to combat harmful child labor, it is important to consider that hazardous activities (construction, manufacturing, and retail) are frequently performed by children directly for family members or to earn needed family income. Moreover, construction and manufacturing offer among the highest average salaries. Involving children or adolescents in these types of jobs has been an important family economic strategy to make small family-operated businesses more feasible and thus more profitable in the long run. Policies that support family businesses—such as subsidized loans—could reduce the need for child labor in developing countries. From a broad perspective, long-term policies that reduce family poverty, decrease rates of adult unemployment, and improve adults' income also are likely to reduce the need for child labor (ILO, 1997a).

In 1996, in a partnership with ILO/IPEC, Brazil launched an official program to eradicate and control child labor, giving families scholarships or other incentives if their children keep attending school and stop working. The program ends child labor and rehabilitates child workers, and the family is provided with benefits in cash, which partially compensate for its loss of income if a child stops working. The economic incentives include monthly allowances paid to parents of child workers between 7 and 14, school access, free books, school meals, and school support in the after-class period. The program also includes job training for adults to facilitate employment and prevent the need for child labor (ILO, 1997a). The program is now widely applied in Brazil. The 30% decrease in child labor suggests that the program has been a success (Instituto Brasileiro de Geografia e Estatística, 2001).

In the state of Rio Grande do Sul in Brazil, the Program for Child Labor Eradication and Prevention (PETI) offers a scholarship to each eligible child of $30 per month that lasts until the child is 14 years old. The program also creates school supports and activities in the period before and after school. For each child, regular attendance at school and regular participation in extraclass activities, including homework, are mandatory to maintain the scholarship. The program also enrolls the parents in courses and workshops focused on the development of professional skills. The goal is to facilitate the adults' access to labor market opportunities and to reduce the pressures on children to work.

Table 3–4 shows an impressive increase in the number of children admitted to the Program for Child Labor Eradication and Prevention since it began in 1996, when 3710 children in throughout the country were enrolled. By 2001, the program had increased to include almost 750,000 children (Brasil, 2002).

An ILO survey on the impact of these kinds of economic incentives, which were offered in 18 developing countries, concluded that poverty makes such incentives necessary, but that in order to be effective they must be combined with other activities—for example, setting up schools, improving teaching, awareness-raising, and community development. The organizations involved pointed to a number of problems, such as the risks of corruption and cheating; creation of family dependence on the program concerned; and the danger that parents might make their children work in order to benefit from the program or put them back to work when the benefits ceased. Care must be taken because these incentives potentially can lead to the need

Table 3–4. Program for Child Labor Eradication and Prevention, Brazil, 2002

Year	Number of children admitted	R$ millions
1996	3,710	0.9
1997	37,025	14.4
1998	117,200	37.8
1999	145,507	82.7
2000	394,969	182.6
2001	749,353	300.4

Note: In 2002, one dollar is equivalent to three reais. R$300.4 million represents about US$100 million.
Source: Brasil (2002).

for a never-ending stream of funds. They may, however, sometimes be the only way to break the vicious circle of poverty, especially in extreme cases of child labor such as bonded labor and prostitution (ILO, 1997a). The experience acquired with such programs seems to indicate that the type of economic incentive in each situation needs to be carefully selected, and families must be asked to help rehabilitate their children to prevent them from becoming dependent. Even more significant is the fact that these experiments have shown that economic incentives are vital for child workers whose survival is threatened once they have been removed from work (ILO, 1997a).

To be most effective, this policy approach needs to be coupled with broad access to public schools and strong efforts to improve the quality of schools. More analyses of this and other alternatives are needed not only so that policy makers and researchers can better understand the impact of child labor on children's health and development, but also so that they can establish efficient strategies to combat the harmful aspects of child labor while boosting poor families' incomes.

Developing Better Methodologies and Broader Policy Approaches

Both research and action are needed. To date, the great majority of the studies on child labor have been cross-sectional and non-population-based. Another drawback of these designs is the potential for selection bias, as in nonrandom samples, because healthier children are more likely to be able to work, and those children who become sick or injured on the job are likely to stop working. In addition, it is important to note that many occupational exposures may lead to ill health effects that are not measured for months or years (Kleinbaum, Kupper, and Morgenstern, 1982; Rothman and Greenland, 1998). Longitudinal studies are needed not only to control for sources of bias but also to gather data on the long-term health outcomes experienced by child workers. Longitudinal data—in fact, data in general on the extent and kinds of work done by children worldwide—are critically important to expand our understanding of the mechanisms by which occupational hazards affect children.

But the causes and consequences are well enough understood to allow us to take action to address many of the problems. Most parents want to do what is in their children's best interest. While parents sometimes are not aware of the risks associated with child labor, it is crucial to recognize that children sometimes work even when parents are aware of the risks or costs, because the families feel they have no other choice. In those cases, the child labor problem must be understood in relation to social class and circumstances such as family disruption or chronic unemployment. Therefore, reform efforts must be multipronged. It is important to inform parents, employers, and children about existing legislation regarding child workers, and to tell them about work-related hazards and the impact that work can have on children's health and education. But it is also essential to increase the availability of social supports, law enforcement, and economic resources that strengthen the society's ability to solve child labor problems related to poverty and social exclusion (BILA, 1998).

References

Amnesty International. 2000. War children tell their stories. *Amnesty* 104: 4–7.

Bequele, A., and W. E. Myers. 1995. *First things first in child labour: Eliminating work detrimental to children.* Geneva: International Labor Organization.

Black, M. 1997. *Child domestic workers: A handbook for research and action.* Child Labour Series No. 15. London: Anti-Slavery International.

Brasil, R. F. d. 2002. Indicadores sócio-econômicos—Programa de Erradicação do Trabalho Infantil, República Federativa do Brasil.

Bureau of International Labor Affairs. 1994. *By the sweat and toil of children: The use of child labor in U.S. manufactured and mined imports.* Washington, D.C.: U.S. Department of Labor.

Bureau of International Labor Affairs. 1998. By the sweat and toil of children, Vol. 5: Efforts to eliminate child labor. Washington, D.C.: United States: U.S. Department of Labor.

Committee on the Health and Safety Implications of Child Labor, National Research Council and Institute of Medicine. 1998. *Protecting youth at work: Health, safety, and development of working children and adolescents in the United States.* Washington, D.C.: National Academy Press.

Cruz Neto, O., and M. R. Moreira. 1998. Child and adolescent labor: Factors, legal aspects, and social repercussions [in process citation]. *Cadernos de Saude Publica* 14(2): 437–41.

ECACL. 2002. Child labor country briefs system: Child labor database, education to combat abusive child labor. Available at: www.beps.net/ChildLabor/Database.htm

Fassa, A. G. 2000. *Trabalho infantil e saúde: Perfil ocupacional e problemas músculo-esqueléticos.* Pelotas, Brazil: Departamento de Medicina Social, Universidade Federal de Pelotas: 140.

Fassa, A. G., L. A. Facchini, M. M. Dall'agnol, and D. C. Christiani. 2000a. *Characteristics of child labor in a city in southern Brazil.* Pelotas, Brazil: Departamento de Medicina Social, Universidade Federal de Pelotas.

Fassa, A. G., L. A. Facchini, M. M. Dall'agnol, and D. C. Christiani. 2000b. *Child labor and musculoskeletal disorders: The Pelotas (Brazil) epidemiological survey.* Pelotas, Brazil: Departamento de Medicina Social, Universidade Federal de Pelotas.

Fausto, A., and R. Cervini. 1996. *O Trabalho e a Rua: Crianças e adolescentes no Brasil urbano dos anos 80.* São Paulo, Brazil: Cortez Editora.

Forastieri, V. 1997. *Children at work: Health and safety risks.* Geneva: International Labor Organization.

Instituto Brasileiro de Geografia e Estatística (IBGE). 1992. *Censo demográfico 1991: Resultados preliminares.* Rio de Janeiro: IBGE: 95.

Instituto Brasileiro de Geografia e Estatística (IBGE). 2001. *Pesquisa Nacional por Amostra de Domicílios—PNAD 1999.* Rio de Janeiro: IBGE.

International Labor Conference. 1999. Convention 182: Convention Concerning the Prohibition and Immediate Action for the Elimination of the Worst Forms of Child Labor, Geneva: International Labor Organization.

International Labor Organization (ILO). 1973. C138 Minimum Age Convention. Geneva: ILO.

International Labor Organization. 1997a. Child labor: How the challenge is being met. *International Labor Review* 136(2): 233–57.

International Labor Organization. 1997b. *Combating the most intolerable forms of child labor: A global challenge.* Child Labor Conference, Amsterdam.

International Labor Organization (ILO). 1997c. *Trade union action against child labour: Brazilian experience.* Brasília: ILO.

International Labor Organization (ILO). 1998a. *Child labour: Targeting the intolerable.* Geneva: ILO.

International Labor Organization (ILO). 1998b. *Statistics on working children and hazardous child labour in brief.* Geneva: ILO.

International Labor Organization (ILO). 2002. Every child counts: New global estimates on child labour. Geneva: ILO.

Kleinbaum, D., L. Kupper, and C. Morgenstern. 1982. *Epidemiologic research: Principles and quantitative methods.* New York: Wiley.

Landrigan, P., and McCammon, J. B. 1997. Child labor: Still with us after all these years. *Public Health Report* 112: 466–73.

Layne, L. A., D. N. Castillo, N. Stout, and P. Cutlip. 1994. Adolescent occupational injuries requiring hospital emergency department treatment: A nationally representative sample. *American Journal of Public Health* 84(4): 657–60.

Ministério do trabalho e emprego. 2000. *Proteção integral para crianças e adolescentes -Fiscalização do trabalho saúde e aprendizagem.* Florianópolis, Brazil: Ministério do trabalho e emprego.

Parker, D. 1997a. Child labor: The impact of economic exploitation on the health and welfare of children. *Minnesota Medicine* 80(7): 10–13, 52–55.

Parker, D. 1997b. Health effects of child labor. *Lancet* 350(9088): 1395–96.

Rothman, K. J., and S. Greenland. 1998. *Modern epidemiology*, 2nd ed. Philadelphia: Lippincott-Raven.

Scanlon, T. J., V. Prior, L. M. N. Lamarao, M. A. Lynch, and F. Scanlon. 2002. Child labor. *British Medical Journal* 325(7361): 401–3.

Somasundaram, D. 2002. Child soldiers: Understanding the context. *British Medical Journal* 324: 1268–71.

UNICEF. 1997. *The state of the world's children 1997.* Oxford: Oxford University Press.

UNICEF. 2001. *Beyond child labor, affirming rights.* New York: UNICEF.

United Nations High Commisioner for Human Rights. 1996. *Rights of the child: Report of the special rapporteur on the sale of children, child prostitution and child pornography.* Geneva: United Nations.

Wunsch Filho, V. 1995. Variações e tendências na morbomortalidade dos trabalhadores. In Velhos e novos males da saúde no Brasil: A evolução do país e de suas doenças, edited by CA Monteiro. São Paulo, Brazil: Editora Hucitec.

Part II

The Broader Impact of Global Working Conditions: The Effect on Families

4

Labor Conditions and the Health of Children, Elderly and Disabled Family Members

JODY HEYMANN, ARON FISCHER,
AND MICHAL ENGELMAN

Historical Transformations

In an unprecedented number of the world's families, both parents now work in the paid labor force. The historical transformation in the nature and location of work has seen its fullest expression in industrialized countries, where the large majority of men and then women entered the modern labor force in the nineteenth and twentieth centuries. Similar processes are now underway in much of the developing world. The twin trends of urbanization and rising levels of paid nonagricultural labor force participation in most of the world's developing regions mean that fewer adults are now regularly working near their children or other family members. Even in rural areas, the transformation of the agricultural economy is pulling the spheres of work and home apart and dramatically changing how children and other family members are cared for.

Urbanization

Marked changes in urbanization have occurred worldwide over the past century. Whereas 18% of the world's population lived in urban areas in 1910, 47% did so in 2000 (Brockerhoff, 2000; McNeill, 2000). In the developing world, urbanization was particularly rapid, more than doubling from 18% to 40% in the second half of the twentieth century. And some individual countries saw even more drastic change. In Botswana, for instance, urbanization increased from 2% to 50.3% between 1960 and 2000 (World Bank Group, 2002). The rapid urbanization that has been occurring in all of the world's regions is expected to continue. The United Nations (UNPD, 1999) has predicted that by the year 2030, 60.3% of the world's population—including 56.2% of the developing world's population—will live in urban areas.

Urbanization can affect the availability of people to help provide routine and sick care for their family members in at least two ways. First, urbanization can influence whether *extended* family members are available to provide sick and well care. Ethnographic studies in several regions have shown that migration from rural to urban areas often separates nuclear families from their extended families (Aja, 2001; Bolak, 1997; Holmes-Eber, 1997; Salaff and Wong, 1981). While urban working families continue to rely on social networks for economic or emergency assistance, they often lack the daily support necessary to care for children and other family members.

Second, urbanization is generally accompanied by a shift away from agricultural work and toward formal sector jobs. The percentage of the world's labor force working in agriculture decreased from 62% in 1960 to 39% in 1995, with declines in every country and region during that time period (World Bank Group, 2002). Between 1960 and 1990, the percentage of the world's adult population involved in the formal labor sector rose from 30% to 39%, with rises in every region (World Bank, 2000). Urban work is more likely than agricultural work to require adults to leave their children and elderly family members at home during the day. Similarly, parents working at formal sector jobs generally are less available to attend to family needs during the workday. Informal sector urban jobs such as street vending are more likely to be compatible with simultaneous care for children and family members than formal ones, but often only with limited or marginal care (Sethuraman, 1998).

Concurrent Shifts in Labor Force Composition

While urbanization has been transforming where families live and work, dramatic shifts have also been occurring in who works for pay. In North America, there has been a steady climb in female labor force participation over the past half century.[1] While 36.4% of working-age women participated in the U.S. labor force in 1960, by 2000 that figure had risen to 59% (World Bank Group, 2002). Over the same period, the rise in Canada was even more marked: in 1960, 28.7% of women were employed or seeking paid work; in 2000, 59.8% were. Western Europe saw similarly rapid growth in female labor force participation, although, in some countries, such as France (48.6%) and Germany (48.4%), not quite to the same levels as in North America. While research to date has focused on the effects of this transformation in North America and Europe, these are not the only regions where women have been rapidly entering the labor force.

In Latin America in 1960, only 24.3% of working-age women participated in the labor force. By 2000, 42.9% of Latin American women were working, and the female share of the labor force had risen in nearly every country. In South America, Uruguay, Nicaragua, Colombia, and Bolivia all had well over 50% of women in the labor force (World Bank Group, 2002). In addition, female labor force participation is well above 50% in Caribbean countries such as Jamaica, Barbados, the Bahamas, and Haiti.

In southern Africa in 1960, the proportion of the female population in the labor force ranged from a low of nearly 36.6% in South Africa to a high of over 90% in Botswana. In the next four decades, the rates increased where they had been the lowest. By 2000, women made up at least 44% of the labor force in every southern African country (World Bank Group, 2002).

The east Asian labor force presented a heterogeneous picture in 1960, although women accounted for nearly 50% of the total regional labor force. Whereas fewer than 30% of women worked for pay in Brunei, South Korea, and Singapore, 88.5% of women were economically active in Cambodia, 86.8% in Thailand, and 81.6% in Vietnam. During the ensuing decades, female labor force participation rates rose in those countries where rates had been low in 1960. By 2000, 69.8% of women in East Asia and the Pacific were in the labor force (World Bank Group, 2002).

In summary, high female labor force participation rates became the world norm in the second half of the twentieth century. In countries where women's labor force participation had been low it increased, often rapidly. By 2000, 56.6% of the world's women were in the labor force (World Bank Group, 2002).

As Heymann (2000a) described in a study of demographic changes in the United States, the transformation of the relationship between work and family is not solely a product of women's entry into the paid labor force but rather of both *men's and women's* entry into the industrial and postindustrial labor force. In the United States, the change in nonagricultural labor force participation rates between 1840 and 1940 among men was similar to the change in those rates among women between 1950 and 2000. Similarly, in the developing world, it is long-term increases in both *men's and women's* paid nonagricultural employment that have resulted in the majority of children being raised in families in which all adults work for pay. These increases have posed new challenges for working families and have changed how families manage their economic and caregiving responsibilities.

The Developing World: Greater Burdens, Fewer Resources

Given these trends, working families in the developing world are, not surprisingly, now facing work–family challenges similar to those faced by families in industrialized countries—but those in the developing world are doing so with significantly higher caregiving burdens and far fewer resources. The age dependency ratios—that is, the ratios of children and elderly to working-age adults—tend to be 50% to 100% higher in the developing world than in industrialized countries (World Bank Group, 2002). In England and the United States, for example, these dependency ratios were .53 and .52, respectively, while in Pakistan, Guatemala, and Yemen they were .83, .89, and 1.05, respectively. In addition, rates of illness involving both common and serious diseases—from childhood diarrhea to pneumonia—are higher in the developing world, further adding to the caregiving responsibilities of working adults (WHO, 1999).

In addition to bearing greater caregiving responsibilities, working adults in the developing world have far fewer resources to help them meet family needs than do their counterparts in developed nations. Not only are family incomes far lower, but governments in the developing world have less to invest in social services than do those in Europe and North America—both in absolute dollars and as a percentage of total public expenditures (World Bank, 2000).[2]

What do these trends and transformations mean for the well-being of families in developing countries? A limited amount of previous research has begun to examine the relationship between parental labor and family health and well-being in developing countries, but the studies have been few and the findings inconsistent because only employment status was examined; working conditions were ignored (Defo, 1994; Fikree and Gray, 1996; Lijestrand and Bergstrom, 1984; Tawiah, 1989).

In previous research in the industrialized world, Heymann and colleagues found that working and social conditions critically affect how the transformations in labor force participation and urbanization influence family health. Working and social conditions mediate the effects of parental work on children's health, children's development and education, the well-being of elderly and disabled family members, and the ability of adults to get and keep a job that could lift their families out of poverty (Heymann, 2000a, 2000b, 2002; Heymann and Earle, 1996, 1998, 1999, 2000, 2001; Heymann, Earle, and Egleston, 1996; Heymann, Toomey, and Furstenberg, 1999). In recent research, Heymann's team has explored whether the same relationships hold true in other nations. In this chapter, we examine conditions in North America, Latin America, Africa, and Asia. We begin with a review of the theoretical and empirical basis for a link between parental working conditions and children's health. We then review similar arguments in relation to the health of elderly and disabled family members. In the core of this chapter, we report new findings from a series of studies conducted as part of the Project on Global Working Families, founded and directed by Heymann, including in-depth interviews of working caregivers from around the world.

Parental Working Conditions and Children's Health

The leading killers of children worldwide are vaccine-preventable diseases (15%), diarrhea (17%), respiratory infections (18%), and perinatal problems (20%) (UNICEF, 2001). Parents can play an important role in preventing and diminishing the toll taken by these and other diseases in at least four ways: for mothers, breast-feeding their infants and for both parents, ensuring that their children receive the full complement of immunizations, ensuring proper adult supervision of their children, and providing care when their children are recuperating from illnesses. Parents' ability to ensure that their children have these basic safeguards against childhood diseases is, however, influenced by working conditions and social supports.

Breast-Feeding among Employed Mothers

Breast-feeding plays a critical role in preventing two of the four leading causes of child mortality: diarrheal diseases and respiratory infections. In developing countries, studies have revealed a 1.5- to 5-fold lower relative risk of mortality among breast-fed children (Feachem and Koblinsky, 1984; Habicht, DaVanzo, and Butz, 1986; Hobcraft, McDonald, and Rutstein, 1985; Jason, Nieburg, and Marks, 1984). Breast-fed infants have lower rates of gastrointestinal infections (Dewey, Heinig, and Nommsen-Rivers, 1995; Feachem and Koblinsky, 1984; Howie et al., 1990; Lepage, Munyakazi, and Hennart, 1982), respiratory tract infections (Cerqueriro et al., 1990; Howie et al., 1990; Watkins, Leeder, and Corkhill, 1979; Wright et al., 1989), otitis media (Aniansson et al., 1994; Duncan et al., 1993), meningitis (Arnold, Makintube, and Istre, 1993), and other infections (Cunningham, Jelliffee, and Jelliffee, 1991; Feachem and Koblinsky, 1984). While deaths from diarrheal diseases are much less common in industrialized countries, a higher fatality rate from diarrhea has been documented among bottle-fed children in the United States, Canada, and the United Kingdom, as well as in developing countries (Cunningham, Jelliffee, and Jelliffee, 1991).

While the benefits of breast-feeding are many and well established, as Yimyam and Morrow (Chapter 5) show, many working women are unable to breast-feed for long. Working away from one's infant while maintaining breast-feeding can be difficult to achieve. However, there is no inherent conflict between employment and breast-feeding. A variety of measures can make it possible for working women to breast-feed. For example, formal workplace policies such as paid parental leave, on-site child care, and breast-feeding breaks can enable working women to breast-feed, and all of these measures have been called for by the International Labour Organization's (ILO) Convention 183.[3]

Access to Immunizations

Avoiding vaccine-preventable diseases requires that children promptly receive the full complement of recommended immunizations. The notion that working conditions can impact child immunizations is supported by research in which parents were directly asked what factors affected their ability to vaccinate their children. Studies in Haiti, Indonesia, and the United States (Coreil et al., 1994; Fielding, Cumberland, and Pettitt, 1994; Lannon et al., 1995; McCormick et al., 1997) have all found that women report conflict with work schedules as a significant barrier to getting their children immunized.

Research from the Project on Global Working Families reveals that parents' ability to ensure proper immunizations depends on the structure of immunization programs, as well as the degree to which those programs take parental work schedules and demands into account. When immunization campaigns occur in child-care centers and preschools, and on weekends or evenings, the children of working parents can be reached. However, immunization programs in many parts of the world are currently structured so that parents or other adult care providers must take time off from work to bring their children to clinics or physicians' offices for immunizations or be home during the day when immunization campaigns occur (CDC, 2001; WHO, 2000). When outreach programs are not in place, our studies suggest that immunization rates depend on whether parental work conditions such as paid leave and schedule flexibility are present that enable parents to be available to take children to clinics and doctors' offices. Because of poor parental working conditions, children in low-income families are more likely to lack immunizations. We will report more on these findings in subsequent sections of this chapter.

Exposure to Illnesses and Injuries

Just as social conditions can influence disease prevention and health promotion for children, they can also affect children's exposure to illnesses and injuries. When children are left alone or in the care solely of other young children, they are more likely to lack clean food and water, and therefore to face a higher risk of getting infections.

Only a few studies have examined the impact of poor child care on children's exposure to infections in developing countries. Iroegbu and colleagues (2000), focusing on Nigeria, measured the bacterial content of foods given to children younger than 2 years old and compared the contamination levels for children who accompanied their mothers to work as street merchants with the levels for children who were left at home. They found that while the contamination levels for both groups of children were dangerously high, contamination was worse for children who stayed at home with older siblings or household helpers. In a study of Haitian mothers who worked as merchants, Devin and Erickson (1996) found that nutritionally deprived children were more likely to be left with male caregivers when their mothers went to the market than were well-nourished children. Follow-up interviews showed that many of the children reportedly left with male caregivers actually had been left alone while the men were working in the fields during the day.

Lack of quality care can also leave children exposed to injuries, but prior to the Project on Global Working Families, this risk factor had not been addressed extensively outside of wealthy countries. Children left alone or without adult supervision are likely to face a higher risk of injury. The Project on Global Working Families has conducted a series of in-depth studies that focus on the challenges that low- and middle-income face in finding adequate care for children, the elderly, and other dependents while working.

Care of Sick Children

While parents play a significant role in preventing children's illnesses and injuries, they also play a critical role in caring for children as they recover from illnesses and injuries. Young children who are sick need their parents or other care providers to take them to the physician, obtain and administer medicines, and provide daily care when they cannot go to child-care facilities or schools. A series of studies have demonstrated that children recover more rapidly from illnesses and injuries when their parents are present (Mahaffy, 1965; Palmer, 1993; van der Schyff, 1979). The presence of parents has been shown to reduce the duration of children's hospital stays by 31% (Taylor and O'Connor, 1989). When parents are involved in children's care, children recover more rapidly from outpatient procedures as well (Kristensson-Hallstron, Elander, and Malmfors, 1997). Because of the importance of parental care, pediatricians have increasingly been offering parents the chance to become involved in different aspects of their children's care (George and Hancock, 1993; LaRosa-Nash and Murphy, 1997).

Research has shown that parents play important roles in the care of children with chronic as well as acute conditions (Hanson et al., 1992; Wolman et al., 1994). For example, the importance of parental involvement has been demonstrated for children with epilepsy (Carlton-Ford et al., 1995), asthma, and diabetes (Anderson et al., 1981; Hamlett, Pellegrini, and Katz, 1992; La Greca et al., 1995). As far as mental health is concerned, the benefits of receiving their parents' care (Sainsbury et al., 1986; Waugh and Kjos, 1992) and the detrimental effects of separating ill young children from their parents have long been demonstrated (Bowlby, 1953; McGraw, 1994; Roberston, 1958). When parental involvement in the care of sick children is increased, children's anxiety decreases (Cleary et al., 1986; Gauderer, Lorig, and Eastwood, 1989; Hannallah and Rosales, 1983; Sainsbury et al., 1986).

Studies conducted as part of Heymann's Work, Family, and Democracy Initiative in the United States have shown that, as in the case of disease and injury prevention and health promotion, care of sick children is affected more by the conditions that working parents face than by the mere fact that they work. When young children are given high-quality child care, the adults providing that care can attend promptly to unanticipated injuries or illnesses, and they can help ensure that children will receive prompt medical care. It is when children are left alone, in the care of other children, or in poor-quality child care that they are likely to fail to receive prompt medical attention (Heymann, 2000a). Efforts to ensure that working parents' children, when sick, will have access to prompt, high-quality medical treatment and parental care are mediated by the social supports families receive and the working conditions they face (Heymann and Earle, 1996; Heymann, Toomey, and Furstenberg, 1999). When parents are able to take leave from work to care for their sick or injured children during the day, their children's health is unlikely to suffer. However, prior to the Project on Global Working Families, research in this field outside the United States and Europe was limited.

Working Conditions and the Health of Elderly and Disabled Family Members

Older individuals live enormously varied lives.[4] Some are in excellent health, continuing to work for pay or to care for children or grandchildren full time, and leading a physically and mentally active life. Because of chronic conditions or disabilities, however, others face significant limitations and must rely on healthier individuals to help them with everything from meeting daily needs (such as bathing, dressing, or eating) to obtaining medical care (Heymann, 2000a). The challenges for working adults in meeting the caregiving needs of elderly and disabled family members will continue to grow due to the confluence of three trends. First, occupational and residential changes to urban environments have been accompanied by the increasing separation of nuclear families from elderly and disabled relatives, and by a decrease in multigenerational households (Chattopadhyay and Marsh, 1999; Chow, 1999; Jamuna, 1997). Second, increasing numbers of women are working full-time, but women still constitute the vast majority of care providers for elderly and disabled family members in developing and industrialized nations alike (Davis et al., 1995; Doress-Worters, 1994; Hashizume, 2000; Ineichen, 1998; Long and Harris, 2000; Medjuck, Keefe, and Fancey, 1998; Rawlins, 2001; Restrepo and Rozental, 1994). Third, medical successes are leading to increased survival rates of disabled and elderly adults. The population of persons aged 80 or over—those likely to need the most care—is expected to grow even faster, increasing more than 5.5 times and reaching 379 million by 2050. The numerical increase in currently developing nations will be dramatic, as the population of people aged 60 or older will go from 374 million in 2000 to 1.6 billion in 2050—more than quadrupling (UNPD, 2001). By 2020, 70% of the total worldwide population aged 60 or older will live in the developing world (Banoob, 1992).

While income transfers have become increasingly common as an alternative to direct elder care (Chattopadhyay and Marsh, 1999), family members remain a major source of social support for older individuals throughout the world. Researchers have reported, for example, that in China (Arnsberger et al., 2000; Ikels, 1991), India (Kumar, 1997), Korea (Kim, 1999), Malaysia (Chen, 1987), Nepal (Niruaula, 1995), and Taiwan (Chattapadhyay and Marsh, 1999; Shyu, Lee, and Chen, 1999), large majorities of the elderly, particularly in rural areas, live with their children and, when ill, turn to them for care. Similar findings regarding preferences for intergenerational coresidence or nearby residence and care were reported for the English-speaking nations of the Caribbean (Rawlins, 1999; Serow and Cowart, 1998), Saudi Arabia (Mufti, 1998), Turkey (Aytac, 1998), and Botswana (Clausen et al., 2000; Draper and Keith, 1992).

While studies in the developing world have documented caregivers' role in shaping the health and well-being of older persons, research has not focused on how working affects caregivers' ability to provide high-quality care. Furthermore, remarkably little research has been done on caregiving for disabled adults globally.

The Project on Global Working Families

Founded and directed by Jody Heymann, the Project on Global Working Families is the first program devoted to understanding and improving the relationship between working conditions and family health and well-being globally. The project currently involves research in North America, Europe, Latin America, Africa, and Asia. In addition to analyzing data on thousands of closed-ended surveys, Heymann, Fischer, Engelman, and others on the project staff have conducted and analyzed nearly 1000 in-depth interviews in Mexico, Botswana, Vietnam, the United States, Russia, and Honduras.[5]

Working families, teachers, child-care providers, health-care providers, and employers have been interviewed in a wide variety of global settings in order to examine the differences and commonalities among the experiences of working adults across social class, occupation, ethnicity, region, and economic and public policy contexts. Semistructured, open-ended interview instruments were used to analyze the complex mechanisms by which families' work and social conditions affect health.

Mexico

From 1999 to 2000, the Project on Global Working Families conducted in-depth interviews in Mexico. Working caregivers attending public clinics in Mexico City and in San Cristóbal de las Casas, Chiapas, were invited to participate. San Cristóbal has a population of 128,000 (Instituto de Salud, 1999), while the state of Chiapas has a population of 3.9 million. Thirty percent of the inhabitants of Chiapas are younger than 10 years of age. One out of five inhabitants is illiterate. One-third live in homes without running water, and one out of five has no electricity (INEGI, 1999). The Mexico City metropolitan area has a population of 16.7 million, while the city proper has a population of 8.5 million (INEGI, 1999, 2000). Twenty-eight percent of the residents are 14 years old or younger (INEGI, 1999). Clinics in the two locations were chosen to ensure variation in occupation, socioeconomic status, family structure, and ethnicity. The sample included clinics serving public and private sector workers, low- and middle-income families, and indigenous and Latino populations.

The overall response rate was 87%. The average age of the respondents was 33 years, with a range from 17 to 60. The average number of children respondents had was 2.6, with a range from 1 to 9; and the average age respondents had been upon having their first child was 21, with a range from 14 to 38. Fifty-five percent of the respondents worked in the formal sector (e.g., teachers, employees of government agencies), 39%

worked in the informal sector (e.g., domestic servants, street vendors), and 5% worked in both. Twenty-three percent of those interviewed were of indigenous ethnicity, primarily Tzeltal and Tzotzil.

Botswana

From 2000 to 2001, the Project on Global Working Families conducted interviews in Botswana. Participants were recruited at government health clinics in Gaborone, Lobatse, and Molepolole. Gaborone is Botswana's largest city and its capital, Lobatse is a small town, and Molepolole is characterized by the census as an urban village (Central Statistics Unit, 1998). As with Mexico, the selected clinics provided care to populations that were diverse in occupation, socioeconomic status, family structure, and ethnicity (including Bakwena, Bangwato, Bangwaketse, and Bakalanga peoples, among others). The selected sites included a large urban public hospital that served urban poor and middle-class outpatients, a small health facility that served a wide range of residents living in a small town, and a government-run medical center that served as the main referral center for the approximately 30 area clinics and outlying health posts in a rural area.

The response rate in Botswana was 96%. Of those interviewed, 49% had never been married, 29% were married, 14% were cohabiting, and 7% were divorced, widowed, or separated. Seventy percent of the respondents worked in the formal sector, 18% worked in the informal sector, and 12% worked in both.

With 38.8% of those between the ages of 15 and 49 infected with the human immunodeficiency virus (HIV), Botswana is at the epicenter of the acquired immunodeficiency syndrome (AIDS) epidemic, which presents the gravest health-caregiving burdens globally (UNAIDS, 2002). Caregiving for HIV/AIDS-infected and -affected family members was a critical focus of the Botswana interviews. Forty-seven percent of the respondents interviewed were not only working but also caring for a family member or friend with HIV/AIDS by providing physical, financial, and emotional support in ways that ranged from cleaning, cooking, and feeding to visiting and providing counseling. The caregivers we interviewed also often reported taking over the HIV patient's household and caregiving responsibilities.

Vietnam

The Project on Global Working Families conducted interviews at three medical centers in Ho Chi Minh City, Vietnam, from 2000 to 2001. Ho Chi Minh, Vietnam's largest city, had a population of 5 million (World Bank, Asian Development Bank, and UNDP, 2000). Thirty-four percent of Ho Chi Minh's residents were 14 years of age or younger, and the city had the largest average household size of any urban area in Vietnam, with 5.5 people per household (General Statistics Office of Vietnam, 1994). To obtain a sample of working parents with a wide range of economic and living situations, the

Project on Global Working Families conducted and analyzed interviews from three sites in Ho Chi Minh City, including a large hospital for children that serves both urban and rural residents, a government-owned general hospital serving a population with diverse economic backgrounds, and the largest public teaching obstetrics and gynecology hospital.

The response rate was 77% for the sample of mothers and 89% for the sample of fathers. The average age of the respondents was 34, with a range from 21 to 51. The average number of children that respondents had was two, with a range from one to four. Fifty-nine percent of the respondents were from Ho Chi Minh City, 32% were from neighboring towns, and 9% had recently migrated to the city. Ninety-four percent of the respondents were Vietnamese, 5% were ethnically Chinese, and 1% were ethnically Cambodian. Ninety-five percent of the respondents were married. Sixty-one percent of the respondents worked in the formal sector, while 35% worked in the informal sector, and 4% worked in both.

Honduras

Working parents, teachers, doctors, and other caregiving professionals were interviewed in Honduras in 2001. Participants were recruited at medical clinics, public day-care centers, shelters, and people's homes in the capital, Tegucigalpa, and in the rural towns of Sabana Grande, Montegrande, Adurasta, San Lorenzo, Laure Abajo, Rosario, and El Chiflon. In addition to examining work and social conditions and their effect on family health, the interviews in Honduras explored the long-term impact on working families of a natural disaster, Hurricane Mitch, which had devastated Central America in October 1998. In Honduras, 14,600 people had died as a result of the hurricane, and an additional 2.1 million had been affected in a manner requiring medical attention or immediate assistance with essentials such as food, water, or shelter (CRED, 2002). Of the 661,760 individuals (82,720 families) whose housing had been affected by the hurricane, 265,760 had been forced to relocate to temporary housing, while 396,000 had continued to live in substandard, hazardous conditions (Programa de las Naciones, 1999).

The United States

From 1996 to 1998, the Project on Global Working Families interviewed working parents, child-care providers, and employers in the United States. Interviews were conducted at a city's public clinics, as well as in public housing projects, at after-school programs, at child-care centers, and at places of employment. Eighty-two percent of the parents who were invited to participate in the representative public clinic sample agreed to do so, and of those, 95% completed both the closed-item survey and the in-depth semistructured interview. Of the families interviewed, 43% described themselves as white, 35% as black or African American, 14% as Hispanic or Latino, 4% as Asian or Pacific Islander, and 4% as multiracial or multiethnic. Sixty percent had household incomes at or below 150% of the federal poverty line. Seventy-two percent had been born in the United States.

The Project on Global Working Families: Early Health-Related Findings

The experiences reported by the respondents interviewed for these studies document how working conditions and the availability, accessibility, affordability, and quality of social supports shaped the impact of work on family health.

Balancing Work and Preventive Care for Children

In Mexico, Botswana, Vietnam, Honduras, and the United States, parents spoke compellingly about how poor working conditions and inadequate social supports threatened the health of their children. Comparisons of respondents' experiences in different countries further demonstrated two key facts. First, parents faced strikingly similar types of work–family problems across all regions. Second, while these problems and their impact on health were significant everywhere, their magnitude was far greater in developing countries, where families were facing significantly greater burdens with far fewer resources.

Impact of social and working conditions on disease prevention. As discussed earlier, two of the most important factors in preventing infectious diseases among infants, toddlers, and preschool children are ensuring that infants are breast-fed and ensuring that each child receives a full set of immunizations. We found that parents' ability to provide both safeguards was dramatically affected by working and social conditions. Respondents repeatedly reported that in the absence of adequate maternity leave, they had been forced to end breast-feeding dangerously early and often had not been able to afford or obtain safe substitutes.

The family of Maria Gonzalez,[6] who lived in Buenas Nuevas, Honduras, had an all too common experience. Neither Maria nor her husband had had the opportunity to learn to read or write, but they managed to put their daughters through school. Their oldest daughter, Leti Marta, aged 23, was working as a bilingual secretary. Leti had a 7-month-old baby, whom Maria was helping to raise while Leti worked to support her baby. The baby's father had abandoned Leti during her pregnancy. Leti's job provided her with only 42 days off after her daughter's birth. Maria Gonzalez explained that when Leti's official maternity leave ended, so did the breast-feeding. Leti tried to express milk, but she was not able to sustain that practice while working. Maria fed her granddaughter milk "from a can," but by the age of 7 months, the girl was pale as a ghost from anemia. Having been weaned too young, she suffered from acute malnutrition and was falling off the growth chart—weighing, as a 7-month-old, what she should have weighed as a 4-month-old.

Working conditions also affected parents' ability to get their children immunized, since many parents could not take leave from work to bring their children to clinics for immunizations. Some vaccination campaigns tried to go out to immunize children, but such efforts often proved ineffective for children left home alone or in inadequate care. Dr. Marcelo Javaloyas, the director of a neighborhood health clinic in Honduras, explained that his clinic was in the midst of a home-vaccination campaign, and he spoke of the impediments to effectively immunizing children who were home alone because their families could not find affordable care:

> We find children home alone, playing in conditions that are dangerous. We go to vaccinate, but the [vaccination record cards] aren't available. . . . The children don't have the information. They can't come to the health center because no one can bring them.

The barriers to breast-feeding and vaccinations that many respondents described were not due to parental work per se, but rather to the conditions working parents found themselves in. Had adequate maternity leave been available, mothers would have been able to breast-feed their children longer. Similarly, if children had been cared for in quality child-care centers instead of being left home alone, they could have been immunized at the centers, which would also have been able to keep accurate records. Moreover, if parents had received paid family leave or had some flexibility in their work schedules, they could have taken their children to doctors for immunizations.

Impact of social and working conditions on injury prevention. When quality child care for preschool and school-age children is available, children fare well. All too often, however, the low-income parents we interviewed found themselves without any affordable, decent care for their children and therefore had no choice but to leave their children home alone. The lack of adult supervision frequently resulted in accidents and injuries.

Caroline Hardin, an American school social worker, described an accident that took place during the 20 minutes that her children spent alone after school while waiting for her to return from work:

> There's some glass doors that go between here and the living room. [The children] were fooling around together. Cassie tried to lock Troy out, and he pushed against the glass door. There must have been a fissure in the glass or something, but it broke and his arm went right through. He really cut himself. . . . When I got home, I rushed him to the hospital.

When children were left alone for longer periods of time with the added responsibility of caring for themselves, the potential for accidents and injuries increased markedly. In Botswana, Nunko Ndebele, a 56-year-old mother of seven children, was also caring for her two grandchildren. She worked as a maid in a church near her home. In 1996, the one-room hut she shared with her family burned to the ground while her children were home alone. She recalled the disastrous experience:

> The children were cooking while I was at work, using the gas stove. I think they switched one button on but didn't light the stove. I can't say what happened, but whatever they did, the whole house was in flames. Everything was burned out. We didn't take a single item out of the house, and when I got back from work, I found that what used to be a house was now in ashes.

At the time of her interview, Nunko still did not have a roof for her rebuilt house.

Of the respondents who discussed the issue[7] in Botswana, half reported leaving their children home alone because they could find no adults to supervise them. In Mexico, nearly two out of five parents had left children home alone. In half of the cases in Mexico where the age of the child left alone was reported, the oldest child in the group left home alone was 7 years old or younger. In Vietnam, 20% reported that they had to leave children home alone.

Unsupervised children were at a heightened risk of injury. Eighteen percent of all respondents in Mexico, 29% of all respondents in Vietnam and 33% of all respondents in Botswana reported that while they were at work, their children had experienced accidents or other emergencies.[8] Virtually all of those interviewed felt that leaving their children in order to work and not having adequate caregiving supports jeopardized the children's health and well-being. Still, economic necessity forced them to make untenable decisions. One Mexican mother summed up the sentiments of many when she explained, "If I don't work, my children will die of hunger."

Barriers to promoting a developmentally healthy environment. Among the parents we interviewed in Mexico, more than half had regularly taken their children to work. Thirty-three-year-old Henrietta Leon had spent 8 years working in a Mexican pants factory. Though she worked until 8:00 P.M., her daughter's day-care center closed at 4 P.M., so Henrietta took her daughter to the factory for the remainder of the afternoon and evening.

The greatest hazard to the development of children in the working families we interviewed was the lack of affordable, quality care for their children while they worked. Moreover, in the absence of access to affordable, quality care, many children were left home alone at young ages or in the care of other young children, often with disastrous consequences. After Hurricane Mitch hit Honduras, for example, many families lost their homes and moved into makeshift rooms at temporary shelters. Without enough money to rebuild their ruined houses, however, some families stayed in small barracks for years. At the time of our interviews, 18-month-old Laurita had lived since birth in a single shelter room shared by her nine-person family. Laurita's father worked long hours as an electrician, and her mother cooked and sold food in the streets for 12 hours a day, 6 days a week. While her parents were away from the family's room, Ramon, Laurita's 10-year-old brother, was charged with caring for Laurita, their three sisters younger than 6, and their 5-month-old brother. But at age 10, Ramon could not keep up with adequately feeding and caring for his five younger siblings. Severely malnourished, Laurita could barely move. Her legs were thin and bent—she had never learned to use them. Ramon explained that Laurita could not yet walk and that he did not know how to get her out of the chair and encourage her to walk.

Such experiences were not limited, however, to families living in poverty after a natural disaster. More than one-third of the parents we spoke with in Mexico, Botswana, and Vietnam reported having to leave their children alone or in the care of other young children without adult supervision. This pattern had severe consequences not only for the young children in need of care but also for the older children who were called on to provide that care. Ten percent of the parents who discussed impacts in Botswana reported that their older children had had to forgo school in order to care for younger siblings. While child labor is a recognized problem affecting both boys and girls in the developing world, home-based work often remains unaddressed due to its informal nature. Studies conducted throughout the world have found that children engage in household work from an early age, even before they are capable of doing wage-earning work (King and Hill, 1993; Wazir, 2000). In western Africa, where girls shoulder a larger share of the caregiving and household work burden, studies have documented the negative effect of such responsibilities on their school participation through school attendance records that showed a significantly higher rate of absences and late arrivals for girls than for boys (World Bank Population and Human Resources Division, 1996).

While it is clear that the healthy development of children involves both physical and cognitive processes that require adults' active involvement and support, we found that many children were spending a large number of their waking hours without adults. The absence of adequate care was affecting whether their basic needs were met, the safety of their surroundings, and the opportunities they had to gain the stimulation necessary for healthy development.

Balancing Work with the Care of Sick Children

In all of the countries we studied, when children became ill, working caregivers who lacked decent working conditions often found it impossible to care adequately for them. Without some flexibility in their work schedules, parents could not take their children to doctors' appointments, nor could they stay home to care for them. Without paid leave, taking time off was difficult for the poorest workers, who could ill afford to forgo even a day's income. Without flexibility at the workplace, caregivers in higher-paying formal jobs worried about placing their jobs in jeopardy if they asked for consideration. The network of social supports that barely managed to hold up under normal circumstances proved to be even more fragile when children became ill.

Barriers to obtaining professional medical care. Respondents in all countries reported that their work responsibilities had impeded their ability to access professional health care when their children needed it. Inadequate early care often resulted in worsened health conditions. Asthma, the most common chronic health condition among children in the United States, significantly affected a number of the families in our study (Heymann, 2000a). Agnes Charles, one of our U.S. respondents, knew her 2-year-old daughter's asthma was flaring up, but Agnes, the sole provider for her family, feared losing her job if she took her daughter to the doctor. Lacking paid leave and workplace flexibility, Agnes went to work and left her daughter with a baby-sitter, leaving the care provider with instructions regarding the child's asthma medication and what to do if her daughter grew more ill. During the day, the toddler grew progressively ill and cried frequently, but the baby-sitter thought she was simply cranky. When Agnes picked her daughter up in the evening, she recognized immediately that the child was in serious respiratory distress; she was retracting the front of her chest as far back as she could toward her spine just to get air into her lungs. Agnes took her daughter straight to the emergency room, where she was immediately admitted to the hospital. Had Agnes been able to take leave from work for the day, the hospitalization probably would have been avoidable through early treatment.

In Vietnam, Khanh Truong Vu, a weaver, explained what happened when her 18-month-old daughter became ill:

> My husband and I had to work long hours every day, and we left the child with my mother-in-law to look after her. She was old and had eight or nine children, so when she saw the child having fever, she thought it was nothing serious and gave her herbal medicine. This continued and the fever got higher. . . . [Later] I took the child to the doctor's, then to Nhi Dong, this pediatric hospital. The doctor took her temperature. The child's fever was above 40 degrees Celsius. They took a test of her [spinal fluid] and said she suffered from meningitis.

The experiences of adults in every country underscored the fact that there are no substitutes for working conditions that allow caregivers to monitor their children's health and rapidly address the children's need for professional care.

Obstacles to parental care. In every country we studied, we met many parents who could not care for their sick children without risking job loss and loss of essential income. Our findings pointed to the failure of social supports and working conditions worldwide to ensure that adults could reasonably manage the demands of both work and caregiving.

In Botswana, we interviewed Tlotlo Gaetsewe, who was charged with the care of her 10-year-old son and three of her sister's children. Tlotlo worked in a factory as a sorter, a low-paying job that barely enabled her to earn enough to pay for basic living expenses, much less afford child care. Tlotlo was luckier than many other employees we interviewed in that she had some paid leave. But the 5 days she received amounted to just one per child she cared for and one for herself per year. Moreover, the company's policy allowed Tlotlo to use this leave only for the duration of documented doctors' visits, not for home care. She explained:

> At work, I am allowed to take the child to the hospital and [then I have to] go back to work, irrespective of how the child is. I have to leave the sick child at home [alone].

She reported that her children suffered from common illnesses frequently and recovered from them slowly.

When children have special health needs or chronic conditions, the toll exacted by inadequate social supports is even greater. In Mexico, we talked with Romona Garciga, a 35-year-old domestic worker. She described her struggles to care for her 12-year-old daughter, who had been suffering from a recurring urinary infection for 2 years:

> The doctor says, "You should drink at least two liters [of water]." But she doesn't when I'm not there, when I am not telling her, "Drink." I come home at five and I see the water there.

Romona could not afford after-school care because she was deeply in debt from her daughter's medical expenses. Moreover, she could not take additional time off, both because she could not afford to lose more pay and because her once-understanding boss had threatened to fire her if she missed further work. The cycle of inadequate supports, limited caregiving, and poor health formed a virtually inescapable trap.

We found children's health problems to be at the center of many work–family conflicts, as parents described whenever they found themselves caught between their obligations at work and their need to care for their children. In Mexico, 42% of the respondents who spoke about this issue had had difficulty caring for their sick children due to work responsibilities, and 20% reported that their working conditions had negatively affected their children's health. In Vietnam, 49% of the respondents reported having difficulty caring for sick children due to work obligations, and 25% felt that their working conditions negatively affected their children's health. In Botswana, 59% of the respondents noted that work had made it difficult for them to care for their sick children, and 34% felt that their working conditions had negatively affected their children's health. Forty-one percent of American respondents said that their working conditions had negatively affected their children's health.

When good policies were not in place, families paid a high price—either leaving children home alone or losing wages. In Mexico, the lack of alternative caregiving options had caused 15% of the respondents we spoke with about this issue to leave their sick children at home alone. In Botswana, half of the families we interviewed spoke about this dilemma, and of those, 27% had left their sick children home alone. Since paid leave was often not available, caring for sick children frequently resulted in a high financial cost for families that were barely making ends meet. Forty-seven percent of Mexican and 20% of Botswanan respondents who discussed the issue with us reported losing pay due to caregiving responsibilities when their children were sick. The lower rate in Botswana reflects the help of government policies regarding paid leave. In Vietnam, two-thirds of respondents discussed the issue. Of those, 7% reported leaving sick children home alone. The proportion of respondents who lost pay when their children were sick was much higher, however, reaching more than 50%.

Balancing Work with Care for Elderly and Disabled Adults

Across all regions, working adults told us stories of how parents, aunts, uncles, and others went from being able to assist with child care to needing substantial care themselves as they aged. As a result, working caregivers often were left with responsibilities for multiple generations that were difficult or impossible to meet adequately while working.

After Hurricane Mitch in Honduras, Nicole Labiosa and her husband had to rebuild their damaged house while continuing to care for family members and conduct paid work. Nicole quickly learned that the hurricane had flooded her parents' small farm, destroying all of their crops and, therefore, their livelihood. For more than 2 months, Nicole, who washed and ironed other people's clothes for pay, and her husband, a bricklayer, struggled to provide food for both their children and Nicole's parents. At the same time, they strove to save enough money to rebuild their ruined home.

With adequate working conditions, illnesses were less likely to be aggravated and caregiving responsibilities were less likely to leave adults unemployed or in poverty. Nguyen Thi Sau, a 39-year-old accountant from Vietnam, reported that her employers were understanding when she had to leave work to care first for her father and later for her aunt. Sau's supervisor at the bank allowed her to take 3 months to care for her father full-time at the end of his life and return to her job after his death. When her aging aunt (who in previous years had provided vital child-care support to Sau) became ill, Sau was able to check up on her regularly from work, an ability that one morning helped head off a potential disaster:

> At ten o'clock that morning I called. The phone rang for a long time. Then my aunt picked up the phone. Her voice was faint; I couldn't hear her well. I asked her if she had eaten her porridge. She replied that she was very tired and put

down the phone. At that moment, I became very worried and scared. I ran out of the office to my motorbike and drove home immediately.

She found her aunt alone, not having eaten or taken necessary medicine. Before returning to work, Sau was able to feed her aunt, give her medications, and arrange for a cousin to look in on her later. Her supervisor supported her familial vigilance.

While Sau's experience was good, when working conditions were poor and social supports few—as was far more commonly the case for the low-income working families we interviewed—the multiple pressures placed on caregivers had serious consequences for the health of dependent family members.

In Mexico, for at least 12% of respondents, caregiving responsibilities for adult relatives or friends had led to difficulties at work, at least 10% had lost pay, and at least 6% had had difficulty retaining a job or had lost an opportunity for promotion due to such caregiving activity.[9]

Policy Implications

The experiences of the working caregivers we studied in Mexico, Botswana, Vietnam, Honduras, and the United States make it clear that poor working conditions and inadequate social supports undermine the ability of low-income adults to care well for their families' health and for their own while working. Adequate working conditions and social supports need to include paid leave and flexibility for working adults, adequate educational opportunities for their school-age children, and decent care for their preschool children and their elderly and disabled family members.

Adequate Workplace Policies

Substantial international consensus has been achieved—in theory, at least—on the need for decent working conditions and adequate social supports. For example, more than 50 nations are signatories to the international agreements and conventions that address the need for reasonable working hours, work schedules, paid vacation, and child care. Within the United Nations, those include the Universal Declaration of Human Rights, the International Covenant on Economic, Social, and Cultural Rights, and the Convention on Human Rights. Within the ILO, those include the Weekly Rest Convention (Convention 14) and the Hours of Work Convention (Convention 1).[10] However, in practice, far less has been done to enact policies that meet these needs.

Paid leave. Adequate paid leave is needed that allows workers to take time off from work to care for the health of children or elderly family members, address children's educational needs, or attend to their own health. Numerous international agreements have affirmed the right of workers to paid time off from work for a variety of reasons connected to caregiving. Paid maternity leave is called for in the United Nations' International Covenant on Economic, Social, and Cultural Rights[11] and the Convention on the Elimination of All Forms of Discrimination Against Women.[12] These agreements have been accepted by 145 and 168 nations, respectively. Paid leave is supported more broadly by the Universal Declaration of Human Rights,[13] accepted by 171 countries, which affirms the right of workers to paid time off from work.

Though paid leave is essential for enabling workers to balance their multiple responsibilities, 37% of respondents who discussed the issue in Botswana and 55% of those who discussed it in Mexico did not have paid leave. Since employment under informal terms is difficult to regulate, paid leave was much scarcer among the informal sectors workers in Botswana and Mexico. Of the informal sector workers who spoke to us on this subject in Botswana and Mexico,[14] 64% and 83%, respectively, lacked paid leave. In the United States, many working parents cannot consistently rely on paid sick leave or paid parental leave. While inadequate working conditions disadvantage all families, the poor are worst off. Forty-five percent of those living below the poverty line lacked paid sick leave all of the time compared to 24% of nonpoor families (Heymann, 2000a).

No adults should have to neglect their children or older family members in order to keep a job or afford necessities. In accordance with accepted international conventions, paid leave should be established and made available to all families globally.

Flexibility. Flexibility at work can enable employed caregivers to manage their multiple responsibilities more successfully by allowing them to arrange their work time so as to accommodate both predictable activities and unpredictable demands. In contrast to paid leave, flexibility appears to be more widely available to workers in the informal sector than to those in the formal sector, where employment terms are often more prescribed. In fact, as many of our respondents indicated, a lack of flexibility in formal sector jobs is often a decisive factor in a caregiver's decision to work in the informal sector. In Mexico, 62% of informal sector workers who discussed this issue with us reported consistent flexibility in their employment. In contrast, among formal sector workers who spoke about flexibility with us, only 18% reported having flexibility whenever they needed it. Among those who discussed flexibility in Vietnam, 64% of the informal sector workers reported being able to alter their work schedule when they needed to do so. In contrast, only 23% of respondents working in the formal sector reported having flexibility whenever they needed it. In Botswana, 34% of informal sector workers and 29% of formal sector workers reported having consistent flexibility at work. In the United States, 44% of working parents living above the poverty line and 55% of those living below the poverty line reported lacking flexibility.

While the informal sector offered greater flexibility, in general, than the formal sector, the difference was small in some countries. Moreover, informal sector jobs varied greatly with some being quite inflexible, as time off led to significant income loss. The degree of flexibility in formal sector work likewise varied significantly both between and within nations.

Care and Educational Opportunities for Children

Outside of work, formal social supports—such as child care, early childhood education programs, and school-age programs that match parents' work calendars—are crucial mediating factors in the relationship among work, caregiving, and family health and welfare. The United Nations' Convention on the Rights of the Child, which has been accepted by 191 countries, calls on states to "render appropriate assistance to parents and legal guardians in the performance of their child-rearing responsibilities and . . . ensure the development of institutions, facilities, and services for the care of children."[15] As mentioned earlier, 168 nations also have accepted the Convention on the Elimination of All Forms of Discrimination against Women, which calls for the "provision of necessary supporting social services," in particular "a network of child-care facilities," which would "enable parents to combine family obligations with work responsibilities and participation in public life."

Throughout the crucial period from birth to age 3 years, children especially need adult care that will foster healthy development (Phillips and Adams, 2001). Across the world, the high percentage of households in which all adults must work full-time to meet their families' basic needs has led to an urgent need to find solutions for infant and toddler care through a combination of paid parental leave and affordable, high-quality child care. Children aged 4 to 5 years need daily care and educational opportunities that promote both their physical and cognitive growth and enable them to develop skills essential for later learning. Numerous studies of early childhood education programs' developmental benefits have shown that children who have access to high-quality preschool education are more likely to develop stronger language skills, read well, perform well on achievement tests, and graduate from secondary school than peers who lack access to early education programs (Andrews et al., 1982; Barnett, 1995; Campbell and Ramey, 1994; Currie and Duncan, 1995; Garber, 1988; Johnson and Walker, 1991; McKay, Condell, and Ganson, 1985) . Decades of research have further established that the benefits of early childhood education are especially striking for children from low-income homes and for marginalized children (Barnett, 1996).

As our findings from around the world have indicated, affordable early education programs that promote children's development are not sufficiently available to many low-income families, and the need to establish such programs is great. For school-age children, supervision and enrichment are needed for the out-of-school hours that do not overlap with their parents' time off from work. Improving the quality and increasing the length of schooldays and the school year would both provide more educational opportunities for children and help working parents ensure that their children would receive careful supervision and educational support in a safe place. The Work, Family, and Democracy Initiative[16] headed by Heymann is currently gathering data for an index measuring the progress of nations in addressing these issues.

Care of Elderly and Disabled Adults

The simultaneous rise in the aging population and in urbanization is creating a caregiving gap for the elderly and disabled. The migration of the younger working population away from their homes of origin in search of work is weakening the family's traditional role as the main source of financial, instrumental, and emotional support for older people (Chattopadhyay and Marsh, 1999; Jamuna, 1997). In the cities, high rents and lack of space pose further serious obstacles to the multigenerational coresidence or proximate residence arrangements that many older persons prefer (Aytac, 1998; Chattopadhyay and Marsh, 1999; Chow, 1999). As more women and men move into the formal workforce, fewer family members are available to provide full-time care for the elderly (Cornman, 1996). Nonetheless, working adults still hold the majority of the responsibility for assisting elderly people financially or instrumentally. Working caregivers who maintain the responsibility of financial support or direct care for elderly relatives are often taxed by multiple obligations that reduce their ability to provide high-quality care.

In the 1995 document "The Economic, Social, and Cultural Rights of Older Persons," the United Nations calls on nations to "make all the necessary efforts to support, protect and strengthen the family and help it, in accordance with each society's system of cultural values, to respond to the needs of its dependent ageing members."[17] The United Nations' Principles for Older Persons assert that "older persons should have access to adequate food, water, shelter, clothing and health care through the provision of income, family and community support and self-help."[18] As a global community, we need to put substance behind those aspirations. To begin with, if low-income working adults are to care for their parents and other older sick family members, they need to be able to take leave to provide that assistance. Their leave needs to be paid and protected from the risk of job loss. For elderly and disabled adults who require regular assistance in order to meet basic and health-care needs, affordable and accessible supports that do not require their children to quit work—an option too many cannot afford—are needed.

Conclusion

In the absence of decent working conditions and adequate social supports, the impact of worldwide dramatic demographic shifts in the nature and location of work on the health of employees' children or elderly and sick family members, as well as on the welfare of families as a whole, can be dire. Yet these problems are addressable. They require, first, that we recognize that the quality of working conditions can be as important to the health of families as to workers themselves; second, that we pay as much attention to the creation of decent working conditions as to the creation of jobs globally; and, finally, that we match social supports to the conditions working families face in the twenty-first century.

Notes

1. Statistics on female labor force participation rates refer to the ratio of the number of women in the labor force divided by the total population of adult women. Female labor force composition rates refer to the proportion of the total labor force that is composed of women. Thus, a statistic noting that female labor force composition was 50% would indicate that an equal number of men and women were engaged in paid work.

2. Exceptions to this generalization include South American countries such as Uruguay and Chile.

3. ILO Conventions are available online at http://ilolex.ilo.ch:1567/english/convdisp1.htm

4. Improved standards of living and better access to medical care have reduced mortality, leading to greater longevity throughout the world. In developed nations, the chronological age of 65, roughly equivalent to retirement age, has been used to define individuals as older. In the developing world, however, age classification varies among countries, rendering a parallel chronological definition more limited in applicability (WHO, 2002). Poverty, malnutrition, poorer health care, and greater health risks are only some of the factors that result in a lower life expectancy. In addition to chronological age, an appropriate definition of older age in the developing world should incorporate changes in social roles and changes in functional capabilities (such as changes in physical and mental health). While there is no standard criterion, in this chapter we follow the UN practice of using the age of 60 or older to refer to the older population.

5. In this chapter, we report qualitative findings from the United States, Mexico, Botswana, Vietnam, and Honduras. Findings from Russia are currently being analyzed. For Mexico, Botswana, and Vietnam we report summary statistics to describe the experiences of the representative sample of respondents. Since the United States studies were conducted using different surveys, we report U.S. statistics when they are available in a form parallel to findings from Mexico, Botswana, and Vietnam. No summary statistics are reported for Honduras due to the small sample size and different methodology.

6. All names have been changed to protect respondents' confidentiality. While we recognize cultural difference in the practice of referring to individuals by name, for consistency we introduce each person by full name and then use the first name only in subsequent references to that person.

7. As described earlier, a semistructured, open-ended interview instrument was used. With this method, respondents are encouraged to describe their experiences in narrative fashion, and follow-up questions are asked. In some cases, time constraints prevent every topic in the instrument from being discussed. The percentages reported throughout this chapter refer to those interviews addressing the specified topic except where otherwise noted. (In the few cases where topics were discussed with less than two-thirds of respondents, this is noted.)

8. The reported figures provide conservative estimates. In Mexico, of families leaving children home alone, 28% reported that their children experienced accidents or other emergencies while the respondents were at work. Twenty-three percent reported that their children

did not experience injuries when home alone, and half did not address the issue directly. In Botswana, of the 64% who discussed the issue of accidents with us, 51% reported that their children experienced accidents while the respondents were at work. In Vietnam, of the 76% who discussed the issue, 38% reported that their children experienced emergencies while the respondents were at work.

9. The figures reported provide conservative estimates. In Mexico, of the 42% of respondents who discussed the issue, 28% reported that caregiving responsibilities for adult relatives or friends had led to difficulties at work. Of the 39% of respondents who discussed the issue, 26% had lost pay for similar caregiving activities. Half of the respondents discussed job retention and promotion, and of those, 12% reported having difficulties due to caring for an adult.

10. United Nations declarations and conventions are available online at http://www.unhchr.ch/html/intlist.htm ; ILO conventions are available online at http://ilolex.ilo.ch:1567/english/convdisp1.htm

11. The full text is available online at http://www.unhchr.ch/html/menu3/b/a_cescr.htm

12. The full text is available online at http://www.un.org/womenwatch/daw/cedaw/

13. The full text is available online at http://www/un.org/Overview/rights.html

14. In Botswana, 24% of all informal sector workers received paid leave, 43% did not receive paid leave, and the remaining third did not address the question. Sufficient data was not available on this question from the Vietnam sample to establish paid leave rates.

15. The full text is available online at http://www.unicef.org/crc/crc.htm

16. The Work, Family, and Democracy Index Initiative is a project systematically defining and measuring the extent to which national public policies throughout the world meet the needs of working families.

17. The full text is available online at http://www.globalaging.org/resources/infopackets/hr-afe2.htm

18. The full text is available online at http://www/un.org/esa/socdev/iyop/iyoppop.htm

References

Aja, E. 2001. Urbanization imperatives in Africa: Nigerian experience. *Philosophy and Social Action* 27(1): 13–22.

Anderson, B. J., J. P. Miller, W. F. Auslander, and J. V. Santiago. 1981. Family characteristics of diabetic adolescents: Relationship to metabolic control. *Diabetes Care* 4(6): 586–94.

Andrews, S., J. Blumenthal, D. Johnson, A. Kahn, C. Ferguson, T. Lasater, P. Malone, and D. Wallace. 1982. The skills of mothering: A study of parent–child development centers. *Monographs of the Society for Research in Child Development,* serial no. 198, 47(6).

Aniansson, G., B. Alm, B. Andersson, A. Hakansson, P. Larsson, O. Nylen, H. Peterson, P. Rigner, M. Svanborg, and H. Sabharwal. 1994. A prospective cohort study on breast-feeding and otitis media in Swedish infants. *Pediatric Infectious Disease Journal* 13(3): 183–88.

Arnold, C., S. Makintube, and G. Istre. 1993. Daycare attendance and other risk factors for invasive *Haemophilus influenzae* type B disease. *American Journal of Epidemiology* 138(5): 333–40.

Arnsberger, P., P. Fox, X. Zhang, and S. Gui. 2000. Population aging and the need for long term care: A comparison of the United States and the People's Republic of China. *Journal of Cross-Cultural Gerontology* 15(3): 207–27.

Aytac, I. A. 1998. Intergenerational living arrangements in Turkey. *Journal of Cross-Cultural Gerontology* 13: 241–64.

Banoob, S. N. 1992. Training needs and services for elderly care in developing countries: Models from Romania, Barbados and Kuwait. *International Journal of Aging and Human Development* 34(2): 125–34.

Barnett, W. 1995. Long-term effects of early childhood programs on cognitive and school outcomes. *The Future of Children* 5(3): 25–50.

Barnett, W. 1996. *Lives in the balance: Age 27 benefit-cost analysis of the High/Scope Perry Preschool Program.* Ypsilanti, MI: High/Scope Press.

Bolak, H. C. 1997. Marital power dynamics: Women providers and working-class households in Istanbul. In *Cities in the developing world: Issues, theory, and policy,* edited by J. Gugler. New York: Oxford University Press.

Bowlby, J. 1953. *Child care and the growth of love.* Baltimore, MD: Penguin Books.

Brockerhoff, M. P. 2000. An urbanizing world. *Population Bulletin* 55(3): 3–44.

Campbell, F., and C. Ramey. 1994. Effects of early intervention on intellectual and academic achievement: A follow-up study of children from low-income families. *Child Development* 65: 684–98.

Carlton-Ford, S., R. Miller, M. Brown, N. Nealeigh, and P. Jennings. 1995. Epilepsy and children's social and psychological adjustment. *Journal of Health and Social Behavior* 36(3): 285–301.

Centers for Disease Control and Prevention (CDC). 2001. *National Immunization Program. Estimated vaccination coverage with individual vaccines and selected vaccination series among children 19–35 months of age by state.* Atlanta, GA: CDC.

Central Statistics Unit. 1998. *1995/96 labour force survey.* Gaborone, Botswana: Labor Statistics Unit, Republic of Botswana.

Centre for Research on the Epidemiology of Disasters (CRED). 2002. *Natural disaster profiles: Honduras.* Brussels: Université Catholique de Louvain.

Cerqueriro, M., P. Murtagh, A. Halac, M. Avila, and M. Weissenbacher. 1990. Epidemiologic risk factors for children with acute lower respiratory tract infection in Buenos Aires, Argentina: A matched case-control study. *Reviews of Infectious Diseases* suppl. 8, 12: S1021–28.

Chattopadhyay, A., and R. Marsh. 1999. Changes in living arrangement and familial support for the elderly in Taiwan: 1963–1991. *Journal of Comparative Family Studies* 30(3): 523–37.

Chen, P. C. 1987. Psychosocial factors and the health of the elderly Malaysian. *Annals of the Academy of Medicine, Singapore* 16(1): 110–14.

Chow, N. W. S. 1999. Aging in China. *Journal of Sociology and Social Welfare* 26(1): 25–49.

Clausen, F., E. Sandberg, B. Ingstad, and P. Hjortdahl. 2000. Morbidity and health care utilisation among elderly people in Mmankgodi village, Botswana. *Journal of Epidemiology and Community Health* 54(1): 58–63.

Cleary, J., O. P. Gray, D. J. Hall, P. H. Rowlandson, C. P. Sainsbury, and M. M. Davies. 1986. Parental involvement in the lives of children in hospitals. *Archives of Disease in Childhood* 61(8): 779–87.

Coreil, J., A. Augustin, N. A. Halsey, and E. Holt. 1994. Social and psychological costs of preventive child health services in Haiti. *Social Science and Medicine* 38(2): 231–38.

Cornman, J. C. 1996. Toward sustainable development: Implications for population aging and the wellbeing of elderly women in developing countries. *Population and Environment* 18(2): 201–17.

Cunningham, A. S., D. B. Jelliffee, and E. F. P. Jelliffee. 1991. Breast-feeding and health in the 1980s: A global epidemiologic review. *Journal of Pediatrics* 118(5): 659–66.

Currie, J., and T. Duncan. 1995. Does Head Start make a difference? *American Economic Review* 85(3): 341–64.

Davis, A. J., I. Martinson, L. C. Gan, Q. Jin, Y. H Liang, D. B. Davis, and J. Y. Lin. 1995. Home care for the urban chronically ill elderly in the People's Republic of China. *International Journal of Aging and Human Development* 41(4): 345–58.

Defo, B. K. 1994. Determinants of infant and early-childhood mortality in Cameroon—the role of socioeconomic factors, housing characteristics, and immunization status. *Social Biology* 41(3–4): 181–211.

Devin, R., and P. Erickson. 1996. The influence of male caregivers on child health in rural Haiti. *Social Science and Medicine* 43(4): 479–88.

Dewey, K., M. Heinig, and L. Nommsen-Rivers. 1995. Differences in morbidity between breastfed and formula-fed infants. Part 1. *Journal of Pediatrics* 126(5): 696–702.

Doress-Worters, P. B. 1994. Adding elder care to women's multiple roles: A critical review of the caregiver stress and multiple roles literatures. *Sex Roles* 31(9–10): 597–616.

Draper, P., and J. Keith. 1992. Cultural contexts of care—family caregiving for elderly in America and Africa. *Journal of Aging Studies* 6(2): 113–34.

Duncan, B., J. Ey, C. Holberg, A. Wright, F. Martinez, and L. Taussig. 1993. Exclusive breast-feeding for at least 4 months protects against otitis media. *Pediatrics* 91(5): 867–72.

Feachem, R. G., and M. A. Koblinsky. 1984. Interventions for the control of diarrhoeal diseases among young children: Promotion of breast-feeding. *Bulletin of the World Health Organization* 62(2): 271–91.

Fielding, J. E., W. G. Cumberland, and L. Pettitt. 1994. Immunization status of children of employees in a large corporation. *Journal of the American Medical Association* 271(7): 525–30.

Fikree, F. F., and R. H. Gray. 1996. Demographic survey of the level and determinants of perinatal mortality in Karachi, Pakistan. *Paediatric and Perinatal Epidemiology* 10(1): 86–96.

Garber, H. 1988. *The Milwaukee Project: Prevention of mental retardation in children at risk.* Washington, D.C.: American Association on Mental Retardation.

Gauderer, M. W., J. L. Lorig, and D. W. Eastwood. 1989. Is there a place for parents in the operating room? *Journal of Pediatric Surgery* 24(7): 705–6.

General Statistics Office of Vietnam. 1994. *Vietnam living standards survey, 1992–1993.* Hanoi.

George, A., and J. Hancock. 1993. Reducing pediatric burn pain with parent participation. *Journal of Burn Care and Rehabilitation* 14(1): 104–7.

Habicht, J. P., J. DaVanzo, and W. P. Butz. 1986. Does breastfeeding really save lives, or are apparent benefits due to biases? *American Journal of Epidemiology* 123(2): 279–90.

Hamlett, K. W., D. S. Pellegrini, and K S. Katz. 1992. Childhood chronic illness as a family stressor. *Journal of Pediatric Psychology* 17(1): 33–47.

Hannallah, R. S., and J. K. Rosales. 1983. Experience with parents' presence during anaesthesia induction in children. Part 1. *Canadian Anaesthetists Society Journal* 30(3): 286–89.

Hanson, C. L., M. J. DeGuire, A. M. Schinkel, S. W. Henggeler, and G. A. Burghen. 1992. Comparing social learning and family systems correlates of adaptation in youths with IDDM. *Journal of Pediatric Psychology* 17(5): 555–72.

Hashizume, Y. 2000. Gender issues and Japanese family-centered caregiving for frail elderly parents or parents-in-law in modern Japan: From the sociocultural and historical perspectives. *Public Health Nursing* 17(1): 25–31.

Heymann, S. J. 2000a. *The widening gap: Why America's working families are in jeopardy—and what can be done about it.* New York: Basic Books.

Heymann, S. J. 2000b. What happens during and after school: Conditions faced by working parents living in poverty and their school-age children. *Journal of Children and Poverty* 6(1): 5–20.

Heymann, S. J. 2002. Low-income parents and the time famine. In *Taking parenting public: The case for a new social movement,* edited by S. A. Hewlett, N. Rankin and C. West. Lanham, MD: Rowman & Littlefield.

Heymann, J., and A. Earle. 1996. Parental availability for the care of sick children. *Pediatrics* 98(2): 226–30.

Heymann, J., and A. Earle. 1998. The work–family balance: What hurdles are parents leaving welfare likely to confront? *Journal of Policy Analysis and Management* 17(2): 312–21.

Heymann, J., and A. Earle. 1999. The impact of welfare reform on parents' ability to care for their children's health. *American Journal of Public Health.* 89(4): 502–5.

Heymann, J., and A. Earle. 2000. Low-income parents: How do working conditions affect their opportunity to help school-age children at risk? *American Educational Research Journal* 37(4): 833–48.

Heymann, J., and A. Earle. 2001. The impact of parental working conditions on school-age children: The case of evening work. *Community, Work and Family* 4(3): 305–25.

Heymann, J., A. Earle, and B. Egleston. 1996. Parental availability for the care of sick children. *Pediatrics* 98(2): 226–30.

Heymann, J., S. Toomey, and F. Furstenberg. 1999. Working parents: What factors are involved in their ability to take time off from work when their children are sick? *Archives of Pediatrics and Adolescent Medicine* 153: 870–74.

Hobcraft, J. N., J. McDonald, and S. Rutstein. 1985. Demographic determinants of infant and early child mortality: A comparative analysis. *Population Studies* 39(21): 363–85.

Holmes-Eber, P. 1997. Migration, urbanization, and women's kin networks in Tunis. *Journal of Comparative Family Studies* 28(2): 54–72

Howie, P., J. Forsyth, S. Ogston, A. Clark, and C. Florey. 1990. Protective effect of breast feeding against infection. *British Medical Journal* 300(6716): 11–16.

Ikels, C. 1991. Aging and disability in China: Cultural issues in measurement and interpretation. *Social Science and Medicine* 32(6): 649–65.

Ineichen, B. 1998. Influences on the care of demented elderly people in the People's Republic of China. *International Journal of Geriatric Psychiatry* 13(2): 122–26.

Instituto Nacional de Estadistica Geografiae Informatica (INEGI). 1999. *Anuario estadistico del distrito federal: Edicion 1999.* Aguascalientes, Mexico: INEGI.

Instituto Nacional de Estadistica Geografiae Informatica (INEGI). 2000. *Indicadores sociodemograficos: 1930–1998.* Aguascalientes, Mexico: Instituto Nacional de Estadistica, Geografia y Informatica.

Instituto de Salud en el Estado de Chiapas. 1999. *Diagnostico de Salud: San Cristobal de las Casas.* Jurisdiccion Sanitaria no. 11. San Cristobal de las Casas, Mexico.

Iroegbu, C. U., H. N. Ene-Obong, A. C. Uwaegbute, and U. V. Amazigo. 2000. Bacteriological quality of weaning food and drinking water given to children of market women in Nigeria: Implications for control of diarrhoea. *Journal of Health Population and Nutrition* 18(3): 157–62.

Jamuna, D. 1997. Stress dimensions among caregivers of the elderly. *Indian Journal of Medical Research* 106: 381–88.

Jason, J., P. Nieburg, and J. S. Marks. 1984. Mortality and infectious disease associated with infant-feeding practice in developing countries. Part 2. *Pediatrics* 74(4): 702–27.

Johnson, D., and T. Walker. 1991. A follow-up evaluation of the Houston Parent Child Development Center: School performance. *Journal of Early Intervention* 15(3): 226–36.

Kim, I. K. 1999. Population aging in Korea: Social problems and solutions. *Journal of Sociology and Social Welfare* 26(1): 107–23.

King, E. M., and M. A. Hill, eds. 1993. *Women's education in developing countries: Barriers, benefits, and policies.* Baltimore, MD and London: Published for the World Bank by the Johns Hopkins University Press.

Kristensson-Hallstron, I., G. Elander, and G. Malmfors. 1997. Increased parental participation in a pediatric surgical day-care unit. *Journal of Clinical Nursing* 6(4): 297–302.

Kumar, V. 1997. Ageing in India—an overview. *Indian Journal of Medical Research* 106: 257–64.

La Greca, A., W. Auslander, P. Greco, D. Spetter, E. J. Fisher, and J. Santiago. 1995. I get by with a little help from my family and friends: Adolescents' support for diabetes care. *Journal of Pediatric Psychology* 20(4): 449–76.

Lannon, C., V. Brack, J. Stuart, M. Caplow, A. McNeill, W. C. Bordley, and P. Margolis. 1995. What mothers say about why poor children fall behind on immunizations—a summary of focus groups in North Carolina. *Archives of Pediatrics and Adolescent Medicine* 149(10): 1070–75.

LaRosa-Nash, P. A., and J. M. Murphy. 1997. An approach to pediatric perioperative care: Parent-present induction. *Nursing Clinics of North America* 32(1): 183–99.

Lepage, P., C. Munyakazi, and P. Hennart. 1982. Breastfeeding and hospital mortality in children in Rwanda. *Lancet* 1(8268): 403.

Lijestrand, J., and S. Bergstrom. 1984. Characteristics of pregnant women in Mozambique—parity, child survival and socioeconomic status. *Upsala Journal of Medical Sciences* 89(2): 117–28.

Long, S. O., and P. B. Harris. 2000. Gender and elder care: Social change and the role of the caregiver in Japan. *Social Science Japan Journal* 3(1): 21–36.

Mahaffy, P. R. 1965. The effects of hospitalization on children admitted for tonsillectomy and adenoidectomy. *Nursing Research* 14(winter): 12–19.

McCormick, L. K., L. K. Bartholomew, M. J. Lewis, M. W. Brown, and I. C. Hanson. 1997. Parental perceptions of barriers to childhood immunization: Results of focus groups conducted in an urban population. *Health Education Research* 12(3): 355–62.

McGraw, T. 1994. Preparing children for the operating room: Psychological issues. *Canadian Journal of Anaesthesia* 41(11): 1094–103.

McKay, R., L. Condell, and H. Ganson. 1985. *The impact of Head Start on children, families and communities: Final report of the Head Start evaluation, synthesis, and utilization project.* Washington, D.C.: CSR, Inc.

McNeill, J. R. 2000. *Something new under the sun: An environmental history of the twentieth-century world.* New York: Norton.

Medjuck, S., J. M. Keefe, and P. J. Fancey. 1998. Available but not accessible: An examination of the use of workplace policies for caregivers of elderly kin. *Journal of Family Issues* 19(3): 274–99.

Mufti, M. H. 1998. Status of long term care in Saudi Arabia. *Saudi Medical Journal* 19(4): 367–69.

Niraula, B. B. 1995. Old-age security and inheritance in Nepal—motives versus means. *Journal of Biosocial Science* 27(1): 71–78.

Palmer, S. J. 1993. Care of sick children by parents: A meaningful role. *Journal of Advanced Nursing* 18(2): 185–91.

Phillips, D., and G. Adams. 2001. Child care and our youngest children. *The Future of Children* 11(1): 35–51.

Programa de las Naciones Unidas para el Desarrollo (PNUD). 1999. Informe Sobre Desarrollo Humano Honduras. *El impacto humano de un huracan.* Tegucigalpa, Honduras: PNUD.

Rawlins, J. M. 1999. Confronting ageing as a Caribbean reality. *Journal of Sociology and Social Welfare* 26(1): 143–53.

Rawlins, J. M. 2001. Caring for the chronically ill elderly in Trinidad: The informal situation. *West Indian Medical Journal* 50(2): 133–36.

Restrepo, H. E., and M. Rozental. 1994. The social impact of aging populations: Some major issues. *Social Science and Medicine* 39(9): 1323–38.

Robertson, J. 1958. *Young children in hospitals.* New York: Basic Books.

Sainsbury, C. P., O. P. Gray, J. Cleary, M. M. Davies, and P. H. Rowlandson. 1986. Care by parents of their children in hospitals. *Archives of Disease in Childhood* 61(6): 612–15.

Salaff, J. W., and A. K. Wong. 1981. *Women, work and the family under conditions of rapid industrialization: Singapore Chinese women.* Toronto: American Sociological Association.

Serow, W. J., and M. E. Cowart. 1998. Demographic transition and population aging with Caribbean nation states. *Journal of Cross-Cultural Gerontology* 13: 201–13.

Sethuraman, V. S. 1998. *Gender, informality and poverty: A global review.* Washington, D.C.: World Bank.

Shyu, Y. I. L., H. C. Lee, and M. L. Chen. 1999. Development and testing of the Family Caregiving Consequences Inventory for home nursing assessment in Taiwan. *Journal of Advanced Nursing* 30(3): 646–54.

Tawiah, E. O. 1989. Child mortality differentials in Ghana: A preliminary report. *Journal of Biosocial Science* 21(3): 349–55.

Taylor, M. R., and P. O'Connor. 1989. Resident parents and shorter hospital stay. *Archives of Disease in Childhood* 64(2): 274–76.

United Nations Children's Fund (UNICEF). 2001. *The state of the world's children, 2001.* New York: UNICEF.

United Nations Development Program (UNDP). 2000. *Human development report.* New York: Oxford University Press.

United Nations Population Division (UNPD). 1999. *World urbanization prospects: The 1999 revision.* New York: Department of Economic and Social Affairs, UN.

United Nations Population Division (UNPD). 2001. *World population prospects: The 2000 revision highlights.* New York: Department of Economic and Social Affairs, UN.

United Nations Programme on HIV/AIDS (UNAIDS). 2002. *The report on the global HIV/AIDS epidemic.* Barcelona: XIV International Conference on AIDS.

van der Schyff, G. 1979. The role of parents during their child's hospitalization. *Australian Nurses Journal* 8(11): 57–61.

Watkins, C. J., S. R. Leeder, and R. T. Corkhill. 1979. The relationship between breast and bottle feeding and respiratory illness in the first year of life. *Journal of Epidemiology and Community Health* 33(3): 180–82.

Waugh, T., and D. Kjos. 1992. Parental involvement and the effectiveness of an adolescent day treatment program. *Journal of Youth and Adolescence* 21: 487–97.

Wazir, R., ed. 2000. *The gender gap in basic education: NGOs as change agents.* New Delhi: Sage.

Wolman, C., M. Resnick, L. Harris, and R. Blum. 1994. Emotional well-being among adolescents with and without chronic conditions. *Adolescent Medicine* 15: 199–204.

World Bank. 2000. *World development report.* New York: World Bank.

World Bank, Asian Development Bank, and United Nations Development Program (UNDP). 2000. *Vietnam 2010: Entering the twenty-first century.* Hanoi: World Bank, Asian Development Bank, and UNDP.

World Bank Group. 2002. *World development indicators, 2002.* Washington, D.C.: World Bank.

World Bank Population and Human Resources Division. 1996. *Guinea: Beyond poverty: How supply factors influence girls' education in Guinea.* Western Africa Department, Africa Region. Washington, D.C.: World Bank.

World Health Organization (WHO). 1999. *World health report 1999: Making a difference.* Geneva: WHO.

World Health Organization (WHO). 2000. *WHO vaccine preventable diseases: Monitoring system.* Geneva: Department of Vaccines and Biologicals, WHO.

World Health Organization (WHO). 2002. *Information needs for research, policy, and action on ageing and older persons: Definition of an older or elderly person.* Geneva: WHO.

Wright, A., C. Holberg, F. Martinez, W. Morgan, and L. Taussig. 1989. Breast feeding and lower respiratory tract illness in the first year of life. *British Medical Journal* 299(6705): 946–49.

5

Maternal Labor, Breast-Feeding, and Infant Health

SUSANHA YIMYAM AND MARTHA MORROW

Reconciling the conflicting rights and demands of women's productive and reproductive roles poses an increasing challenge to health policy formulation. Conflicts between these roles are intensified by rapid development and social change. International conventions concur that women have a right to offer optimum nutrition to their babies through breast-feeding and that babies have a right to be breast-fed. Simultaneously, women are entitled to seek gainful employment. For many, furthermore, employment is essential to the economic survival of their families. It is essential that a false dichotomy not be permitted to arise between these various rights.

Breast-Feeding's Benefits for Both Mothers and Infants

Breast-Feeding as the Best Alternative for Infants' Health

Breast-feeding has long been recognized as superior to artificial feeding in a variety of ways. The evidence of the nutritional, immunological, behavioral, economic, and environmental benefits of breast-feeding for both developed and developing countries is overwhelming and indisputable (American Academy of Pediatrics, 1997; Cunningham, Jelliffe, and Jelliffe, 1991; Enger, Ross, and Bernstein, 1997; Mitra and Rabbani, 1995; Newcomb et al., 1994; Newman, 1995; Palmer and Kemp, 1996; Riordan and Auerbach, 1993; Short, 1993; Smyke, 1993; Sterken, 1998; WABA, 1998; WHO, 2001a; Yoon et al., 1996). Many studies have emphasized the particular benefits for infant health and child survival in developing countries (Cunningham, 1995; Jelliffe and Jelliffe, 1989; Palmer and Kemp, 1996; Villalpando and Lopez-Alarcon, 2000; WHO, 1998, 2001b; Wilmoth and Elder, 1995). The United Nations Children's Fund (UNICEF) noted that if all infants were exclusively breast-fed, about 1.5 million lives would be saved annually (UNICEF, 1999). Breast milk is uniquely suited to the human infant's digestive system because it is perfectly balanced with protein, fat, minerals, and vitamins. Its composition changes throughout the day and over the months (Lawrence, 1995; Reeder, Martin, and Koniak-Griffin, 1997; Woolridge, 1995), providing optimal nutrition to promote growth and development (Palmer and Kemp, 1996; Reeder, Martin, and Koniak-Griffin, 1997; Sweet and Tiran, 1997; WHO, 1994; Woolridge, 1995), even permitting catch up growth for infants reared in unfavorable circumstances (Villalpando and Lopez-Alarcon, 2000). Apart from being highly nutritious, breast milk contains important immunological factors that provide protection against infections of the gastrointestinal tract and respiratory system (Borgnolo et al., 1996; Cunningham, 1995; Palmer and Kemp, 1996; Reeder, Martin, and Koniak-Griffin, 1997; WHO, 2001a), otitis media (Cunningham, 1995; Walker et al., 1994; WHO, 2001a), obesity, certain metabolic and other diseases (Cunningham, 1995; Mitra and Rabbani, 1995; Wang and Wu, 1996), and hypertension later in life (Singhal, Cole, and Lucas, 2001). Breast-feeding also seems to decrease children's chances of developing allergies (Halken et al., 1995; Palmer and Kemp, 1996; Shaheen et al., 1996), cancer (Davis, 1998; Shu et al., 1995), and other problems such as atopic disease in later life (Saarinen and Kajosaari, 1995; WHO, 2001a).

Breast-feeding may enhance psychomotor development (Koopman-Esseboom et al., 1996), promote brain growth and intellectual development (Reeder, Martin, and Koniak-Griffin, 1997), heal the effects of trauma at birth, and enhance interpersonal relationships and the child's sleeping patterns (McKenna and Bernshaw, 1995; Wang and Wu, 1996). Many researchers have argued that breast-feeding offers psychological benefits because it facilitates bonding between mother and child (Dettwyler, 1995; Reeder, Martin, and Koniak-Griffin, 1997; WHO, 1993). Exclusive or almost exclusive breast-feeding helps to space births, with health benefits to both mother and child (Ellison, 1995; Reeder, Martin, and Koniak-Griffin, 1997; Palmer and Kemp, 1996; WHO, 2001a, 2001b).

Breast-feeding is economical at personal, family, and national levels. For one child, the costs for bottles, breast milk substitutes, and preparation and storage of those substitutes total at least several hundred dollars per year (Palmer and Kemp, 1996; WABA, 2000a; WHO, 1998; Wilmoth and Elder, 1995). For the family, Meershoek (1993) has suggested that breast-feeding costs include the mother's increased food intake, time devoted to feeding, and possible lost employment opportunities. Bottle feeding requires time and fuel (such as electricity) to prepare the formula, and in poor countries, the high relative cost of formula may lead to reduced expenditures on food for other family members (Riordan and Auerbach, 1993). Breast-feeding is one of the most cost-effective child survival interventions because morbidity is lower in breast-fed children and, consequently, money is saved for health services and home care (Meershoek, 1993; Palmer and Kemp, 1996; Riordan and Auerbach, 1993). At the national level, breast-feeding has substantial cost benefits (Coates, 1993; Palmer and Kemp, 1996; WHO, 1998; Wilmoth and Elder, 1995). Breast-feeding is environmentally friendly, whereas packaging, bottles, teats, and fuel for sterilization all create pollution and waste (Palmer and Kemp, 1996).

Breast-feeding and Women's Health

Breast-feeding offers an array of benefits for mothers. Oxytocin, a hormone released during breast-feeding, stimulates contractions that return the uterus to its normal size, thus decreasing the likelihood of postpartum hemorrhage (Dettwyler, 1995; WHO, 1993). Breast-feeding helps mothers return to their normal weight faster (Sweet and Tiran, 1997; WHO, 1998) and reduces fertility (Sweet and Tiran, 1997; WHO, 2001a). If menstruation has not resumed, women who exclusively breast-feed on demand have 98% pregnancy protection in the first 6 months postpartum. Inhibiting the return of menstruation allows women to build up stores of iron and alleviate anemia (WHO, 1994). Women who have breast-fed seem to be less likely to develop not only cancer of the breast, ovaries, or cervix but also osteoporosis (Enger et al., 1998; Michels et al., 1996; Newcomb et al., 1994; Riordan and Auerbach, 1993; Rosenblatt and Thomas, 1995; WHO, 1993). Lower rates of illness in breast-fed babies mean that mothers are less likely to carry the burden on their own health of looking after a sick child (UNICEF, 1999).

In psychological terms, breast-feeding brings many mothers a sense of achievement in providing sustenance they alone can offer (Dermer, 1998; Dettwyler, 1995; Laufer, 1990). It also enables the mother and infant to have close physical contact, even as hormonal messages are transferred between them (Dettwyler, 1995). Breast-feeding makes it easier for a mother to provide security, warmth, and comfort to her child (Dettwyler, 1995).

Global Breast-Feeding Prevalence and Trends

The twentieth century saw large variations and swings in breast-feeding practices across time and geographical region. Breast-feeding rates plummeted in Western countries between the 1940s and early 1970s. This dramatic fall was succeeded by a sharp increase in prevalence for about a decade, followed by plateaus or declines in some countries, such as the United States, in the second half of the 1980s (Losch et al., 1995). By contrast, exclusive breast-feeding in Poland rate rose from 1.5% in 1988 to 17% in 1995, and, in Armenia, exclusive breast-feeding of infants under four months of age rose from 0.7% in 1993 to 20.8% in 1997 (WHO, 2002). In the developing world, rates of initiation and duration have periodically risen and fallen over the past several decades, with large variations within and between countries and regions. Generally speaking, breast-feeding duration has fallen as urbanization has increased, and optimal breast-feeding practices are rare (UNICEF, 2002; WHO, 1993).

The World Health Organization (WHO) maintains a global database on breast-feeding initiation and duration and the prevalence of exclusive breast-feeding (WHO, 1996). Based on these data and on partial updates (WHO, 1998), a picture has emerged of practices in the past two decades. Initiation rates ranged from 63% to 89% in the

Western Pacific region and from 73% to 94% in the Southeast Asia region, which together cover Asia and the Pacific. Relatively higher rates were found in Latin America and the Caribbean (77% to 94%) and Africa (92% to 99%). In all regions, rural women were more likely than urban women to initiate breast-feeding. The median duration was longest in Southeast Asia (25 months) and Africa (21 months), shorter in the Western Pacific region (14 months), and shortest in the Americas (10 months). The percentage of infants exclusively breast-fed for the first 4 months of age ranged from 49% in Southeast Asia to just 16% in Europe, with the Western Pacific region, at 33%, close to the world average of 35%. In May 2001, an expert review panel reported to the fifty-fourth World Health Assembly its conclusion that 6 months is the optimal duration of breast-feeding, overturning the more flexible previous recommendation of 4 to 6 months (WHO, 2001a).

Surveys have shown consistently that breast-feeding prevalence and duration are higher among educated, more affluent mothers in industrialized countries but higher among rural, poorer, and less educated women in developing countries (Donath and Amir, 2000; Kocturk and Zetterstrom, 1989; WHO, 1993; Wilmoth and Elder, 1995). Rural occupations are usually more compatible with child care, including breast-feeding (Wongboonsin and Ruffolo, 1993). Wilmoth and Elder (1995) suggested that the urban reduction in breast-feeding has stemmed from media portrayals of bottle feeding as modern and convenient, as well as from declines in the number of extended family households that can care for the growing number of women in paid employment. For instance, Melville (1990) described earlier weaning among urban Jamaican women as related to the lack of family assistance with household tasks that mothers received, making them busier and less likely to suckle frequently. Other variables often associated with infant feeding have been ethnicity, marital status, age, parity, and employment status, but the directions of the associations have been inconsistent within and between countries and regions (Gabriel, Gabriel, and Lawrence, 1986; Hills-Bonczyk et al., 1993; Kocturk and Zetterstrom, 1989; Kurinij et al., 1989; O'Campo et al., 1992; Richardson and Champion, 1992; Scott and Binns, 1999).

Associations between Breast-Feeding and Maternal Employment

Investigations into the relationship between infant feeding and maternal paid work have produced contradictory findings, thus posing challenges for health promotion and policy design. Much of the confusion is an artifact of differences in study objectives; methodology; terminology; normative patterns of infant feeding and female workforce participation; and variations in the level of social, cultural, and governmental support offered to mothers in different populations. Frequently, findings are presented without discussion of their broader context. Confounding may also occur if researchers have not controlled for other factors (such as age, education, or parity) known to influence infant-feeding practices. Where data analysis is not explained precisely, results must be viewed cautiously. Auerbach, Renfrew, and Minchin (1991) presented compelling evidence that conclusions drawn from studies related to infant feeding have been compromised regularly by imprecise, inconsistent terminology; in particular, lines have been blurred between exclusive, predominant, and partial breast-feeding, or data on duration have not been gathered. These limitations may have contributed to the inconsistency in the literature on employment, especially where studies have been treated as equivalent, even though they examined different outcomes (for instance, when and whether formula was introduced or the timing of the mother's return to the workplace).

In their review of 82 studies worldwide, Van Esterik and Greiner (1981) noted that women rarely attributed weaning or formula use to employment; however, as Wright, Clark, and Bauer (1993) pointed out, many studies did not ask explicitly whether working interfered with breast-feeding. Furthermore, these authors commented that the term *work* is conflated with *employment*, although women's productive unpaid work has important economic implications for households and may be compatible with breast-feeding. Conversely, "working outside the home (or other activities that separate mother and infant) can interfere with lactation . . . [because] nursing occurs less frequently, resulting in a lack of stimulation of the nipples and a decline in milk production" (262).

Wright, Clark, and Bauer presented an alternative, more reflective approach to these complexities. Using ethnographic and structured interviews, they found that Navajo Indian women who delayed employment for 3 months breast-fed longer than those who resumed work earlier or those who remained unemployed, even after controlling for socioeconomic variables. The authors' explanation focused on the fact that a very early separation from the infant was more damaging to lactation's physiological demand-supply mechanism, while a "desire for intimacy" might have induced a relatively greater determination to continue breast-feeding among the subgroup returning to work after 3 months.

Scott and Binns (1999) reviewed factors associated with initiation and duration of breast-feeding among Western women, as documented in English-language publications between 1985 and 1997. They suggested that the variance in associations found with employment usually could be attributed to study design. Some researchers had examined the association between specific predelivery variables—such as mothers' intention to resume employment or their infant-feeding intentions—and breast-feeding initiation and duration after childbirth, whereas other researchers had tracked the practices after mothers actually returned to work. Overall, Scott and Binns concluded that intending to return to work was not negatively associated with either intending to breast-feed or actually initiating breast-feeding. However, resumption of employment was related to premature weaning. They cited a large cross-sectional American study that found a higher incidence of breast-feeding among employed than among unemployed women in 1984 compared to 1980, but the proportion of women breast-feeding their infants aged 5 to 6 months was higher among the unemployed. They added that the most recent North American studies using multivariate analysis had found the resumption of employment to be negatively associated with both the initiation and the duration of breast-feeding.

Our review of recent literature indicated that the relationship between employment and breast-feeding is generally negative in both industrialized and developing countries. Gielen and associates (1991), after controlling for demographic characteristics in a heterogeneous urban American sample, interviewed twice in the first 3 months postpartum, concluded that intending to work in the first 6 months did not influence initiation, but being employed was significantly associated with early cessation of breast-feeding. Avery and associates (1998), in a prospective study among American primiparas, used multivariate analysis to determine that planning to work outside the home was one predictive variable (among others) for premature weaning. A smaller intervention study found that those who planned to return to work or attend school in the first 3 months postpartum weaned earlier than those who planned to stay at home (Arlotti et al., 1998). Another prospective American investigation (Skinner et al., 1997) found that mothers who gave their infants cereal before 4 months of age were more likely to be employed.

Noble (2001) reported on a longitudinal United Kingdom study of 10,530 mothers of full-term singleton infants. Adjusted logistic regression found no relation between work intentions and breast-feeding intentions, but it showed that planning to return to employment prior to 6 weeks postpartum reduced the likelihood of initiating breast-feeding. An analysis of focus groups among low-income people (of both sexes and different ages) in South Australia (McIntyre, Hiller, and Turnbull 1999) revealed a widespread belief that breast-feeding could not be combined with paid employment.

For Southeast Asia, a secondary data analysis of representative national surveys was undertaken to identify individual and community characteristics influencing the duration of breast-feeding in Vietnam, a country with a very high female workforce participation rate (Swenson, Thang, and Tieu, 1993). Duration was found to be longer among more highly educated women. The authors speculated that these women were more likely to work in settings where it is easier to continue breast-feeding and were more likely to be more affluent, thus facing less pressure to resume paid work. A telephone survey of breast-feeding practices was undertaken in 1996 with 120 Singapore women who attended public talks given by the Breast-Feeding Mothers' Support Group (Fok, 1997). Sixty-two percent breast-fed for a shorter time than planned (67% weaned by 2 months), and the intended resumption of work was the most commonly cited reason. An analysis of questionnaires completed by 235 Hong Kong breast-feeding mothers in the postpartum period in 1995 showed similar findings (Chee and Horstmanshof, 1996). In Malaysia, 500 mothers with healthy singleton infants were interviewed at 6 weeks postpartum (Chye et al., 1997). Twenty-six percent were exclusively formula feeding, and only 25% were exclusively breast-feeding; logistic regression analysis showed that those in the latter group were less likely to be in paid employment postnatally.

Clearly, the maintenance of lactation among employed women is more difficult in some settings than in others. Thus, simply looking at statistical associations and drawing conclusions about the impact of work on breast-feeding may be misleading if the underlying social realities are ignored. In the United States and Australia, maternity leave, nursing breaks, and on-site child care are available only in a few professional workplaces. As Frank (1998) has noted, breast-feeding takes time, and full-time working mothers in countries without these provisions have fewer opportunities to suckle their infants. A study of American women's experiences with combining breast-feeding and employment found that the most successful women were older and more highly educated, and tended to work in professional jobs that offered greater flexibility (Hills-Bonczyk et al., 1993).

A crucial distinction that often remains unclarified (as Wright, Clark, and Bauer, 1993, noted) is the nature of employment—specifically, whether it involves separation from the infant. Home-based work, flexible hours, or the capacity to bring the child to the workplace create a situation starkly different for the feeding dyad than a rigid 8- to 10-hour job undertaken apart from the infant. Winikoff and Castle (1988) discussed the importance of this distinction in their landmark study, utilizing ethnographic methods and cross-sectional household surveys, in four cities in the developing world (Bangkok, Thailand; Bogota, Colombia; Nairobi, Kenya; and Semarang, Indonesia).

> [E]mployment per se does not emerge consistently as a significant independent predictor of breastfeeding duration and use of infant formula. This is not surprising, given the different contexts of female economic activities . . . and the diverse cultural and social norms in the four cities. Thus, the impact . . . must be assessed with reference to other factors that may modify its effects on infant feeding choices. (121)

The authors presented ethnographic data to explain the longer breast-feeding duration among employed Indonesian women than among those in the other locations, citing "the acceptance of female economic activity and socio-cultural supports which enable the continuation of breastfeeding when women leave their homes to work for pay" in Java (134).

This chapter reports on a study delving into the experiences of employed women as mothers in Thailand, which has an estimated population of 62 million. The focus is on the effects of employment on breast-feeding among women from various work sectors and on women's perceptions of themselves as they attempt to balance their roles. The chapter concludes with comments on the implications of the study findings in terms of the current international discourse on health promotion, particularly in the context of basic human rights.

Infant Feeding in Thailand: Breast-Feeding Patterns and Maternity Protection Provisions

While Thailand boasts nearly universal initiation of breast-feeding, national surveys have shown declines in duration, plus extremely low rates of exclusive breast-feeding (virtually unknown by 2 months of age) (Family Health Division, 1994). Theoretically, paid maternity leave of 3 to 4 months would allow mothers to practice exclusive breast-feeding before returning to work (WHO, 1994). However, few Thai women are guaranteed lengthy benefits, and other necessary supports such as breast-feeding breaks are not mandated by law.

Changes were made to maternal leave legislation in Thailand in 1993. Prior to May of that year, government and state enterprise employees were authorized 60 days of fully paid leave, with the option of a further 30 days of personal leave if approved by the employers. For the private sector, "permanent" employees (defined as those who have worked at least 180 days) were entitled to 30 days with pay and another 60 without pay. The Labour Protection Law of May 1993 gives public sector employees 90 days with full pay and an additional 180 days of unpaid personal leave for "child rearing." Private sector permanent employees are authorized 90 days with pay, 45 days covered by employers and 45 claimed from the national social security fund to which the employees have also contributed. The component covered by social security has been available only since March 30, 1995 (Pruekpongsawalee, 1995).

Studies that looked at utilization of maternal leave and correlations with infant feeding in Thailand, particularly in urban areas, were undertaken prior to the enactment of these laws. Boonwanich (1993), examining breast-feeding patterns among 790 public employees in Bangkok, found that about half of the babies were weaned by the time of women's completed maternity leave. In their 1991 investigation in Bangkok, Richter and colleagues (1992) found that most private sector employees took 30 days or less, while most government workers took 31 to 45 days. About one-quarter of manufacturing employees stopped working for at least 2 months, probably (they speculated) because many were dismissed—in contravention of labor laws—when their pregnancies became known. Most informal sector employees are hired on 3- and 6-month contracts or on a daily basis, and thus are ineligible for leave because they are not "permanent" employees, and provisions do not apply to the informal sector. The study found that 45% of those in the informal sector who worked outside the home ceased work for 16 to 30 days. Those working in the home usually took little time off, probably because it was easier for them to combine work and child care.

In a review of others' studies, Richter and colleagues (1992) found that formal child care (as with creches) in Bangkok, especially in the workplace, was extremely rare: only 1 out of 80 factories surveyed had a child-care facility for its workers. Most mothers, when asked, said they preferred to care for their young children themselves, with relatives, particularly grandmothers, being the second choice. However, demographic shifts toward more nuclear families, housing shortages, and rural–urban migration meant that many women had to seek other care options when relatives were unavailable. More affluent women could hire a nanny or send their children to the few centers that existed; but poorer women, especially migrants, often were forced to leave their infants in their home villages, with obvious implications for breast-feeding. Richter and colleagues found such village-based care for a large percentage of infants of manufacturing employees and informal sector workers employed outside the home. Children of home-based informal sector employees generally were cared for by their mothers. Factory workers living apart from their infants voiced enthusiasm at the notion of on-site child care.

Richter and associates (1992) found that infant feeding in Bangkok was closely related to type of employment. Breast-feeding rates among women who worked at home for pay were about the same as those for unemployed women, replicating Winikoff and Castle's (1988) results from their Bangkok study undertaken around 1980, although their rate at 6 months was lower than that found by the earlier researchers (about 51% versus about 61%). Self-employed and family workers who worked outside the home had the shortest duration of breast-feeding (37% breast-fed for 1 month or less and 22% did not breastfeed at all), perhaps (Richter et al. suggested) because financial pressures impelled them to resume work early. At 2 months postpartum, government employees (who were more likely to take relatively longer leave) had higher breast-feeding rates than private employees (52% versus 42%) (Richter et al., 1992). These studies are useful in delineating the nature and range of practices among Bangkok women, whose differences (work groups, workplace benefits, and living situations) have important implications for their options and behaviors.

The Study of Women in Chiang Mai

Increasing urbanization and female workforce participation around the world create new dynamics for women as mothers. Global economic downturns, as well as structural adjustment programs and reductions in public services, have led to longer working hours for women, both at home and in the workplace, with impacts on health and parenting (Jiggins, 1994:32–4; Lim, 1993). A multidisciplinary investigation in Chiang Mai, Thailand's second largest city (estimated population 1.4 million in 2001), enabled us to explore issues facing employed mothers within a country in transition.

Between 1985 and 1995, Thailand was the world's fastest-growing economy (8.4% real average annual gross domestic product [GDP] growth), followed by three other Asian countries: China, South Korea, and Singapore (Phongpaichit and Baker, 1998). This unexpected boom was fueled primarily by massive new Japanese investment, mainly in export-oriented industries. Phongpaichit and Baker argue that, despite the crash of the economy during the Asian currency crisis (starting in 1996), the boom "changed Thailand forever" (6), among other things turning it into one of the world's most inequitable societies (partly through the lag in creating appropriate legal controls on business and the state). Elsewhere, Phongpaichit and Baker (1997) cite a 1990 survey that found that up to 44% of Thai workers were paid less than the minimum wage. Studies in the 1980s and 1990s found that firms commonly renewed employees' probation or shifted to temporary hiring to evade legal requirements about worker entitlements. Overall, there was a dramatic increase in the number of insecure jobs. In 1987 the garment industry employed about 17,000 employees in factories and 780,000 subcontracted pieceworkers. About two-thirds of workers in large textile, engineering, electrical, and chemical factories were paid on a daily, piecework, or casual basis in 1993 (201).

During the 1970s, 70% to 90% of new jobs on a global level were filled by women aged 14–24 (Bell, 1992). The feminization of labor dramatically changed the lives of women and families in Thailand in the boom period in much the same way as it did in neighboring Asian countries during the previous two decades (Lim, 1993). Bell (1992) asserted that "indeed this [economic] development has been literally built in large measure on the backs of Thai women" (61). The influx into the new manufacturing industries also meant greatly increased migration by young women to urban centers and into jobs "characterised by poor working conditions, exploitation, and low wages" (Whittaker, 2000:37).

Chiang Mai has been one of the epicenters of Thailand's boom. By the late 1980s, the demand for manufacturing land and labor could not be satisfied within metropolitan Bangkok, and investors turned to the relatively populated Chiang Mai valley. Factories were built around the suburbs of the city, and subcontracting in garment production even spread to neighboring villages (Phongpaichit and Baker, 1998). The most recent statistics put female labor force participation rates in Chiang Mai at 64.5% (just above the national average), representing more than 45% of the total workforce aged 15 and over (National Statistics Office, 2000). The study site included the central area and periurban districts within 30 kilometers.

Chiang Mai, in many ways, is a prototype of a rapidly changing urban center. Thailand's boom, its high female employment levels, and its increased urbanization were closely replicated at the same time by its near neighbors, especially Malaysia, Indonesia, China, and the Philippines (World Bank, 1998).

Data Collection

Data gathering was undertaken in two stages between mid-1994 and late 1995. Stage 1 was a pilot study including interviews with key informants, observation of health facilities, review of references to breast-feeding in the media, interpretation of policy documents, and in-depth interviews. Stage 2 consisted of interviews with 313 employed mothers using a semistructured questionnaire.

Behavioral health studies such as this one are typically either prospective or retrospective. The benefits of a prospective design include avoiding long recall periods and having the capacity to detect change over time by making repeated measures. The disadvantages include greater cost, a prolonged data collection phase, and "the risk that behavior and attitudes of respondents will be modified by repeated interviewing" (Campbell et al., 1999, 26), known as the *Hawthorne effect* (Berg, 1998). Retrospective studies, while less useful for following change over time, do not share this risk. We chose a retrospective study. We felt that ethically we could not refuse to give advice (based on professional training) during interviews if it was requested, and that fact could have affected the outcomes. Another important consideration was the nature of the topic, especially our focus on a dynamic decision-making process and experiences over time. We felt these were better explored with methods that allowed for reflection after the event.

To minimize the potential for confounding that could arise if women wrongly recalled their breast-feeding practices, we used multiple methods of data collection (triangulation). Cross-checks of hospital records were available and were undertaken for about 85% of the sample. These covered parity, birth date and weight, type of delivery, type of feeding at discharge, and infant age at complete weaning. We found high congruence (95%) between recall during interviews and the records.

Employed mothers were recruited if they had been in paid employment prior to giving birth, currently had infants aged between 4 months and 3 years, had initiated breast-feeding, and had completely weaned by the time of interviewing. Infants' age range was decided on the basis of Thai urban breast-feeding patterns current at that time, when virtually all women initiated breast-feeding, with a median duration of 8.5 months (Family Health Division, 1994, 33). This span permitted scope for different types of decisions to have been made, and consequences considered, without being too far removed from the events of interest. Total weaning was important because it was only after weaning that we could gauge breast-feeding *duration*, as well as the *impact of employment on infant feeding*, among those wanting to combine these activities. Studies that rely on interviews with women who are currently breast-feeding, cannot establish duration reliably.

We approached women consecutively as they arrived at the University Hospital Growth Monitoring Clinic or the University Child Care Center. Those meeting the criteria were invited to participate, and only one declined.

A quota system was used and updated daily to ensure that our sample reflected the occupational profile of women delivering at the University Hospital (based on the previous year's records). This institution serves about two-thirds of the Chiang Mai population, offers both public (55%) and private (45%) care, and caters to people from all social classes. The 313 women we recruited included those from both the formal sector (white- and blue-collar workers) and the informal sector (such as pieceworkers at home, street or market vendors, and domestic workers in private homes). The sample closely matched the range and proportion of employment types among Thailand's female workforce, as estimated by national and international surveys (National Statistics Office, 2000; World Bank, 1998).

Data Analysis

In this chapter, we have summarized the findings in relation to infant-feeding practices and experiences during the first 6 months postpartum. Because mixed feeding and the giving of complementary foods to even young infants are normative in Thailand (a 1993 national survey estimated that just 1% of Thai infants were exclusively breast-fed at 4 months [Family Health Division 1994]), we categorized practices as (*1*) *no breast-feeding*, (*2*) *breast-feeding with formula*, or (*3*) *breast-feeding without formula*. Our classification system enabled us to gauge practices as *relatively* better or worse in relation to the optimal standard of exclusive breast-feeding and in relation to national norms. Employment was classified into four work groups: (*1*) *public sector*, (*2*) *private sector*, (*3*) *pieceworker at home*, or (*4*) *self- or family-employed*.

Findings and Discussion

Patterns of combining employment and breast-feeding. Most women in our sample faced enormous challenges in attempting to balance their productive and reproductive roles. Sixty-nine percent returned to work within the first 6 months postpartum, and reported that they strongly wished to satisfy the bulk of their infants' nutritional needs with their own milk during and after this critical early period. Of the original 313 respondents, 295 (94%) breast-fed for at least 1 month. Of this subgroup, 203 had resumed paid employment by 6 months postpartum. Of these, 53 (26%) had stopped breast-feeding before or at the time of resuming employment, while 150 (74%) had continued to breast-feed. But within a month after returning to work, another 36 (24%) of the 150 had totally weaned their infants (Fig. 5–1).

Table 5–1 summarizes the demographic and employment characteristics of the women who had breast-fed for at least 1 month postpartum.

The overall mean breast-feeding duration was 8.3 months, which closely matched the mean found in national surveys among urban Thai women in 1993 (Family Health Division, 1994). Those who stopped work for at least 6 months had an average duration of 12.8 months, compared to 6.9 months for those who resumed employment within this period. Figure 5–2 illustrates the negative relationship between outside employment and breast-feeding found in this study.

Difficulties in combining breast-feeding and employment. Most formal sector—especially public sector—workers in our sample were in relatively stable, highly paid, high-status positions with maternity leave rights. However, these benefits came at a cost: inflexible maternity leave regulations that forced employees to return early in order to retain their jobs. Public sector professionals reported that taking off more than their normal leave would have been difficult. One respondent, Umpa,[1] said, "My boss suggested I return to work at two months after delivery because he would promote me to a new position which was better than my old one." Perceived or explicit

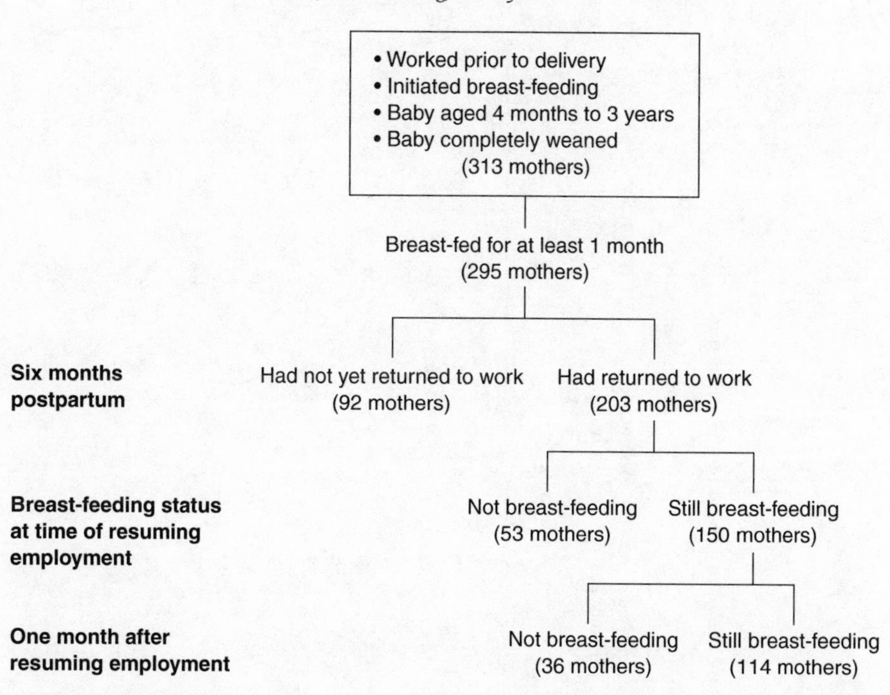

Figure 5–1. Breast-feeding and employment status of the sample in the first 6 months.

pressure related to future prospects and current job security led some women to take even less than their allocated leave, particularly in situations requiring them to seek permission to take more than 2 months off. Some expressed guilt if their absence created extra burdens for colleagues.

Informal sector workers, who had few thoughts of advancement and had no maternity leave, often stopped working and stayed home to care for their babies for a few years, but only if doing so was affordable. The low pay and insecurity of such work meant that many felt compelled by financial need to resume employment earlier than they wished. Some self-employed women returned early if no one could take over their business. Sudthida, who owned a stationery shop, said:

> I had to go back to work only 2 weeks after delivery since no one else could take care of my shop. We need this income to support my family. Also, if I closed the shop longer than 2 weeks it would reduce our customers in the future.

Across the sample, almost all those who resumed employment early attempted to combine it with breast-feeding. Among those who did wean when they went back to work, no significant relationship was found on the basis of infant age, social class, or work group, as noted in Table 5–2. However, these factors were related to whether women used formula when they rejoined the workplace.

Table 5–1. Demographic and Work Characteristics of Employed Women by Work Group

			Formal sector				Informal sector				
	Total (N = 295)		Public employee (n = 67)		Private employee (n = 152)		Pieceworker at home (n = 25)		Self/family employed (n = 51)		
Characteristics	N	%	N	%	n	%	n	%	n	%	χ^2 (p value)
Maternal age (years)											
<30	163	**55**	17	**25**	106	**70**	18	**72**	22	**43**	42.96
≥30	132	**45**	50	**75**	46	**30**	7	**28**	29	**57**	(<0.001)
Maternal education[a]											
Primary	98	**33**	2	**3**	55	**36**	19	**76**	23	**45**	
Secondary	94	**32**	15	**22**	55	**36**	6	**24**	19	**37**	82.99
Tertiary	103	**35**	50	**75**	42	**28**	0	**0**	9	**18**	(<0.001)
Family income (baht)[b]											
<10,000	119	**40**	10	**15**	72	**47**	18	**72**	19	**37**	
10,000–19,999	115	**39**	26	**39**	65	**43**	7	**28**	17	**33**	57.52
≥20,000	61	**21**	31	**46**	15	**10**	0	**0**	15	**30**	(<0.001)
Work location											
Inside the home	50	**17**	0	**0**	0	**0**	25	**100**	25	**49**	204.46
Outside the home	245	**83**	67	**100**	152	**100**	0	**0**	26	**51**	(<0.001)

Nature of job											
Salaried with inflexible hours	220	75	67	100	130	86	0	0	23	45	130.78
Regular office hours	177	60	45	67	109	72	0	0	23	45	(<0.001)
Shift work	43	15	22	33	21	14	0	0	0	0	
Nonsalaried with flexible hours	75	25	0	0	22	14	25	100	28	55	
Piecework	47	16	0	0	14	9	22	88	12	24	
Seasonal work	28	9	0	0	8	5	3	12	16	31	
Right to take maternity leave											
No	150	51	1	2	74	49	25	100	51	100	139.12
Yes	145	49	66	98	78	51	0	0	0	0	(<0.001)
Returned to work within 6 months											
No	92	31	1	2	58	38	15	60	19	37	40.89
Yes	203	69	66	98	94	62	10	40	32	63	(<0.001)

[a]The most recent data on school enrollments for northern Thailand shows a primary:seconday:tertiary ratio of 4:4:3 (combined rural and urban) (National Statistics Office, 2000).

[b]Family income is monthly in the national currency (baht). Average monthly income at the time of the study was approximately 10,000 baht.

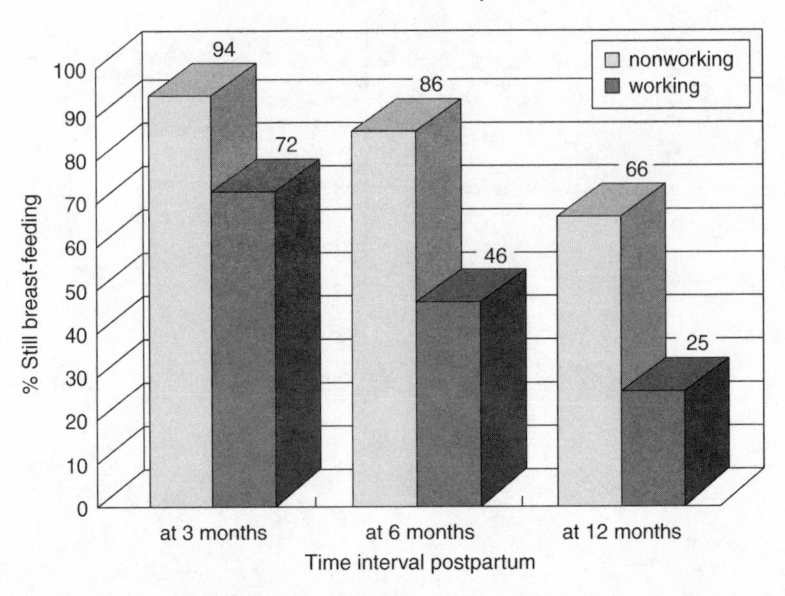

Figure 5–2. Comparisons of breast-feeding rates between nonworking and working women.

For those who worked outside the home, workplace support and the presence of a convenient child-care center were important in maintaining lactation. Of the 203 respondents who resumed employment within 6 months, 168 worked outside the home. Of the women whose infants were put into a child-care center (mainly at or near the workplace), 90% were breast-feeding when they went back to work, versus 76% of those whose infants were at their own homes and 48% of those whose infants went to another household ($p < .01$). A child-care center clearly made a difference to Pimporn, a university lecturer:

> I returned to work when my baby was 3 months old. I sent her to the child-care center in my faculty . . . [so that] I could breast-feed her twice a day. I could continue breast-feeding without giving a bottle until she was nearly 2 years old.

Once back in the workforce, women faced serious difficulties in sustaining lactation, particularly if they had rigid working environments and long hours of separation from their infants. Among the 154 formal sector workers who resumed employment within 6 months, less than a quarter reported any workplace support for maintaining breast-feeding (primarily in terms of breast-feeding breaks or permission to bring infants to work). Worst off were private sector employees, only 9% of whom received any support (versus 42% of those in the public sector) ($p < .001$).

We have noted the problems that arise in research on employment and breast-feeding if no distinctions are made between how different types of work relate to breast-feeding. Table 5–3 demonstrates the marked differences we found in relation to work

Table 5–2. Associations between Social Class and Breast-Feeding at the Time of Resuming Employment

	Not breast-feeding (n = 53)		Breast-feeding: Total (n = 150)		Breast-feeding: With formula (n = 105)		Breast-feeding: Without formula (n = 45)			
Age of infant (months)	N	%	n	%	N	%	n	%	χ_2^2 (p Value)[a]	χ_1^2 (p Value)[b]
Maternal age										
<30	25	25	75	75	59	79	16	21	5.36	0.13
≥30	28	27	75	73	46	61	21	39	(0.02)	(0.72)
Maternal education										
Primary	7	17	35	83	19	54	16	46	6.53	2.77
Secondary	19	26	53	74	37	70	16	30	(0.04)	(0.25)
Tertiary	27	30	62	70	49	79	13	21		
Work group										
Public sector employee	15	23	52	77	45	87	7	13	52.03 (<0.001)	1.95 (0.58)
Private sector employee	27	31	60	69	51	85	9	15		
Pieceworker at home	2	20	8	80	2	25	6	75		
Self/family employed	9	23	30	77	7	23	23	77		

[a]χ_1^2 = comparison between mothers who were and were not breast-feeding at the time of resuming employment.

[b]χ_1^2 = comparison between two subgroups: (*1*) those breast-feeding with formula and (*2*) those breast-feeding without formula at the time of resuming employment.

group at the 6-month point. Had we looked only for correlations between paid employment and (any) breast-feeding, our results would have had little meaning; instead, the significance of the nature of employment is indisputable.

Effects of employment on breast-feeding. Among those in our sample who continued breast-feeding after resuming work in the first 6 months postpartum, half said employment had negative impacts on breast-feeding; this perception was more common among formal than informal sector workers ($p < .001$). Some mothers turned to mixed feeding; however, probably because formula use typically interferes with the physiological demand–supply lactation mechanism, these women experienced more breast-feeding problems (mainly a reduced milk supply) than those who avoided formula ($p < .05$). Umporn described this vicious circle:

> I planned to continue breast-feeding after returning to work because I knew that breast milk was best for my baby. You know, it's just so hard to maintain a sup-

Table 5–3. Associations between Resuming Employment, Work Group, and Infant Feeding at 6 Months

	Not breast-feeding ($n = 123$)		Breast-feeding: Total ($n = 172$)		Breast-feeding: With formula ($n = 62$)		Breast-feeding: Without formula ($n = 110$)		χ_2^2	χ_2^2
	n	%	n	%	N	%	n	%	(p Value)[a]	(p Value)[b]
Stopped work ($n = 92$)	13	14	79	86	9	11	70	89	38.30	41.64
Resumed work ($n = 203$)	110	54	93	46	53	57	40	43	(<0.001)	(<0.001)
Work group ($n = 203$)										
Public sector employee	42	63	25	37	22	88	3	12	45.15 (<0.001)	15.08 (0.002)
Private sector employee	53	61	34	39	27	79	7	21		
Pieceworker at home	2	20	8	80	1	12	7	88		
Self/family employed	13	33	26	67	3	11	23	89		

[a]χ_1^2 = comparison between those who were and those who were not breast-feeding for at least 6 months.
[b]χ_2^2 = comparison between two subgroups: (*1*) those breast-feeding with formula and (*2*) those breast-feeding without formula for at least 6 months.

> ply. During my busy times at work, I didn't have enough time to express. . . . This may have caused a decrease in my supply. I felt that I didn't have enough milk for my baby. She would always cry when I breast-fed her, and I had to give her a bottle after that. Eventually, my baby refused to be breast-fed anymore. So, she had only bottle milk 3 weeks after I returned to work.

In order to stimulate the breasts to maintain the milk supply, working women must either breast-feed or express their milk during working hours. However, doing either was difficult for most women in our sample, and expressing at work was largely avoided due to lack of time and suitable facilities. There appeared to be little employer awareness, much less support.

Yupin, a worker in an electronics company, like many other women in modern factories, had restricted toilet breaks:

> It was impossible for me to express during my working period because the only place is the mixed-sex toilets. And you know it takes time to express, so I couldn't finish within the 3 minutes we are allowed to go the toilet. . . . You would be asked why you took so long by the foreman.

Sadly, most (79%) of those who expressed did not actually give this milk to their infants, primarily because they lacked suitable storage facilities. Buaboon, who worked in a garment factory, said, "I didn't give expressed milk to my baby because it might give her diarrhea. There is no refrigerator for storing the milk in the factory." About 41% of women who worked outside the home breast-fed during working time. Not surprisingly, those who were self- or family-employed were more likely to maintain this practice, given the greater flexibility of their work and their greater autonomy. Some brought their baby to the workplace or breast-fed at the child-care center if it was nearby. Those who breast-fed during working hours were also less likely to use formula ($p < .001$).

Those who did not breast-feed during working hours usually cited geographical separation: *long distance from the maternal workplace and place of child care*, 78%); *limitation of time*, 8%; *not allowed to go outside the workplace during working hours*, 10%. Some actually went without lunch to breast-feed during their hour-long break, a practice hardly sustainable over the long term. For most, an hour was simply not long enough to travel, breast-feed, and return to work. Some workplace policies presented fundamental obstacles to mother–baby interaction. Several factory workers were not permitted to leave the premises during the day, as Buaboon noted: "My house is not far from the factory, just five minutes by motorcycle. Unfortunately, they didn't allow me to go outside. So, I gave formula to my baby during working hours." Only one workplace (a hospital) in this study provided on-site child care.

Effects of breast-feeding on employment. Our study also revealed that maintaining lactation (especially without formula supplementation) had negative impacts on employment for 27% of the 150 breast-feeding women who resumed work by 6 months postpartum. The main difficulties were decreased productivity (73%) and exhaustion (20%). Once again, there was also a strong association with work group ($p < .001$), but in this case informal sector employees were more likely than formal sector employees to encounter problems. As Pannee, a home-based pieceworker, said: "Of course, with having a baby around and breast-feeding, I could not work much. I might work while the baby was sleeping. But I often could not concentrate fully on my work; my mind was always with the baby." Although informal sector workers more easily maintain lactation because typically they are less often separated from their infants, breast-feeding competes with work outputs, especially for those paid by the piece. Their low income status exacerbates these dilemmas.

Dilemmas of conflicting demands: women's emotional health. Resuming employment in the first year after childbearing often results in pronounced stress as the mother attempts to fulfill the complicated requirements of her roles as mother and worker (Morse and Bottorff, 1989). In our study, most women said they had experienced some type of conflict or anxiety, no matter how they had chosen to combine their roles. The delicate balancing act often posed severe emotional and physiological strains.

Table 5–4 shows that those who resumed work early were least satisfied, overall, with the way they managed infant feeding. The table also shows that those who continued breast-feeding after resuming work were more satisfied, perhaps because they felt they

Table 5–4. Infant Feeding Satisfaction in the First 6 Months by Resumption of Employment and Feeding Practices

	Stopped work for at least 6 months		Returned to work within 6 months							
			Total		Stopped breast-feeding ($n = 53$)		Continued breast-feeding ($n = 150$)			
Felt satisfied	N	%	n	%	n	%	n	%	χ_2^2 (p Value)[a]	χ_1^2 (p value)[b]
Yes	77	84	114	56	13	24	101	67	29.00	20.96
No	15	16	89	44	40	76	49	33	(<0.001)	(< 0.001)

[a]χ_1^2 = comparison between mothers who stopped work and those who resumed employment early.
[b]χ_2^2 = comparison between two subgroups: (*1*) those who stopped breast-feeding and (*2*) those who continued breast-feeding at the time of resuming employment.

had succeeded at both roles. While 84% of those who stopped paid work and continued breast-feeding felt satisfied with their infant-feeding experiences, some faced conflict because they were no longer making a financial contribution to the family.

In addition, many of the 53 women in our study who had weaned by the time they returned to work—that is, for a shorter period than they had hoped to breast-feed—said that they had experienced sadness, depression, or guilt about not having met their breast-feeding goals. Jumrieng was a worker in a textile factory in Chiang Mai who moved with her husband from her hometown to work in the city.

> I took 2 months of maternity leave. When it was over, I returned to work because we needed more income for the family. I had to send my baby to my mother, who lived in Lumphun [another province] during weekdays and take her home on Friday evening, because there were no other adults at my home. . . . I introduced bottle feeding when she was 1 month old and stopped breast-feeding 2 weeks before returning to work. I felt guilty but I didn't have any other choice. It seemed that I was not a good mother.

Others who tried to combine employment and breast-feeding, but then experienced a low milk supply, expressed regret at weaning earlier than planned.

Dilemmas of conflicting demands: physiological health. Fulfilling multiple demands has physical as well as emotional implications. In our study, exhaustion and fatigue were commonplace, especially among those who had the double burden of paid and unpaid work. Sida, who worked the night shift in an electronics company for more than 60 hours a week, told us:

> I usually work 6 nights a week . . . from 7 P.M. to 7 A.M. I have to sit in a row with others the whole night. Usually we have a half-hour break at midnight for

a meal. Then we work until a quarter to six and we have another half-hour for breakfast. I usually arrive home at 7:30 A.M. In the first week I breast-fed my baby before going to bed about 8 A.M. and woke up to feed her again at midday, but then I couldn't sleep well after that. I felt very tired from lack of sleep. . . . It's just too much for me. In the end, I stopped breast-feeding a week after returning to work.

This mother was dealing with a work schedule that would likely leave any worker sleep deprived. In such situations, any sort of child care or infant feeding may well have been perceived as an unwelcome demand on inadequate rest time. Although most mothers complained about fatigue, some had more flexibility in coping with this problem.

The exhaustion that accompanied various women's attempts to fulfill their various roles also affected their nutritional status. While some lacked time to eat, others, like Julai, complained about loss of appetite. "Because I was breast-feeding, I had to wake up many times each night. I was so tired I had no appetite. I lost more than 5 kilograms."

Conclusions and Recommendations

In the face of rapid social change, Thai women have almost universally continued to initiate breast-feeding, despite high labor force participation rates while their infants are young. In this study of 295 Chiang Mai mothers who fully established lactation, breast-feeding continued to be the norm during the early postpartum period, but it declined dramatically as they returned to paid employment, particularly outside the home. Our results resemble those found previously in urban Thailand (Richter et al., 1992; Winikoff and Castle, 1988) and elsewhere (Hills-Bonczyk et al., 1993; Scott and Binns, 1999). Taken together, these studies make a compelling argument that for women employed outside the home, lengthy separation from their babies quickly leads to formula use and weaning. Combining productive and reproductive roles is complicated, and speaking of employment or infant feeding as a choice ignores the many constraints impinging on women. Decision making in these matters is often less a question of free choice than of compulsion because of financial pressures, the demands and characteristics of work, and normative social patterns, including child-rearing customs, idealized concepts of the "good mother," and lack of support from husbands (Morrow, 1992; Morrow and Barraclough, 1993; Rodriguez-Garcia, 1990; Whittaker, 2000). The physiological toll of trying to meet internally and externally imposed expectations was evident in a lack of self-care, fatigue, and exhaustion.

Our results add to the growing body of evidence that *employment itself* is less important than working conditions, including the opportunity for frequent suckling or expressing of breast milk to maintain the supply of breast milk (Hills-Bonczyk et al., 1993; Morse and Bottorff, 1989; Valdes et al., 2000; Winikoff and Castle, 1988; Wright,

Clark, and Bauer, 1993). This study demonstrated that *intentions* to breast-feed were inadequate in the face of compelling obstacles arising from the circumstances of employment, not the fact of seeking paid work per se. This distinction is crucial but too often omitted from studies purporting to find few or no associations between infant feeding and "working". We believe this imprecision has contributed to the contradictory findings reported elsewhere. Our interpretation echoes that of Winikoff and Castle (1988), who concluded that meaningful explications of links between employment and breast-feeding must take into account prevailing social, cultural, and workplace norms. The review article by Scott and Binns (1999) and the study among Navajo women by Wright, Clark, and Bauer (1993) make similar assertions.

As in other studies (Hills-Bonczyk et al., 1993; Morse and Bottorff, 1989; Valdes et al., 2000), women in our investigation avoided expressing at work because of the nearly complete lack of appropriate facilities, supportive advice, and breaks to undertake this time-consuming activity. With diminished demand, lactation begins to shut down; this physiological process receives insufficient attention in debates about combining women's roles.

Despite these physiological universals, however, our study also demonstrated that women in different work settings face particular challenges, which further underscores the importance of context in interpreting different decisions and practices. While the formal sector workers (especially in the public sector) in our study had maternity leave, higher-status jobs, and higher rates of pay, such workers (like their Bangkok counterparts a decade earlier [Winikoff and Castle, 1988]) were compelled to resume employment after a (typically) short period of leave if they wanted to keep their jobs. Returning to employment that separates the mother–infant pair for many hours each day, it is hardly surprising that most professional women weaned their infants earlier than they had wished.

Based on our study results, it would be wrong to conclude that women must leave the workforce entirely if they hope to breast-feed successfully. Although those who stopped working did breast-feed relatively longer than those who resumed their formal sector positions, the breast-feeding duration among women who returned to *informal* sector work within 6 months postpartum was virtually the same as it was for those who quit working. This compelling finding again parallels results from the Winikoff and Castle investigation (1988) in Bangkok. The most plausible explanation, corroborated by our qualitative data, was the impact of easy access to the infant to enable frequent suckling. Still, informal sector workers also reported exhaustion and stress as they struggled to earn a living from a low-paid job and make time to breast-feed their infants.

Professional women everywhere are likely to find it difficult to sustain lactation due to lengthy separation and heavy workloads (unless arrangements are made to express at work). The growing informal workforce, in rich and poor countries alike, may be confronted with stark choices about productivity or breast-feeding. In the following sections, we argue that women should not be forced to make such choices, and we consider some approaches that support the health and rights of both women and infants.

Breast-Feeding and Maternal Employment: Basic Human Rights

Breast-feeding and paid work should be compatible. Increasingly, the fulfillment of both reproductive and productive roles is being identified internationally as an inherent right rather than as a dichotomy. This right confers an array of important benefits in terms of health, gender equity, and socioeconomic development. As WHO (1993, 94) has declared:

> The successful integration of women's productive and reproductive lives is the basis for both child survival and economic development. Every infant has the right to be breastfed. Every woman has the right to breastfeed. All human beings have the right to earn their living in order to maintain life and health for themselves and their dependents.

The construction of breast-feeding as a human right rests upon several United Nations conventions. The International Covenant on Economic, Social and Cultural Rights (adopted in 1966) guarantees the rights to work and to health, and the Convention on the Rights of the Child (adopted in 1989) cites "the right of the child to the enjoyment of the highest attainable standard of health" and calls for "appropriate measures to reduce infant and young child mortality." Specific mention is made of the "advantages of breastfeeding." The Convention on the Elimination of All Forms of Discrimination Against Women (adopted in 1979) states that women shall have appropriate services in connection with pregnancy and lactation.[2]

In June 2000, two-thirds of representatives to the eighty-eighth International Labor Organization (ILO) Conference voted in favor of Convention 183 (ILO, 2000). The Maternity Protection Convention specifies the right of employed women to breastfeed. The convention applies to all employed women, including the estimated 250 million in the informal sector who have employers, even if their contracts are only verbal. Convention 183 calls for increases in minimum maternity leave (to 14 weeks), paid breast-feeding breaks, and protection against discrimination on the grounds of breast-feeding. Like its counterpart United Nations treaties, it remains voluntary until formally ratified by individual governments, and transforming its statutes into binding law will be a lengthy process in most countries.[3] While passed in 1952, the predecessor to the Convention 103 was ratified by only 37 member countries, and as of May 2002, only 3 countries had endorsed Convention 183. Breast-feeding and human rights proponents will need to mount a vigorous campaign to ensure that the Maternity Protection Convention does not founder.

Beyond formal ratification and legislation, it is also essential that public awareness be raised about provisions that already exist to ensure that they are fully implemented.

For example, researchers (Friesen et al., 1998) recently found that in Papua New Guinea 64% of the employed women sampled were unaware that their nation's Employment Act entitled them to two daily 30-minute breast-feeding breaks. Our study revealed that women in Chiang Mai were unsure of their rights and sometimes were reluctant to make use of them for fear of jeopardizing future prospects or burdening their colleagues. The International Confederation of Free Trade Unions is spearheading the Maternity Protection Campaign.

The very existence of the new convention offers a platform for advocacy and offers direction to policy makers. If there are nursing breaks and child-care provisions at the workplace, even formal urban employment can be compatible with breast-feeding (Thompson and Bell, 1997; WHO, 1993; Zinn, 2000). Where these benefits have been applied, they have led to higher rates of resumption of employment, decreased absenteeism, and increased staff loyalty in the United States (Thompson and Bell, 1997), Malaysia, and Scotland (WABA, 2000b). Other organizations have joined the effort to disseminate such information and promote new policies. For instance, the 54th World Health Assembly agenda item 13.1 (May 2001) recommended a renewed commitment by governments to breast-feeding promotion, citing the "right of everyone to have access to safe and nutritious food," the Convention on the Rights of the Child, ILO policies, and the revised (6-month) guidelines on the optimal duration of exclusive breast-feeding. In so doing, the assembly brought into prominence existing shortfalls in implementation of current ILO and United Nations conventions and reiterated their crucial importance to public health and human rights.

Overview of Maternity Policies Internationally

Currently, legislation to support employed breast-feeding women varies widely among countries and regions. The World Alliance for Breast-feeding Action (WABA, 2002) has compiled an updated summary of country-specific maternity protection policies and provisions drawing on ILO reports, its own networks, and trade union data. As of January 16, 2002, only 72 out of 160 countries offered at least 14 weeks of maternity leave (some are unpaid), the minimum required under Convention 183. Numbers by region were 8 out of 35 in Asia and the Middle East, 2 out of 5 in Oceania, 6 out of 32 in the Americas, 20 out of 48 in Africa, and 36 out of 40 in Europe. Paid breast-feeding breaks were allowed in some workplaces in 106 countries (27 out of 40 European countries, plus about two-thirds in all other regions: Asia, Oceania, the Americas, and Africa).

Public policy in this matter tends to reflect prevailing sociopolitical and economic philosophies of individual countries. Though it voted for Convention 183, the United States voiced concern over the "prescriptive" provisions and has not ratified either this convention or the related Convention 103, developed in 1952. Although the U.S. Family and Medical Leave Act authorizes 12 weeks of (often unpaid) maternity leave, most private businesses are not required to comply. The issue of protective legislation for American workers is often ignored in published discussions on breast-feeding promotion, which tend to place primary emphasis on education about techniques of maintaining lactation (Bocar, 1997; Corbett-Dick and Bezek, 1997; USAID, 1990; Wyatt, 2002). By contrast, some Latin American countries opposed Convention 183 and even considered it a defeat because they feared that their much stronger existing provisions would be watered down. Chile, for example, offers women fully paid maternity leave for 6 weeks prior to and 12 weeks following delivery, two daily breast-feeding breaks, and mandatory on-site child care where 20 or more women are employed (Valdes et al., 2000). Brazil gives 4 months of leave through social insurance and two daily 30-minute breast-feeding breaks for 6 months after return to employment (UNICEF, 1999). Scandinavian countries are also known for their family-friendly supports, and Norway offers 42 weeks of paid leave (UNICEF, 1999). The Irish government requires employers to provide breast-feeding "facilities" for the first 4 months, and Victoria State, in Australia, has passed legislation outlawing discrimination against women for breast-feeding or expressing breast milk (WABA, 2001a). Bangladesh recently approved 4 months of maternity leave but failed to introduce legislation mandating breast-feeding breaks (WABA, 2001b). In various countries, maternity leave benefits typically are unevenly conferred and apply only to the formal sector. Sometimes these are offered within a specific workplace, such as the new, generous provisions for the Australian Catholic University (WABA, 2001b).

Although it has been shown that technical advice is crucial for exclusive breast-feeding even where excellent benefits exist (Valdes et al., 2000), international opinion, the recent literature, and findings from this study overwhelmingly support the contention that strong public policy is a prerequisite to enable women to combine paid work and lactation.

Optimal breast-feeding is intrinsic to better public health. Enabling this to become a reality in Thailand, as elsewhere, calls for a bold commitment to priorities that may sit uneasily with current economic orthodoxy. It should be remembered that enhanced population health yields economic, social, and development advantages. Moreover, the right of all women to breast-feed and to be gainfully employed has now been endorsed internationally, and it is from this starting point that other decisions should follow. The primary challenge is to reject the false dichotomy between the right to work and the right to breast-feed (and, for infants, to be breast-fed). If workplaces do not facilitate the maintenance of lactation even when infant nutrition is seen solely as the responsibility of individual mothers, the rights of mothers are being abrogated. On the other hand, if nations, societies, and workplaces are held responsible for guaranteeing the rights of infants and mothers—by enacting public policy and raising awareness of social support needs—the putative dichotomy disappears. There need be no trade-off between public health and gender equity. Indeed, they are mutually reinforcing and intertwined, and the achievement of both will confer substantial social and economic benefits on all populations.

Notes

1. All names used in this chapter for our sample's participants are pseudonyms.

2. The full text of these conventions, and ratification status, may be obtained from the Office of the High Commissioner for Human Rights, United Nations, Geneva.

3. For further discussion on the nature of ILO conventions, see Chapter 11 in this volume by K. Elliott and R. Freeman.

References

American Academy of Pediatrics. 1997. Breastfeeding and the use of human milk. *Pediatrics* 100: 1035–39.

Arlotti, J. P., B. H. Cottrell, S. H. Lee, and J. J. Curtin. 1998. Breastfeeding among low-income women with and without peer support. *Journal of Community Health Nursing* 15(3): 163–78.

Auerbach, K. G., M. J. Renfrew, and M. Minchin 1991. Infant feeding comparisons: A hazard to infant health? *Journal of Human Lactation* 7(2): 63–71.

Avery, M., L. Duckett, J. Dodgson, K. Savik, and S. J. Henly 1998. Factors associated with very early weaning among primiparas intending to breastfeed. *Maternal and Child Health Journal* 2(3): 167–79.

Bell, P. F. 1992. Gender and economic development in Thailand. In *Gender and development in Southeast Asia,* edited by P. and J. Van Esterik. Proceedings of the 20th Meetings of the Canadian Council for Southeast Asian Studies, York University, Oct. 18–20, 1991. Montreal: Canadian Asian Studies Association.

Berg, B. L. 1998. *Qualitative research methods for the social sciences.* Boston: Allyn and Bacon.

Bocar, D. L. 1997. Combining breastfeeding and employment: Increasing success. *Journal of Perinatal and Neonatal Nursing* 11(2): 23–43.

Boonwanich, P. 1993. Study of the effect of duration of postnatal maternal leave and other factors on breastfeeding patterns among civil servants. *Journal of Provincial Hospitals* 12(5): 9–17 (in Thai).

Borgnolo, G., F. Barbone, G. Scornavacca, D. Franco, A. Vinci, and F. Iuculano. 1996. A case-control study of *Salmonella* gastrointestinal infection in Italian children. *Acta Paediatrica* 85(7): 804–8.

Campbell, O., J. Cleland, M. Collumbien, and K. Southwick. 1999. *Social science methods for research on reproductive health.* WHO/RHR/HRP/SOC/99.1. Geneva: World Health Organization.

Chee, Y. O., and L. Horstmanshof. 1996. A review of breastfeeding practices in Hong Kong—1994/1995. *Breast-feeding Review* 4(1): 7–12.

Chye, J. K., Z. Zain, W. L. Lim, and C. T. Lim. 1997. Breastfeeding at six weeks and predictive factors. *Journal of Tropical Pediatrics* 43(5): 287–92.

Coates, M. M. 1993. Tides in breast-feeding practice. In *Breastfeeding and human lactation,* edited by J. Riodan and K. G. Auerbach. Boston: Jones and Bartlett.

Corbett-Dick, P., and S. K. Bezek 1997. Breastfeeding promotion for the employed mother. *Journal of Pediatric Health Care* 11(1): 12–19.

Cunningham, A. 1995. Breastfeeding: Adaptive behavior for child health and longevity. In *Breastfeeding: Biocultural perspectives,* edited by P. Stuart-Macadam and K. A. Dettwyler. New York: Aldine De Gruyter.

Cunningham, A., D. B. Jelliffe, and E. F. Jelliffe. 1991. Breast-feeding and health in the 1980s: A global epidemiological review. *Journal of Pediatrics* 118(5): 659–66.

Davis, M. K. 1998. Review of the evidence for an association between infant feeding and childhood cancer. *International Journal of Cancer—Supplement* 11: 29–33.

Dermer, A. 1998. Breastfeeding and women's health. *Journal of Women's Health* 7(4): 427–31.

Dettwyler, K. A. 1995. Beauty and the breast: The cultural context of breast-feeding in the United States. In *Breastfeeding: Biocultural perspectives,* edited by P. Stuart-Macadam and K. A. Dettwyler. New York: Aldine De Gruyter.

Donath, S., and L. H. Amir. 2000. Rates of breastfeeding in Australia by state and socioeconomic status: Evidence from the 1995 National Health Survey. *Breast-feeding Review* 8(3): 23–27.

Ellison, P. T. 1995. Breastfeeding, fertility, and maternal condition. In *Breast-feeding: Biocultural perspectives,* edited by P. Stuart-Macadam and K. A. Dettwyler. New York: Aldine De Gruyter.

Enger, S. M., R. K., Ross, and L. Bernstein. 1997. Breastfeeding history, pregnancy experience and risk of breast cancer. *British Journal of Cancer* 76(1): 118–23.

Enger, S. M., R. K. Ross, A. Paganini-Hill, and L. Bernstein. 1998. Breast-feeding experience and breast cancer risk among postmenopausal women. *Cancer Epidemiology, Biomarkers and Prevention* 7: 365–69.

Family Health Division. 1994. *A study of breastfeeding situation.* Bangkok, Thailand: Family Health Division, Ministry of Public Health.

Fok, D. 1997. Breast-feeding in Singapore. *Breastfeeding Review* 5(2): 25–28.

Frank, E. 1998. Breastfeeding and maternal employment: Two rights don't make a wrong. *Lancet* 352(9141): 1704.

Friesen, H., J. Vince, P. Boas, R. Danaya, D. Mokela, G. Ogle, P. Asuo, A. Kemiki, W. Lagani, T. Rongap, M. Varughese, and W. Saweri. 1998. Infant feeding practices in Papua New Guinea. *Annals of Tropical Paediatrics* 18(3): 209–15.

Gabriel, A., R. Gabriel, and R. A. Lawrence. 1986. Cultural values and biomedical knowledge: Choices in infant feeding. *Social Science and Medicine* 23(5): 501–19.

Gielen, A. C., R. R. Faden, P. O'Campo, C. H. Brown, and D. M. Paige. 1991. Maternal employment during the early postpartum period: Effects on initiation and continuation of breast-feeding. *Paediatrics* 87(3): 298–305.

Halken, S., H. P. Jacobsen, A. Host, and D. Holmenlund. 1995. The effect of hypo-allergenic formulas in infants at risk of allergic disease. *European Journal of Clinical Nutrition* 49(Suppl. 1): S77–83.

Hills-Bonczyk, S. G., M. D. Avery, K. Savik, S. Potter, and L. J. Duckett. 1993. Women's experiences with combining breastfeeding and employment. *Journal of Nurse Midwifery* 38(5): 257–66.

International Labor Organization (ILO). 2000. Convention 183. 88th Session, 30 May–15 June 2000, Report IV (1), Maternity protection at work. Revision of the Maternity Protection Convention (Revised), 1952 (No. 103), and Recommendation, 1952 (No. 95). Geneva: ILO.

Jelliffe, D. B. N., and E. F. P. Jelliffe. 1989. Breastfeeding: General review. In *Programmes to promote breast-feeding,* edited by D. B. N. Jelliffe and E. F. P. Jelliffe. Oxford: Oxford Medical Publications.

Jiggins, J. 1994. *Changing the boundaries: Women-centered perspectives on population and the environment.* Washington, D.C.: Island Press.

Kocturk, T., and R. Zetterstrom. 1989. The promotion of breastfeeding and maternal attitude. *Acta Paediatrica Scandinavica* 78: 817–23.

Koopman-Esseboom, C., N. Weisglas Kuperus, M. A. de Ridder, C. G. Van der Paauw, L. G.

Tuinstra, and P. J. Sauer. 1996. Effects of polychlorinated biphenyl/dioxin exposure and feeding type on infants' mental and psychomotor development. *Pediatrics*, 97(5): 700–6.

Kurinij, N., P. H. Shiono, S. F. Ezrine, and G. G. Rhoads. 1989. Does maternal employment affect breast-feeding? *American Journal of Public Health* 79(9): 1247–50.

Laufer, A. B. 1990. Breastfeeding: Toward resolution of the unsatisfying birth experience. *Journal of Nurse-Midwifery* 35(1): 42–45.

Lawrence, R. A. 1995. Commentary: Breastfeeding is more than just good nutrition. In *Breast-feeding: Biocultural perspectives*, edited by P. Stuart-Macadam and K. A. Dettwyler. New York: Aldine De Gruyter.

Lim, L. L. 1993. The feminization of labour in the Asia-Pacific rim countries: From contributing to economic dynamism to bearing the brunt of structural adjustments. In *Human resources in development along the Asia-Pacific rim*, edited by N. Ogawa, G. Jones, and J. G. Williamson. Singapore: Oxford University Press.

Losch, M., C. I. Dungy, D. Russell, and L. B. Dusdieker. 1995. Impact of attitudes on maternal decisions regarding infant feeding. *Journal of Pediatrics* 126(4): 507–14.

McIntyre, E., J. D. Hiller, and D. Turnbull. 1999. Determinants of infant feeding practices in a low socio-economic area: Identifying environmental barriers of breastfeeding. *Australian and New Zealand Journal of Public Health* 23(2): 207–9.

McKenna, J. J., and N. J. Bernshaw. 1995. Breastfeeding and infant–parent cosleeping as adaptive strategies: Are they protective against SIDS? In *Breast-feeding: Biocultural perspectives,* edited by P. Stuart-Macadam and K. A. Dettwyler. New York: Aldine De Gruyter.

Meershoek, S. 1993. The economic value of breastfeeding. *Breast-feeding Review* 2(8): 354–57.

Melville, B. 1990. Urban–rural differentials and determinants of breastfeeding in western Jamaica. *Breast-feeding Review* 2(2): 82–84.

Michels, K. B., W. C. Willett, B. A. Rosner, J. E. Manson, D. J. Hunter, G. A. Colditz, S. E. Hankinson, and F. E. Speizer. 1996. Prospective assessment of breastfeeding and breast cancer incidence among 89,887 women. *Lancet* 347(8999): 431–36.

Mitra, A. K., and F. Rabbani. 1995. The importance of breastfeeding in minimizing mortality and morbidity from diarrhoeal diseases: The Bangladesh perspective. *Journal of Diarrhoeal Diseases Research* 13(1): 1–7.

Morrow, M. 1992. Breastfeeding and the limits of informed choice: Cultural, social and economic constraints for Vietnamese and Chilean Women in Melbourne. Ph.D. dissertation, Department of Health Administration and Education, Lincoln School of Health Sciences, La Trobe University, Bundoora.

Morrow, M., and S. Barraclough. 1993. Breastfeeding and public policy in Australia: Limitations of a nutritional focus. *Health Promotion International* 8(2):135–46.

Morse, J. M., and J. L. Bottorff. 1989. Intending to breastfeed and work. *Journal of Obstetric Gynecologic and Neonatal Nursing* 18(6): 493–500.

National Statistics Office. 2000. *Report of the labor force survey whole kingdom round 3: August 2000.* Bangkok: National Statistics Office.

Newcomb, P. A., B. F. Storer, M. P. Longnecker, R. Mittendorf, E. R. Greenberg, R. W. Clapp, K. P. Burke, W. C. Willett, and B. MacMahon. 1994. Lactation and reduced risk of premenopausal breast cancer. *New England Journal of Medicine* 300: 81–86.

Newman, J. 1995. How breast milk protects newborns. *Scientific America*n 4: 76–79.

Noble, S. 2001. Maternal employment and the initiation of breastfeeding. *Acta Paediatrica* 90(4): 423–28.

O'Campo, P., R. R. Faden, A. C. Gielen, and M. C. Wang. 1992. Prenatal factors associated with breastfeeding duration: Recommendations for prenatal interventions. *Birth: Issues in Perinatal Care and Education* 19(4): 195–201.

Palmer, G., and S. Kemp. 1996. Breastfeeding promotion and the role of the professional midwife. In *Baby friendly mother friendly,* edited by S. F. Murray. London: Mosby.

Phongpaichit, P., and C. Baker. 1997. *Thailand: economy and politics.* New York: Oxford University Press/ASIA BOOKS.

Phongpaichit, P., and C. Baker. 1998. *Thailand's boom and bust.* Chiang Mai, Thailand: Silkworm Books.

Pruekpongsawalee, M. 1995. Women and the law. In *Perspective policies and planning for the development of women,* edited by the National Commission on Women's Affair. Bangkok: Amarin.

Reeder, S. J., L. L. Martin, and D. Koniak-Griffin. 1997. *Maternity nursing: Family, newborn, and women's health care,* 18th ed. Philadelphia: Lippincott.

Richardson, V., and V. Champion, V. 1992. The relationship of attitudes, knowledge, and social support to breast-feeding. *Pediatric Nursing* 15: 183–97.

Richter, K., C. Podhisita, K. Soonthorndhada, and A. Chamratriothirong. 1992. *Child care in urban Thailand.* Nakhonpathom, Thailand: Institute for Population and Social Research, Mahidol University.

Riordan, J., and K. G. Auerbach. 1993. *Breastfeeding and human lactation.* Boston: Jones and Bartlett.

Rodriguez-Garcia, R. 1990. Breastfeeding and the working mother: The freedom to choose. *Journal of Human Lactation* 6(2): 47–48.

Rosenblatt, K. A., and D. B. Thomas. 1995. Prolonged lactation and endometrial cancer. WHO Collaborative Study of Neoplasia and Steroid Contraceptives. *International Journal of Epidemiology* 24(3): 499–501.

Saarinen, U. M., and M. Kajosaari. 1995. Breastfeeding as prophylaxis against atopic disease: Prospective follow-up study until seventeen years old. *Lancet* 346: 1065–69.

Scott, J. A., and C. W. Binns. 1999. Factors associated with the initiation and duration of breastfeeding: A review of the literature. *Breastfeeding Review* 7(1): 5–16.

Shaheen, S. O., P. Aaby, A. J. Hall, D. J. Barker, C. B. Heyes, A. W. Shiell, and A. Goudiaby. 1996. Measles and atopy in Guinea-Bissau. *Lancet* 347(9018): 1792–96.

Short, R. 1993. *Breastfeeding, fertility and population growth.* Nutrition policy discussion paper no. 11, 20th Session. Administrative Committee on Coordination (ACC), Sub-Committee on Nutrition (SCN) for the United Nations. Geneva: World Health Organization, ACC/SCN.

Shu, X. O., J. Clemens, W. Zheng, D. M. Ying, B. T. Ji, and F. Jin. 1995. Infant breastfeeding and the risk of childhood lymphoma and leukaemia. *International Journal of Epidemiology* 24(1): 27–32.

Singhal, A., T. J. Cole, and A. Lucas. 2001. Early nutrition in preterm infants and later blood pressure: Two cohorts after randomised trials. *Lancet* 357: 413–19.

Skinner, J. D., B. R. Carruth, K. Houck, J. Moran, F. Coletta, R. Cotter, D. Ott, and M. McLeod. 1997. Transitions in infant feeding during the first year of life. *Journal of the American College of Nutrition* 16(3): 209–15.

Smyke, P. 1991. *Women and health.* London: Zed Books.

Sterken, E. 1998. Breastfeeding and intelligence. *INFACT/IBFAN Newsletter* (Winter 1998). Toronto: INFACT Canada. Available at http://www.infactcanada.ca/InfactHomePage.htm

Sweet, B. R., and D. Tiran. 1997. *Mayes' midwifery: A textbook for midwives.* London: Bailliere Tindall.

Swenson, I. E., N. M. Thang, and P. X. Tieu. 1993. Individual and community characteristics influencing breastfeeding duration in Vietnam. *Annals of Human Biology* 20(4): 325–34.

Thompson, P. E., and P. Bell. 1997. Breast-feeding in the workplace: How to succeed. *Issues in Comprehensive Pediatric Nursing* 20: 1–9.

United Nations Children's Fund (UNICEF). 1999. *Breastfeeding: Foundation for a healthy future.* New York: UNICEF.

United Nations Children's Fund (UNICEF). 2002. UNICEF statistics. Breastfeeding and complementary feeding. Available at http://www.childinfo.org/eddb/brfeed/index.htm

United States Agency for International Development (USAID). 1990. *Breastfeeding: A report on A.I.D. programs.* Washington, D.C.: USAID.

Valdes, V., E. Pugin, J. Schooley, S. Catalan, and R. Aravena. 2000. Clinical support can make the difference in exclusive breastfeeding success among working women. *Journal of Tropical Pediatrics* 46: 149–54.

Van Esterik, P., and T. Greiner. 1981. Breastfeeding and women's work: Constraints and opportunities. *Studies in Family Planning* 12(4): 184–97.

Villalpando, S., and M. Lopez-Alarcon. 2000. Growth faltering is prevented by breast-feeding in underprivileged infants from Mexico City. *Journal of Nutrition* 130(3): 546–52.

Walker, A., R. Chernoff, A. Joffe, and M. E. Wilson. 1994. Child abuse, sudden infant death syndrome, infectious disease and vaccinations. *Current Opinion in Pediatrics* 6(2): 225–31.

Wang, Y. S., and S. Y. Wu. 1996. The effect of exclusive breastfeeding on development and incidence of infection in infants. *Journal of Human Lactation* 12(1): 27–30.

Whittaker, A. 2000. *Intimate knowledge: Women and their health in North-East Thailand.* St Leonards, Australia: Allen & Unwin.

Wilmoth, T. A., and J. P. Elder. 1995. An assessment of research on breastfeeding promotion strategies in developing countries. *Social Science and Medicine* 41(4): 579–94.

Winikoff, B., and M. A. Castle. 1988. The influence of maternal employment. In *Feeding infants in four societies: Cause and consequences of mothers' choices*, edited by B. Winikoff, M. A. Castle, and V. H. Laukaran. New York: Greenwood Press.

Wongboonsin, K., and V. P. Ruffolo. 1993. The future of Thailand's population policy: Potential directions. *Asia-Pacific Population Journal* 8(3): 3–18.

Woolridge, M. W. 1995. Baby-controlled breastfeeding: Biocultural implications. In *Breastfeeding: Biocultural perspectives*, edited by P. Stuart-Macadam and K. A. Dettwyler. New York: Aldine De Gruyter.

World Alliance for Breastfeeding Action (WABA). 1998. *WABA Link* 15 (July/August).

World Alliance for Breastfeeding Action (WABA). 2000a. *Breastfeeding: The best investment.* Penang, Malaysia: Jutaprint.

World Alliance for Breastfeeding Action (WABA). 2000b. *WABA Link* 23 (August).

World Alliance for Breastfeeding Action (WABA). 2001a. *WABA Link* 24 (December 2000/January 2001).

World Alliance for Breastfeeding Action (WABA). 2001b. *WABA Link* 26 and 27 (October).

World Alliance for Breastfeeding Action (WABA). 2002. *Status of maternity protection by country—Update 16 January 2002.* Penang, Malaysia: WABA.

World Bank. 1998. *World development indicators 1998.* Washington, D.C.: World Bank.

World Health Organization (WHO). 1993. *Breastfeeding: The technical basis and recommendations for action.* Geneva: WHO.

World Health Organization (WHO). 1994. Infant and young child nutrition (progress and evaluation report on the International Code of Marketing of Breast-milk Substitutes). In *Report by the director-general at the Forty-seventh World Health Assembly.* Geneva: WHO.

World Health Organization (WHO). 1996. *Global data bank on breast-feeding.* Geneva: WHO.

World Health Organization (WHO). 1998. *Complementary feeding of young children in developing countries: A review of current scientific knowledge.* Geneva: WHO.

World Health Organization (WHO). 2001a. *The optimal duration of exclusive breastfeeding: Results of a WHO systematic review.* Geneva: WHO.

World Health Organization (WHO). 2001b. *Infant and young child nutrition* (*Agenda item 13.1*). Fifty-Fourth World Health Assembly (WHA54.2), May 18, 2001. Geneva: WHO.

World Health Organization (WHO). 2002. Global Data Bank on Breastfeeding, updated 13 March 2002. Available at http://www.who.int/nut/db_bfd.htm

Wright, A. L., C. Clark, and M. Bauer. 1993. Maternal employment and infant feeding practices among the Navajo. *Medical Anthropology Quarterly* 7(3): 260–80.

Wyatt, S. N. 2002. Challenges of the working breastfeeding mother. Workplace solutions. *American Association of Occupational Health Nurses Journal* 50(2): 61–66.

Yoon, P. W., R. E. Black, L. H. Moulton, and S. Becker. 1996. Effect of not breastfeeding on the risk of diarrheal and respiratory mortality in children under two years of age in Metro Cebu, the Philippines. *American Journal of Epidemiology* 143(11): 1142–48.

Zinn, B. 2000. Supporting the employed breastfeeding mother. *Journal of Midwifery and Women's Health* 45(3): 216–25.

6

Parental Labor and Child Nutrition Beyond Infancy

PETER GLICK

Women play multiple roles in the family that affect the health and well-being of all family members. In almost all societies around the world, they are assigned by custom to be the primary caregivers to infants and children (UNDP, 1995). Activities carried out by women such as breast-feeding, preparing food, collecting water and fuel, and seeking preventive and curative medical care are crucial for children's healthy development. Women also play important roles as generators of family income, whether in family farms or businesses or as wage employees. In developing countries especially, such work is likely to be essential to family survival.

Whether women's roles as caregivers and as providers of family income conflict with one another or complement each other has important implications for the health and welfare of children. For developing countries, the implications for child nutrition, in particular, have been the subject of much empirical investigation and debate (Glick and Sahn, 1998; Lamontagne, Engle, and Zeitlin, 1998; Leslie, 1989). Mothers who work may lack the time to breast-feed adequately, prepare nutritious foods for their young children, or make use of public services designed to improve child nutrition. Although there will be market substitutes for at least some time-intensive inputs (such as prepared foods or hired domestic help), these may be too costly for many women. Working women may rely on other members of the household to provide child care, but the quality of care provided by these substitutes may be poor, especially if the caregivers are older children. On the other hand, the additions to family income from mothers' employment should benefit children's nutrition and may more than compensate for any reductions in the quantity or quality of care, implying a net improvement in nutrition from maternal work. Furthermore, high quality child-care services can improve child nutrition.[1]

Understanding how women's work affects children's well-being has, if anything, become more important in the past two decades, because women's participation in the labor force has been increasing. Although some of the recorded increase in female participation in developing countries reflects better accounting for unpaid labor, most observers would agree that in many regions of the developing world—for example, Latin America and South Asia—women's economic activity has increased significantly since 1970 (Mehra and Gammage, 1999). In regions where it has stayed the same or fallen slightly, such as East Asia and Africa, female participation rates were already high.

Equally significant have been changes in the nature of women's work, reflecting structural changes as economies develop as well as, increasingly, integration into the global economy. Women, like men, have shifted from agriculture to expanding manufacturing, service, and commerce sectors. These and concomitant changes in the living situations of women and families worldwide—including urbanization and changes in family structure—are changing women's incomes, flexibility of employment, and child-care needs and options. Hence, the relation of women's work to child welfare is itself evolving.

In contrast to the rise in female labor force participation, male participation has declined slightly in the past several decades in much of the world—a result of more time in school for the young and increased pensions for the old. Still, it remains consistently around 90% in all regions of the world for men aged 20 to 59 (Tzannatos, 1999). If they work more in the labor force than women, however, men work much less at home. In most societies in the developing world, men have very limited involvement in child care and child nurturing, at least for very young children and infants (Anandalakshmy, 1994; Evans, 1995b; Olmsted and Weikart, 1995). Nor do they increase their time devoted to these activities when their partners work (see Engle and Breaux, 1994, and references therein).

Although they typically spend much less time than women in caring for and nurturing young children, fathers do play important roles in child development in most cultures, at least for older children and particularly for sons in some societies. Evidence indicates that when fathers participate in child rearing, there are important intellectual, social, and emotional benefits for children (Hoffman, 1989; Ishii-Kuntz, 1995; Rossi, 1983). Still, activities related to the nutrition of young children, which is the focus of this chapter, currently remain overwhelmingly the domain of women and girls. This is the reason for the emphasis on the impacts of women's work in this chapter.

In this chapter, I summarize what is known about the relationship of women's work and child nutrition in developing countries. In the next section, I review the empirical work in this area. Despite methodological differences (and, at times, weaknesses), the literature overall yields a number of consistent findings that are relevant for policy. In the third section, I map out how global trends toward urbanization and international economic integration are affecting women's work in developing countries and its relation to the well-being of young children. I conclude with a discussion of how policies can reduce the potential conflicts and increase the complementarities between women's employment and child welfare.

Empirical Evidence

Effects of Women's Employment on Child Nutrition

The body of empirical research examining the relationship of women's work to child nutrition is now quite substantial. There is enormous variation in terms of methodology and focus among these studies. Largely reflecting data limitations, most do not try to account fully for the relationship of health outcomes to all potential health determinants (such as breast-feeding, child care, or household sanitation). Instead, they directly estimate the effect of mother's work status or hours of work on child nutrition. In some cases, controls are added for other factors that are thought to influence nutrition; in other cases, researchers simply report bivariate correlations of child nutrition and a variable representing the mother's work status. Nutritional outcomes are typically measured using anthropometric indicators such as weight for age or height for age measured against international standards for a healthy population, though occasionally dietary indicators such as caloric intake or intake of specific nutrients are used.

The fact that nutrition and many of its determinants are due, to some degree, to household choices makes it inherently difficult to give a causal interpretation of observed associations of maternal work and child nutrition. In technical terms, the estimated effect of the explanatory variable (work) on the outcome variable (nutrition) is likely to suffer from simultaneity bias. Child health can determine maternal time use and work behavior rather than the reverse, for example if mothers of chronically ill children decide not to participate in the labor force so as to accommodate their children's greater needs for care. Further, there may exist unobserved (to the researcher) differences between women or households in terms of preferences or abilities that influence the work or time allocation of the mother, on the one hand, and health outcomes, on the other. This too will confound estimates of the relationship of mother's work and child nutrition. However, relatively few studies to date have attempted to apply the appropriate statistical techniques (such as instrumental variables) to account for the likely simultaneity of the relation of mother's time use and child nutrition (Blau, Guilkey, and Popkin, 1996; Glick and Sahn, 1998).

Leslie (1989) reviews early bivariate studies of maternal work and child nutrition; more recent research using essentially a bivariate approach includes Abbi and associates (1991), Bamji and Thimayamma (2000), Rabiee and Geissler (1992), and Wandel and Holmboe-Ottesen (1992). In some cases, these analyses are refined by stratifying the sample on factors such as the child's age or maternal workload. Many of these studies found a negative association between mother's work and child nutrition, but for others the correlation was positive or else no significant relationship was found. However, since they lack controls for confounding factors, these simple associations cannot be interpreted as showing a causal relation from work to nutrition. For example, women who work are more likely to be from poor households and hence to have less well-nourished children, all things being equal.

Of greater value, therefore, are multivariate analyses, that is, studies employing regression techniques to control for other household or individual factors that affect nutrition. By way of a preview of the overall findings, no broad conclusion emerges from these studies about the effect of women's work on child nutrition. However, this should not be surprising, given the very different social contexts considered and the variation in the types of women's employment considered. What the literature does effectively is offer insights as to why women's employment may have positive effects in some cases but negative ones in others. To highlight the relevant factors, the following review categorizes the studies by the specific aspects of the work–nutrition relation analyzed.

Factors Mediating the Effects of Women's Employment on Child Nutrition

Nature and intensity of work. A number of studies consider differences either in the type of work or in the level of work effort (i.e., labor supply). The type of work is presumed to matter because the compatibility of work and caring for children is likely to be different for different work activities. Informal sector work is usually considered to be more compatible with child care than formal employment, given the greater flexibility of hours or the possibility of combining work and child supervision in informal employment; work in or near the home should be more child-care compatible than work outside or far from the home. Using instrumental variable methods to predict mother's hours of work in informal and formal employment in Thailand, Chutikul (1986) found a positive effect of informal work on child weight for height and height for age but a negative effect of formal work, consistent with a greater compatibility of informal work and child care. Similarly, for Nicaragua, Wolfe and Behrman (1982) found that children of informal sector workers, but not those of formal sector workers, were taller than children of women who were not employed. In a rural Indian sample, Kumar (1978) found children of women who worked in the fields to be malnourished relative to those whose mothers engaged in income-earning activity at home.

However, differences by type of maternal work have not been universally found. Glick and Sahn (1998) found that predicted maternal informal (self-employment) and formal (wage) employment hours in urban Guinea had statistically equivalent negative effects on child height, controlling for the mother's income. Popkin (1980) found no significant difference in the nutritional status of children whose mothers worked at home and those whose mothers worked away from home in his Philippines sample. Likewise, Smith and colleagues (1980) and Vial and Muchnik (1989) found no effects of distance to work or occupation variables in, respectively, Haiti, and Chile.[2]

These studies differed significantly in the extent to which they controlled for factors such as household income and the use of substitute care providers (to be discussed below). Since each of these factors may be correlated both with health outcomes and with occupation or type of work, the lack of consistent findings regarding the nature of maternal employment is perhaps not surprising. Also, many activities that might be assumed to permit simultaneous work and child supervision or care may not, in fact, do so. This applies to urban self-employment (as will be discussed below), as well as traditional family agriculture. For example, women often find it inconvenient or unsafe to bring their children to the fields while they work (Doan and Popkin, 1993; Gryboski, 1996).

A number of studies, in addition to those of Glick and Sahn and Chutikal cited above, have considered the effects of the level of a woman's labor force activity. Adelman (1983) found for Peru that, controlling for household income, children of women who worked part-time were taller than children of women who worked full-time. Rabiee and Geissler (1992) reported that children of women in their rural Iranian sample who had heavy agricultural workloads had lower weight for age and energy intake, and a higher incidence of diarrhea, than children of women with light workloads. Their sample was very small, and they did not attempt multivariate analysis, but it is noteworthy that children of high-workload women were at a disadvantage in spite of being in families with higher mean incomes than the other group. In contrast to these studies, Franklin (1979), in an analysis that did not control for income, reported for Colombia that children of full-time workers were taller than children of part-time workers.

All things being equal, of course, women who work longer hours earn more income. Therefore, nutrition regressions that include separate variables for the mother's labor supply and her labor income are of particular interest, as they permit direct estimation of the hypothesized trade-off between income effects and time effects. Soekirman (1985) distinguished hours of work and income impacts on nutrition for his Indonesian sample, and found a significant negative effect of maternal work only for children of women who worked more than 40 hours a week and earned less than the minimum wage. Glick and Sahn (1998) also found evidence of a trade-off in Guinea, but the overall effect of work appeared negative for a larger portion of their sample. In urban Guatemala, a negative effect on children's nutritional status of mother's work was found only for children of domestic workers, who worked long hours and received very low pay (Engle and Pederson, 1989). Each of these studies demonstrates the obvious but important point that the effects of maternal work are more likely to be positive for higher-wage women.

Age of the child. Very young children, especially infants, have particularly strong needs for the most time-intensive care. Therefore, if there are any negative effects of mother's work, we would expect them to be felt more strongly by younger children than by older children. This expectation has been borne out by the relatively few studies in which researchers examined samples containing both infants and older children and differentiated by age in the analysis. Haggerty (1981), for Haiti, and Engle and

Pedersen (1989), for Guatemala, found that maternal work was associated with lower nutritional status (relative to children of nonemployed mothers) for children younger than 1 year of age but with superior nutritional status for children 1 to 2 years of age. Popkin (1983), distinguishing between children younger and older than 2 years in his preschooler Philippines sample, found a negative effect of maternal employment on height and weight for age only for the younger group. Similarly, Abbi and associates (1991), who found generally negative associations between maternal work and several dimensions of child health in rural Marasahrtra, India, reported that these correlations were usually stronger for children younger than 3 years of age than for those aged 3 to 6. Since older children are more reliant on purchased foods and less critically dependent on maternal time for breast-feeding and other activities, we might expect mother's *income* to have stronger (positive) effects on older children. This is exactly what Glick and Sahn (1998) report for their Guinea sample, comparing results for children aged 2 to 5 years with those for children younger than 2.

Given the important benefits of breast-feeding for infants in terms of both nutrition and reduced exposure to infection, can these negative associations between maternal work and infant nutrition be explained by work-related differences in breast-feeding? The extensive literature on the relationship of maternal work and infant feeding in the third world does not show a negative association between work and the decision to breast-feed (Leslie, 1989; Ruel, Haddad, and Garrett, 1999). However, while rates of initiation of breast-feeding do not seem to differ, some studies have shown a shorter exclusive breast-feeding duration among employed women, which may raise the nutritional risks for infants of working mothers (see Chapter 5 by Yimyam and Morrow).

Quantity and quality of substitute care. Working mothers in poor countries typically turn to substitute sources of care for their children. Ethnographic studies have indicated the wide range of alternative providers used, including other members of the household, kin or nonkin support networks outside the household, hired domestic help, and formal day care (Joekes, 1989). However, the last two options remain relatively rare in the developing world, as they are unaffordable for most women.

Some of the statistical analyses of maternal work and child nutrition have attempted to account for the effects of mother's work on her own time in child care or household work, as well as on the time of other household members in these activities. Other research has considered the quality of care provided by substitutes. An example of the former is the study of Panama by Tucker and Sanjur (1988). They reported that the mother's time spent on cooking and child care fell with her labor market participation, but the total time of all household members in these activities did not, indicating that others in the household fully made up for the loss of the mother's time. They concluded that the actions of others in the household prevented negative time-related impacts of mother's work, which in their regressions had no significant impacts on their anthropometric indicators (while it had positive impacts on children's dietary intake and hemoglobin level). Popkin (1983) found that mother's predicted labor force participation had no significant effect on her own time in child care (instead, it reduced her leisure time) but did increase the child-care time of siblings, while Engle and Pederson (1989) reported that working mothers in urban Guatemala were more likely than nonworkers to report the use of adult help in child care. It should be noted that reductions in maternal home work time resulting from participation in paid work, if they occur, invariably fail to offset the increased hours spent on market activities; that is, the woman's total hours of work rise at the expense of her leisure time. Evidence for this has come from a wide range of time-use studies (Bunster, 1983; Nieves, 1981; Overseas Education Fund, 1979; Popkin, 1983). The term *double day* aptly describes the situation of most working women in poor countries, whose normal workday is followed by substantial work in the home.

Even if, as in the cases just discussed, intrahousehold substitution in time use ensures that overall child-care time is maintained, the quality of that care may not be adequate. This is especially an issue if young children are entrusted to the care of older siblings who are children themselves—a common practice in developing countries (Joekes, 1989). In a recent review of the literature on care and nutrition, Engle, Menon, and Haddad (1999) conclude that while there is no consistent association between total time spent in care and nutrition outcomes, specific care behaviors (or, more generally, the quality of care) do matter: for example, boiling water, being responsive to signals from the child during feeding and to the amount eaten, and ensuring the cleanliness of the feeding location. Compared with adults, children lack the maturity and knowledge to carry out these tasks effectively, so we would expect nutrition outcomes to be poorer when children are left in charge. This hypothesis has consistently been supported by research that considers the nature of care support in households in which mothers work. When children are used as substitute caregivers, the association between maternal work and child nutrition is either negative or less favorable than when the care is provided by another adult (Bittencourt and DiCicco, 1979; Engle, 1991; Engle et al., 1985; Shah, Walimbe, and Dhole, 1979).

Lamontagne, Engle, and Zeitlin's (1998) study of 12- to 18-month-olds in Nicaragua is a particularly detailed examination of the interactions of mother's work, the quality of care, and child nutrition. They report that "inadequate" care (care by a preteen child or by mothers who took children with them to street-vending jobs) was negatively correlated with both weight for age and height for age, though in regression analysis only the latter negative association remained. In a regression with controls for the adequacy of care and other factors, mother's work had positive effects on weight for height (no significant impacts of work were found for weight for age or height for age). Lamontagne, Engle, and Zeitlin's approach is in some respects similar to that of Blau, Guilkey, and Popkin (1996), who took advantage of very detailed longitudinal Philippine data on infants to examine the effects of mother's labor supply on child nutrition, using statistical controls (instrumental variable fixed effects) for simultaneity in the relation of work and nutrition. They found that, controlling for the time in child care of different members of the household, as well as for infant feeding practices and many other household nutrition determinants, mother's hours of work had no effect on infant weight or height.

On the basis of their findings, Lamontagne, Engle, and Zeitlin, as well as Blau, Guilkey, and Popkin, conclude that fears about negative impacts on children of women working are unfounded. However, both studies included in their regressions not just women's employment variables but also controls for many direct inputs into nutrition that women's work is likely to affect—in particular, child-care time and (in the case of Blau, Guilkey, and Popkin) breast-feeding. Hence, their results actually support a more limited conclusion: if maternal work does not have negative impacts on intervening factors such as total child-care time, it will have no *direct* negative effects on nutrition.

These two studies can be contrasted to the more structural approach of Popkin (1983). Rather than holding other inputs such as total child-care time constant when assessing the impact of maternal work, Popkin first estimated the effect of maternal work on child-care time (as well as on calorie and protein intake) and then estimated the effect of these inputs on child health in his Philippines sample. Predicted labor force participation had no effect on mother's time spent in child care but increased the time siblings spent in child care (as previously noted) and also increased caloric intake. Working through the effects on time and nutrient availability, Popkin ultimately concluded that there is no impact of mother's work on child nutrition. Note that unlike Lamontagne, Engle, and Zeitlin's approach and that of Blau, Guilkey, and Popkin, the estimated impact in this case incorporates the effects of maternal work on key health inputs.

Maternal health. A potentially important aspect of the nexus of maternal work, child care, and nutrition is the effect of work on the mother's own health and, through that, on the quality of caregiving. A number of studies from developing countries indicate that longer working hours or increased work intensity are associated with poorer physical and mental health in women (Floro, 1995; Verbrugge, 1983; Wolfe and Haveman, 1983). Obviously, the type of work performed is a key factor. Where negative effects of work on women's health do occur, they are, of course, of concern in their own right.[3] The further issue of how work-related health stresses on mothers (including simply fatigue), in turn, impact child health and development has not been the subject of much research. Even the more general question of the effects of caregiver health (whether influenced by work or not) on the quality of care or on child health and development has received little attention (Engle, Menon, and Haddad, 1999). One exception is a study on Egypt showing that anemic women were less active caregivers and provided poorer diets to children than did nonanemic women (Rahmanidfar et al., 1992).

More direct pathways from maternal to child health involve work-related health stresses on mothers during pregnancy, which may lead to lower birth weight, or during lactation, which may have negative effects on infant nutrition through a reduced quantity or quality of breast milk. Hernandez-Pena and colleagues (1999) found that the birth weight of children of street vendors in Mexico was negatively associated with maternal work fatigue during pregnancy (see also Chapter 10 of this volume by Denman, Cedillo, and Harlow). Also in Mexico City, Cerón-Mireles and colleagues (1997) found that birth weight was lower for children whose mothers reported long working hours or problems on the job. In rural areas in particular, health stresses on women have a strong seasonal dimension. During peak seasons for labor use (for instance, during the harvest), lactating and pregnant women expend additional energy in agricultural work, often when household food consumption is low (Holmboe-Ottsen, Mascarenhas, and Wandel, 1988). This implies lower birth weights as well as reduced quality or quantity of breast milk (Cornia, 1984).

Control over earnings. The income contributed by mother's work should, controlling for changes in the quantity or quality of child care, benefit child nutrition. The extent or even existence of this benefit, however, depends on how the additional income is spent. If women have strong (relative to their spouses) preferences for child welfare and they have control over their own earnings, the income effects on nutrition will be larger than those from the spouse's or other household income. Several recent careful econometric analyses have indicated that women's income is more likely than men's income to be spent on items that benefit children (such as food)—indicating, at least in the contexts studied, that women have stronger preferences for child welfare. Although most research in this area has not considered the effects specifically of women's work-related income, one can infer that if mothers work *and* control their earnings, the benefits to child welfare (again, controlling for time effects) may be large. Glick and Sahn (1998) did examine this issue directly for their Guinea sample. They reported that increments to maternal income (predicted in a two-stage procedure to control for the simultaneity of mother's work or earnings and child health) had effects on preschooler height for age that were more than 10 times greater than the effects of other household income. Similarly, in Hoddinott and Haddad's (1994) study of rural Côte d'Ivoire, a larger predicted share of household income earned by women led to better child anthropometric outcomes. The same result was found for periurban Guatemala by Engle (1993), using the share of (uninstrumented) maternal income in total family income.

Whether women control their own earnings depends on the specific cultural or social context. In many African societies, women's and men's incomes are not pooled or are only partially pooled within the household, so each member retains control over personal earnings (Fapohunda, 1988; Munachonga, 1988); essentially, there are separate, or partially separate, economic spheres within the household. In these cases, meeting the needs of children typically falls within the women's economic sphere. Where income is instead pooled, the key factor is decision-making power over the use of this income, and this is likely to be a function of each member's contribution or, more generally, his or her economic status. A number of studies have indicated that when women work, they gain greater power in decisions about the use of family resources (Acharya and Bennett, 1982; Blumberg, 1988; Engle, 1993). This may be because working outside the home fosters greater assertiveness or confidence, or because working women have a stronger "fallback position"—that is, they can more credibly threaten to move out on their own if they are not granted greater control. In these situations, the income benefits to children of women's employment may be large. However, control over earnings or increased decision-making power as a result of performing paid work cannot be presumed. In South Asia, for example, a number of studies reveal that many or most wage-earning women are obligated to turn over their pay to their husbands or other male family members (Argawal, 1986; Standing, 1991; Zohir and Paul-Majumder, 1996).

Therefore, the negative association, or lack of a positive association, between mother's work and child health outcomes found in some case studies may reflect women's inability to use their incomes to benefit their children. For example, the studies by Abbi and colleagues (1991) of rural India and those by Rabiee and Geissler (1992) of rural Iran, both of which found a negative association, involved cultural contexts in which we might expect women to have relatively little control over their own agricultural output or income (see Chapter 9 by Ghorayshi). In contrast, in their study of a rural public works program in Niger, Brown, Johannes, and Webb (1994) found that the predicted share of female public works employment raised preschooler weight for age. Male participation in the program, on the other hand, had no effect on child health. These regressions controlled for caloric availability, which male participation was found to reduce; because of this negative effect on calorie consumption, men's participation in the public works program may actually have had a negative effect on nutrition. In this setting, women apparently had stronger preferences for child welfare than men, as well as the ability to control their earnings from the project. These findings echo those of Hoddinott and Haddad (1994) for rural Côte d'Ivoire, previously mentioned.

Prospects and Policies

The foregoing survey of research demonstrates, that posing a broad question such as "What is the effect of mother's work on child nutrition?" is too oversimplified to be useful: the links between maternal work and child outcomes are complex, involving the cultural context, the nature of work, and a range of intervening factors. Instead, the focus should be on providing insights for identifying where risks or benefits to children exist, elucidating the specific reasons for the risks or benefits, and coming up with policies that reduce the risks and enhance the benefits while not perpetuating gender inequalities, either in the overall burden of work or in economic opportunity.

We have some understanding of the conditions under which women's work may be beneficial to nutrition (complementarity) and where it may entail risks (conflict). One factor that emerges strongly is the importance of the quality of alternative child care. Where substitutes for working mothers' care are of poor quality, which is likely to be the case when the substitutes are older siblings, young children's nutrition appears to suffer. More research is needed from different settings on the links between mother's work, the choice and quality of child-care alternatives, and child welfare. A second important care-related factor is the age of the child. Older children are likely to benefit from mother's work because of the additional consumption expenditures made possible by her earnings. On the other hand, infants, who require very intensive caregiving (including breast-feeding), may incur a nutritional risk. Third, the literature suggests that the greater a woman's earning power and the greater her control over what she earns, the more her children will benefit from her employment. The nature of women's work in terms of its compatibility with child-care activities may also be important, though here the evidence is less consistent. Finally, much less understood, and warranting more investigation, are the links between work, a woman's own health, and the quality of child care.

Urbanization, Changes in Families, and Women's Employment

Research and policy on the relation of women's employment to child health must address several important long-term trends in the family and work lives of women and men in developing countries, which were alluded to at the beginning of the chapter. Many of these trends are associated with rapid urbanization. While the population of the developing world is expected to rise by about 60% from 2000 to 2025, the urban population is projected to almost double during that time (Haddad, Ruel, and Garrett, 1999). Urbanization is associated with important changes in family structure: family units in urban areas are smaller and have weaker ties to the extended family.[4] With fewer aunts, grandparents, or other relatives living in the household or nearby, urban households have fewer alternative caregivers for working mothers (Joekes, 1989). At the same time, daughters are less available as substitute care providers because they are more likely to be enrolled in school (especially at the secondary level), a reflection of the easier access to schools in the urban environment.

Urbanization also typically correlates with a higher proportion of female-headed households, in part reflecting patterns of rural-to-urban migration. In Latin America, the majority of such migrants are women without partners. In Africa and much of South Asia, a very different pattern usually exists: men migrate, leaving women and children behind in rural areas (though the men usually provide support through remittances). As a result of these trends, the rate of female-headed households is almost 30% in Latin America and the Caribbean, over 20% in sub-Saharan Africa, and about 15% in East and South Asia (Himes, Landers, and Leslie, 1992). If no spouse is present and remittances or transfers are not adequate, the pressure on a woman to participate in the labor force obviously will be very strong. At the same time, there are usually fewer potential substitute caregivers in female-headed households, which tend to be smaller than male-headed ones. Hence, for many women who are heads of households, the time stresses on them—and, by implication, the health risks to themselves and their children—are likely to be high.

The nature of women's paid work also changes dramatically with urbanization, particularly with respect to the prevalence of formal sector employment. In terms of pay and security, urban jobs represent a step up for women compared with work in rural settings (Horton, 1999). However, urban jobs are generally less flexible with respect to hours and less compatible with child care than agricultural work in rural areas (Ruel, Haddad, and Garrett, 1999). In spite of the increase in formal employment that accompanies urbanization, in many areas of the world the urban informal sector absorbs more women than does the formal sector. This is especially true for Africa. In West African cities, most working women are found in the informal sector (Becker, Jamer, and Morrison, 1994; Glick and Sahn, 1997). Informal work on the whole offers greater possibilities for combining work and child care, and for many women this is the rationale for choosing such work. However, even in urban informal employment, the opportunities for doing this are more limited than in rural work activities. For example, street vending may require working long hours some distance from the home and in an environment that is unsafe for children.

The trends associated with urbanization thus increase the need for substitute care while reducing the availability of traditional sources of such care. More families therefore seek assistance from outside the family. Throughout the developing world, the use of hired domestic help or institutional child care is higher in urban areas than rural areas (Ruel, Hadad, and Garrett, 1999). Still, since domestic help is unaffordable for most households and publicly provided child care remains scarce, the number of families using these alternatives even in urban areas remains low. Community networks among women in urban neighborhoods can serve as a partial replacement for the extended family structure of the rural environment. Overall, however, child care is a particularly pressing problem in urban settings, raising concerns about the health of young children of working mothers who cannot secure adequate care.

Implications of Globalization for Women's Employment and Child Welfare

Increasing integration into the world economy through trade and globalized production networks is profoundly affecting women's and men's livelihoods. For women, the most important change has been the increase in manufacturing employment in export industries (see Chapter 10 by Denman, Cedillo, and Harlow). Women now represent over a third of the manufacturing labor force in the developing world and almost half in some Asian countries (Mehra and Gammage, 1999). In textiles, footwear, or electronics manufacturing in export processing zones,[5] women may account for as much as 70% to 90% of the workforce (Romero, 1995). Whether this trend is beneficial to women is much debated. Poor or dangerous working conditions in export manufacturing jobs have been widely reported, including in articles in the popular press. There is usually very little or no opportunity for advancement for women, and job turnover is very high. At the same time, these jobs usually represent an improvement over the alternatives currently available to women (Mehra and Gammage, 1999; Romero, 1995). Moreover, through the growth of such employment, globalization has reduced occupational and pay differentials of men and women (Tzannatos, 1999).[6]

While manufacturing employment may raise women's earnings, it is usually inflexible with regard to hours and incompatible with child supervision. Even where firms provide on-site child-care facilities, long daily commutes on crowded public transportation make it impractical for many women to take their children to these facilities. The difficulty of combining work and child-care responsibilities for women in modern manufacturing jobs is without doubt a major reason for the prevalence of young, unmarried (and childless) women in firms in export processing zones.[7] Frequently, however, the makeup of the workforce is due to outright discrimination in hiring. Many employers in export processing zones (as well as elsewhere in the formal economy) simply do not hire married women or women with children—or routinely dismiss women once they get married or become pregnant—to avoid the anticipated productivity losses associated with their domestic responsibilities (Pearson, 1995; Seguino, 1997). Others require pregnancy tests or even sterilization certificates. Hence, many women—or, in some cases, most women—are locked out of whatever benefits these jobs have to offer.

Critics of globalization argue that although the rise of women's manufacturing employment implies a significant formalization of female labor relative to women's previous activities, on a global scale it represents an *in*formalization (or feminization) of labor. International competition puts pressure on employers to keep labor costs low, leading them to replace male labor with cheaper and more "flexible" female labor (Standing, 1989, 1999). Similarly, to keep or attract business investment, governments are increasingly reluctant to intervene in the labor market to ensure job protection and other benefits typically associated with formal employment. This provides an explanation for an apparent countertrend in women's work: the informalization of female labor through outsourcing and subcontracting to home-based workers. This process is occurring in both developed and developing countries (Mehra and Gammage, 1999; Standing, 1999). Pay and benefits (if there are any) are low under these arrangements compared with those of employment in factories; with little or no job security offered to workers, employers gain significant flexibility.

Despite its disadvantages, it might seem that such home-based employment could at least ease the tensions between work and child care. However, the implications for children are not necessarily positive. This work is essentially industrial activity carried out in the home (Floro, 1995). Children are potentially exposed to hazardous or toxic materials not associated with more traditional forms of income-generating activity in the home. They are also likely to be put to work helping their mothers with their jobs, increasing the risks to their health and safety. Working in isolation, women are not likely to gain empowerment from their work, which may limit the benefits accruing to children from their income. The actual effects of home-based subcontracting work on child welfare remain largely unknown, however, and deserve further study.

It is important to note that the majority of the population of the developing world still lives in rural areas, and these areas are also being affected by globalization. The agricultural sector experiences structural changes with development and greater integration into the world economy, and these changes have implications for work and children. For example, large-scale mechanized agriculture employing a wage labor force reduces compatibilities between work and child care compared with work on small family farms. Even in the context of the family farm, commercialization can have important implications for men's and women's time allocation and incomes, with ramifications for child welfare. Commercialization shifts household labor from subsistence crop farming, which in many contexts is traditionally under women's control, to cash cropping, the income from which is more likely to be under their husbands' control. This shift in the control of family income may blunt the benefits to children from the increases in household income resulting from the turn to market-oriented production.[8]

Policies to Reduce Conflicts between Women's Dual Roles

The trends outlined in the previous section heighten the importance of policies to address the conflicts women face between their need to generate family income and their need to ensure their children's well-being. Taking center stage in the policy discussion is the provision of decent child-care services for working women. Recent research makes it clear that decent child care entails more than simply child minding and feeding; it includes other activities necessary for a child's development, such as engaging the child in social interaction that fosters cognitive and social development (CGECCD, 1993; Martorell, 1996; Myers, 2000).

The potential benefits of publicly supported child care are numerous. The most compelling one is the benefit to children themselves in situations where mothers must work yet cannot afford adequate care. Accessible child care can reduce nutritional risks to children who otherwise would either receive inferior care in the home (for example, from older children) or have to accompany their mothers to work. Further, recent longitudinal evidence from developing countries has indicated that well-designed early childhood care and development programs have significant long-term benefits for primary school enrollment and academic performance via preschool effects on physical and mental growth (Myers, 1995; Young, 1996). Moreover, the most disadvantaged children appear to experience the largest gains, because these programs supply aspects of care that wealthier parents can provide on their own but poor parents cannot (see Young, 1996, and references therein). By disproportionately improving the future schooling and productivity of poor children, these programs can reduce poverty and inequality in succeeding generations.

Also potentially benefiting from child-care programs are the older children of working mothers, since there will be less pressure on them to curtail their schooling to help out in the home. Since this burden falls much more strongly on girls than boys (see Glick, 2002, and references therein), the availability of subsidized child care will have the greatest benefits for girls' schooling, helping to reduce gender gaps in access to education. This, in turn, implies an efficiency rationale for such programs. From the perspective of the large social returns to educating girls (Strauss and Thomas, 1995), households are likely to underinvest in girls' schooling. This will likely hold true even if parents fully value such schooling. In principle, they could borrow money to pay for the child-care services that would free their daughters to attend school. However, poor households lack the collateral to obtain loans, and credit markets do not function in such a way as to enable them to borrow against the future earnings of their daughters. Subsidized child care can therefore be viewed as a substitute for a poorly functioning credit market or, alternatively, as a form of public investment in girls' education.

Of course, women themselves also benefit from access to subsidized child care, since it reduces their total burden of productive activities in the home and the market. As noted earlier, women who enter the labor force continue to provide substantial amounts of child care and other household work, at the expense of their leisure time as well as their physical and emotional well-being. Case studies of developing countries usually show that, on average (even counting women who are not employed), women's total hours of work on the job and at home exceed those of men, who do much less in the home (UN, 1995). Therefore, an additional rationale for publicly supported child care is that it will lead to greater gender equity in the overall burden of work by spreading the burden of care over the entire society (male and female) through the taxes used to finance the service. Gender equity is also served in a broader sense in that women gain greater choices over their own lives. A handful of studies on developing countries have shown that women's labor force participation responds positively to reductions in the cost of child care (see Lokshin, Glinskaya, and Garcia, 2000, and references therein).

Reducing the domestic work obligation of women is not merely a matter of fairness but also of economic efficiency. Palmer (1991) characterizes this obligation as a *reproduction labor tax* that distorts the allocation of labor in the economy. Rather than a monetary tax, the tax is extracted in the form of the labor of women, who are obligated by social norms to spend a given amount of their time in domestic work. In standard microeconomic theory, allocative efficiency requires that a factor of production such as labor be allocated to different activities so that its productivity at the margin (the output that could be produced by an additional hour of work) is the same in each activity. When women are constrained to spend a given amount of their time in domestic activities, they are unable to allocate their labor between these and market-oriented activities so as to satisfy the efficiency condition. As a result, for many women, marginal productivity will be higher in market work. Their labor will thus be misallocated: it will be undersupplied to the market economy and oversupplied to domestic work. Public policies that increase the accessibility of child care give women greater flexibility in allocating their productive labor across different activities, thus potentially increasing economic efficiency. Instead of imposing the costs of child care directly on women's time, such policies spread the costs over society by financing the service from general taxes on incomes or profits.

Despite the impressive range of potential benefits of child-care services, the provision of these services in developing countries lags well behind the increasing need. A small but growing number of countries, particularly in Latin America and Southeast Asia, have formulated national child-care or work-family policies. Moreover, throughout the developing world, there has been a major growth in early child development interventions (CGECCD, 1993). The problem is the inadequate coverage of these interventions, many of which have not been expanded beyond the pilot program stage (Young, 1996).[9]

Where child-care programs are available, they are frequently limited in that they tend to be focused on "older" children, such as those aged 3 to 6 years (Himes, Landers, and Leslie, 1992). Often this is because the function of these programs is seen as preparation for school. Another reason is the traditional belief that mothers should be with their children during their initial years. Yet the empirical evidence discussed in this chapter indicates that to the extent that nutritional risks to children of working mothers exist, they will be greatest for very young children. Together with evidence of the benefits to this age group of early childhood care and development interventions, this strongly suggests that existing programs need to be reoriented to serve mothers of newborns to 3-year-olds in addition to those with older children.[10] Another shortcoming of many current programs is that they are not set up to take children for the entire day, a reflection again of a focus on early education rather than child care. This obviously limits their usefulness to working women.

Government-supported child care (where it exists) takes many forms across the world. Although this chapter is not the place to review the range of existing policies and programs, a few points can be noted. As Cochran (1993) emphasized in his review of 29 country case studies, the cultural and political contexts, including attitudes toward government and the family, are key factors shaping child-care programs. They will determine the private–public mix as well as the nature of the providers, such as informal family-based care or formal center-based care. Many successful urban programs in the developing world involve informal care, whereby the government trains and partially subsidizes a private provider, usually a woman from the neighborhood working out of her home (Ruel, Hadad, and Garrett, 1999). These approaches are significantly cheaper than formal care centers, and they also may make it is easier to get parents and the community to contribute their own time and money. An effective large-scale application of the home-based approach is the Colombian Community Childcare and Nutrition Project, which was serving 800,000 children 28 months after it was initiated (Evans, 1995a). Another practical strategy, particularly helpful to women in the informal sector, is the setting up of mobile crèches (child-care facilities) near women's worksites. India's mobile crèche system, for example, was designed to serve women in the construction industry. This approach has broad applications to agriculture, where temporary crèches can be used to serve women engaged in harvesting work.

In some developing countries in which there has been national legislation on child care, individual firms are required by law to provide child care to their employees. For the government, this holds obvious appeal from a fiscal point of view, but it has well-known disadvantages compared with public financing. It depends on enforcement, which is usually inadequate or nonexistent. The beneficiaries are likely to be limited to employees of large formal sector firms. To the extent that the legislation is enforced, it raises the costs to firms of employing women relative to men and hence acts as a disincentive to hiring women. In contrast, public financing of child-care services from taxes (on individuals or firms) ensures access for all women, including those who are self-employed or in informal sector wage work, and does not create a hiring disincentive. This principle—endorsed by the International Labor Organization (ILO), among others—extends to other forms of work-family benefits, such as maternity or parental leave. Successful public financing schemes usually avoid reliance on unstable general tax revenues and instead set up a special national fund for child-care programs to which employers and individuals contribute. Variants of this approach are in operation in a number of Latin American countries. In Colombia, for example, the main early child development program is financed through a 3% payroll tax (Waiser, 1998).

Finally, given resource constraints, it may be necessary to target services to women and children who are most in need or for whom nutritional risks are thought most likely to be present. Based on the evidence reviewed in this chapter, this group would include women with infants who must work to support their families, working mothers more generally with very low incomes, and female heads of households. One means of reaching these women (in lieu of administratively difficult individual means testing) would be to target poor neighborhoods by funding service providers in these neighborhoods, as was done, for example, in Mexico's Initial Education Project (Young, 1996).

Among other policies, greater flexibility in work schedules for full-time employees also will potentially benefit both working women and their children. Flextime eases the problem of employer disincentives to hiring women because it does not reduce the total hours of work; instead, it reallocates them over the work day or week. The applicability of flextime to the developing world will probably be restricted because these arrangements are characteristic of formal sector work and often are limited to white-collar occupations. Even given these limits, however, flextime has the potential to expand women's access to formal employment by making such employment easier to balance with child care.

Another policy implication drawn from existing research is that the benefits to children of women's employment may be small if women cannot control how their earnings are spent. Public policy can indirectly affect the balance of power in household decision making and control over resources. Legislation that guarantees women's rights to own and inherit property, that makes divorce and child support easier to obtain, and that provides social assistance to female-headed households will increase a woman's options outside of her marriage, raising her bargaining power within the relationship. Compelling arguments for many of these policies are usually made on the grounds of gender equity. By enhancing a woman's power to determine the allocation of household resources—in particular, her own labor earnings—these policies have the additional advantage of increasing the complementarities of women's work and child welfare.

Even where women do have control over what they earn, the benefits to children are limited by the simple fact that women's earnings are low, and low relative to men's. Significant gender differentials in pay in the developing world persist, though as noted earlier, they appear to be narrowing. Legal measures to reduce gender discrimination in earnings or in access to better-paying occupations will raise women's incomes, helping them to achieve economic parity with men and potentially indirectly benefiting children's health and education. The same applies to programs such as microcredit schemes that target women's self-employment earnings.

Note, however, that while measures to improve women's labor market incentives have the potential to increase children's welfare, they can be expected to raise the participation or labor supply of women, not just their hourly earnings. This will tend to exacerbate the tension between the demands of work and child care, increasing the time stresses on women and potentially limiting the nutritional and other benefits to children. As Leslie and Buvinic (1989) pointed out, programs targeting women's livelihoods have often failed to recognize this dilemma. Therefore, it is important that improvements in incentives for women, while obviously laudable in their own right, be accompanied by measures that address the concomitant increase in the need for child care.

The foregoing policy recommendations are in the spirit of the comprehensive platforms advocated by organizations such as the ILO and the United Nations Commission on the Status of Women. The ILO's *Decent Work for Women* (1996), for example, calls for pay equity and work-family measures including job flexibility, the provision of child-care services, and family leave. However, at the same time that issues of gender equity and work–family balance have been receiving greater international attention, economic globalization and its attendant premium on international competitiveness have discouraged new policies affecting labor markets and social protection. So, too, has the process of economic reform and structural adjustment occurring in many developing countries. The trend has thus been in the opposite direction, toward deregulation of labor markets and downsizing of public sectors.

In the globalized economy, any country that attempts to intervene singly against this trend will find itself at a disadvantage to the extent that its policies raise local labor costs relative to those elsewhere, since this will reduce the relative profitability of exporting and import-competing firms operating within its borders. Firms with a high degree of international mobility, especially foreign enterprises in export processing zones, will move on if they find the costs sufficiently burdensome. On the other hand, if all countries were to act in concert to implement similar policies, none would suffer a relative disadvantage (see Chapter 12 by Elliott and Freeman).

This *collective action dilemma* is usually discussed in the context of direct labor market interventions such as minimum wage legislation. However, it also applies, in principle, to work-family measures such as child-care provision, even when these measures are financed out of public revenues rather than imposed on employers. As noted earlier, this strategy is preferable to mandating that individual firms provide the services as part of employee compensation. In addition to avoiding disincentives specifically to hiring women, a more general aspect of public financing of such services is that it avoids having to raise firms' labor costs; hence it would seem to have no negative implications for international competitiveness. However, the revenue for public programs must come from somewhere. Optimally, both individual workers and firms would contribute, the latter through taxes on profits. The problem governments now face is that globalization is increasing the international mobility of both capital and skilled labor. With more firms and people having the option of moving elsewhere in response to higher taxes, governments are finding it harder to raise revenues to finance social programs (Lee, 1997; Tanzi and Chu, 2000). Indeed, low taxes are one of the main inducements offered by governments to attract firms to export processing zones. A country acting in isolation to finance new programs through an increase in taxes thus incurs a competitive disadvantage; the collective action dilemma remains.

Of course, the extent of the problem will be a function of the size—and, hence, cost—of the social programs envisaged. If child care were just one of a range of services to be provided under comprehensive programs for social protection or work–family balance, this would imply for many countries the need for nontrivial increases in public resources, possibly leading to resistance or flight on the part of capital and labor.[11] It is hard to say to what extent these types of considerations are preventing more effective work-family policies from being instituted in developing countries, but certainly advocates of such policies need to be aware of the issue. In principle, international coordination of policy to get around the collective action problem, which has been advocated in regard to core labor standards (Lee, 1997), is relevant as well for work-family policies.

Changing Gender Norms

Finally, the policies discussed so far have largely taken as given existing gender roles within the household, under which the care of children is the responsibility solely or primarily of women or girls. But social norms regarding gender roles should not be regarded as unchangeable. In the past decade, coordinated international efforts have begun to address this issue in developing countries. Most visibly, the 1994 United Nations International Conference on Population and Development emphasized the need to promote men's shared responsibility for parenthood. As yet, however, there are few examples of programs directed at fathers in developing countries. Advocates of such approaches stress the need to increase fathers' roles in caring for children, especially young children, and to increase their financial support for their children, whether or not they live with them (see, for example, Engle and Breaux, 1998).

If the experience of industrialized countries is any guide, real changes in male attitudes and behavior will take time. In most of these countries, changes in the time contributions of fathers to child care and other domestic work have lagged well behind the rhetoric (Evans, 1995b). Among the few studies of fathers and their children in developing countries are two described by Engle and Breaux (1994) for urbanizing West Africa and China. In the first case, pressures on men for greater financial success reduced the (already little) time traditionally spent with their children. In the second, in contrast, urbanization seems to have increased expectations of closer relations of fathers with their children.

These examples suggest that certain aspects of the development process may act to weaken—or possibly strengthen—the ties (both of time and of income) of fathers to their children. There are a number of forces serving to weaken traditional ties. Gender-selective migration to cities separates men from their children, as does an increased prevalence of divorce. As economies move away from subsistence agriculture to wage employment, men become more subject to unemployment due to national or even international economic cycles. In the extreme, this affects not just income but family cohesion itself, since the likelihood of family abandonment rises when fathers are unemployed (Brown, Broomfield, and Ellis, 1994; Katzman, 1992).

On the other hand, development can lead to favorable transformations in the priorities and expectations of fathers through improvements in income and education, as well as through exposure to alternative role models in the mass media (Engle and Breaux, 1994). Investing in education—and altering curricula to promote different perspectives of family roles while doing so—as well as exploiting the mass media, are means by which public policy can speed up these changes. It is also possible to change priorities more directly by providing financial incentives (or removing disincentives). One example, at least in principle, is the greater flexibility in work schedules, or flextime arrangements, mentioned earlier. If these workplace policies do not entail interruptions in employment or risks to career advancement, they will make it less costly for fathers to assume a larger role in the care of their children. A parental leave policy that is gender neutral and not perceived as damaging to job seniority or status may have the same effect.

Notes

1. Although this chapter, like most of the empirical literature, focuses on children's nutrition, women's work may also have significant impacts on their schooling. For schooling, there is a similar expectation of positive income effects and (for girls especially) negative time-

related effects, the latter due to substitution for the mother in household work. These issues and the available evidence are discussed at length in Glick (2002).

2. In some cases, occupation variables are included in regressions that lack controls for the level of household resources (see, e.g., Engle and Pederson, 1989). In these cases, the estimated effects of occupation are likely capturing differences in income, not just variation in the compatibility of work and child care.

3. It would clearly be incorrect to presume a negative effect of work on women's health, given that work can also improve health by providing income for higher consumption of food or medical care. For many women, this compensates for work-related stresses and energy demands. Research conducted primarily in industrialized countries finds a positive association between employment and health for both women and men (see Ross and Mirowsky, 1995, and references therein).

4. Family size in the developing world has been declining for other reasons as well, such as gender-specific migration (discussed later) and reductions in fertility.

5. Export processing zones are enclaves set up outside a country's normal customs barriers to attract foreign investment. The inducements include exemption from duties on imported intermediate inputs, as well as lower corporate taxes and less regulation than in the normal economy (ILO/UNTC, 1988).

6. This is not an uncontested view; see Joekes (1995). Also, as countries move up the technological ladder, the demand for skilled labor rises, putting women at a relative disadvantage unless they are given equal access to training or education. This may be a factor behind reversals in the trend to close the earnings or occupation gender gaps in countries such as Taiwan and Mexico (Pearson, 1995; Seguino, 1997).

7. Another explanation, offered in the Southeast Asian context, is that such employment is regarded by families as a short-term strategy for generating income from daughters before they are married off (Greenhalgh, 1985; Salaf, 1990). Alternatively, the work may simply be too physically stressful for long-term employment.

8. This is one possible explanation of the finding of Braun and Kennedy (1994) that even though increased cash cropping raised household incomes in a range of country settings, the benefits to child nutrition were quite modest.

9. It is estimated that only 1% of mothers in developing countries get help in raising their infants beyond that provided by family and friends (Young, 1996).

10. Generous maternal or parental leave policies can substitute for publicly provided infant care, as happened in Sweden (Gunnarsson, 1993). However, in developing countries, such a policy would not reach poor women unless they were in formal employment.

11. With respect to child care specifically, estimates of the costs of scaled-up public provision vary enormously, depending on the type of service (formal vs. informal, comprehensive child development programs vs. largely custodial services, etc.) and coverage (e.g., poor women only vs. all women). See Waiser (1998) and Barnett (1997).

References

Abbi, R., P. Christian, S. Gujral, and T. Gopaldas. 1991. The impact of maternal work status on the nutrition and health status of children. *Food and Nutrition Bulletin* 113(1): 20–25.

Acharya, M., and L. Bennett. 1982. Women and the subsistence sector: Economic participation and household decision-making in Nepal. World Bank staff working paper no. 526. Washington, D.C.: World Bank.

Adelman, C. 1983. An analysis of the effect of maternal care and other factors affecting growth of poor children in Lima, Peru. D.Sc. thesis, School of Hygiene and Public Health, Johns Hopkins University, Baltimore, MD.

Anandalakshmy, S., ed. 1994. *The girl child and the family. An action research study.* Delhi: Department of Women and Child Development, Ministry of Human Resource Development, Government of India.

Argawal, B. 1986. Women, poverty, and agricultural growth in India. *Journal of Peasant Studies* 13(4): 165–220.

Bamji, M., and B. V. S. Thimayamma. 2000. Impact of women's work on maternal and child nutrition. *Ecology of Food and Nutrition* 39: 13–31.

Barnett, W. S. 1997. Costs and financing of early child development programs. In *Early child development: Investing in our children's future,* edited by M. E. Young. New York: Elsevier.

Becker, C., A. Jamer, and A. Morrison. 1994. *Beyond urban bias in Africa: Urbanization in an era of structural adjustment.* Portsmouth, NH: Heinemann.

Bittencourt, S., and E. DiCicco. 1979. *Child care needs of low-income women: Urban Brazil.* Washington, D.C.: Overseas Education Fund of the League of Women Voters.

Blau, D. M., D. K. Guilkey, and B. M. Popkin. 1996. Infant health and the labor supply of mothers. *Journal of Human Resources* 31(1): 90–139.

Blumberg, R. L. 1988. Income under female versus male control. *Journal of Family Issues* 9: 51–84 .

Braun, J., and E. Kennedy, eds. 1994. *Agricultural commercialization, economic development, and nutrition.* Baltimore, MD: Johns Hopkins University Press.

Brown, J., R. Broomfield, and O. Ellis. 1994. *Men and their families: Contributions of Caribbean men to family life.* Kingston, Jamaica: Child Care and Development Centre.

Brown, L., Y. Johannes, and P. Webb. 1994. Rural labor-intensive public works: Impacts of participation on preschooler nutrition: Evidence from Niger. *American Journal of Agricultural Economics* 76(5): 1213–18.

Bunster, X. 1983. Market sellers in Lima, Perú: Talking about work. In *Women and poverty in the third world,* edited by M. Buvinic, M. A. Lycette, and W. P. McGreevey. Baltimore, MD: Johns Hopkins University Press.

Cerón-Mireles, P., C. Sánchez-Carrillo, S. D. Harlow, and R. Núñez-Urquiza. 1997. Maternal working conditions and low birth weight in Mexico City. *Salud Publica de Mexico,* 39(1): 2–10.

Chutikul, S. 1986. Malnourished children: An economic approach to the causes and consequences in rural Thailand. East–West Population Institute paper no. 102. Honolulu, HI: East–West Center.

Cochran, M. 1993. *Public child care, culture, and society: Crosscutting themes.* In *International handbook of childcare policies and programs,* edited by M. Cochran. Westport, CT: Greenwood Press.

Consultative Group on Early Childhood Care and Development (CGECCD). 1993. Towards a comprehensive strategy for the development of the young child: An inter-agency policy review. Available at http://www.ecdgroup.com

Cornia, G. A. 1984. A survey of cross-sectional and time-series literature on factors affecting child welfare. *World Development* (special issue, The Impact of World Recession on Children) 12(3): 187–202.

Doan, R. M., and B. M. Popkin. 1993. Women's work and infant care in the Philippines. *Social Science and Medicine* 36: 297–304.

Engle, P. L. 1991. Maternal work for earnings and childcare strategies: Nutritional effects. *Child Development* 62: 954–65.

Engle, P. L. 1993. Influences of mother's and father's income on children's nutritional status in Guatemala. *Social Science and Medicine* 37(11): 1303–12.

Engle, P. L., and C. Breaux. 1994. *Is there a father instinct? Fathers' responsibility for children.* New York: The Population Council.

Engle, P. L., and C. Breaux. 1998. *Fathers' involvement with children: Perspectives from developing countries.* Social Policy Report. *Society for Research in Child Development* 12(1).

Engle, P. L., P. Menon, and L. Haddad. 1999. Care and nutrition: Concepts and measurement. *World Development* 27(8): 1309–37.

Engle, P. L., and M. E. Pedersen. 1989. Maternal work for earnings and children's nutritional status in urban Guatemala. *Ecology of Food and Nutrition* 22: 211–23.

Engle, P. L., M. E. Pedersen, and R. Schmidt. 1985. The effects of maternal employment on children's nutritional status and school participation in rural and urbanizing Guatemala. Washington, D.C.: Report prepared for USAID.

Evans, J. 1995a. *Childcare programmes as an entry point for maternal and child health components of primary health care.* Geneva: Maternal and Child Health and Family Planning Division of Family Health, World Health Organization.

Evans, J. 1995b. *Men in the lives of children.* Coordinator's Notebook no. 16, Consultative Group on Early Childhood Care and Development. Available at http://www.ecdgroup.com

Fapohunda, E. 1988. *The nonpooling household: A challenge to theory.* In *A home divided: Women and income in the third world,* edited by D. Dwyer and J. Bruce. Stanford, CA: Stanford University Press.

Floro, M. S. 1995. Economic restructuring, gender and the allocation of time. *World Development* 23(11): 1913–29.

Franklin, D. 1979. *Malnutrition and poverty: The role of mother's time and abilities.* Chapel Hill, NC: Economics Department, Research Triangle Institute.

Glick, P. 2002. Women's work and its relation to children's health and schooling in developing countries: Conceptual links, empirical evidence, and policies. Cornell Food and Nutrition Policy Program Working Paper no. 131. Available at http://www.he.cornell.edu/cfnpp

Glick, P., and D. Sahn. 1997. Gender and education impacts on employment and earnings in a developing country: The case of Guinea. *Economic Development and Cultural Change* 45(4): 793–823.

Glick, P., and D. Sahn. 1998. Maternal labor supply and child nutrition in West Africa. *Oxford Bulletin of Economics and Statistics* 60(3): 325–55.

Greenhalgh, S. 1985. Sexual stratification: The other side of "growth with equity" in East Asia. *Population and Development Review* 11(2): 265–314.

Gryboski, K. L. 1996. Maternal and non-maternal time-allocation to infant care, and care during infant illness in rural Java, Indonesia. *Social Science and Medicine* 43(2): 209–19.

Gunnarsson, L. 1993. Sweden. In *International handbook of childcare policies and programs,* edited by M. Cochran. Westport, CT: Greenwood Press.

Haddad, L., M. T. Ruel, and J. A. L. Garrett. 1999. Are urban poverty and undernutrition growing? Some newly assembled evidence. *World Development* 27(11): 1891–1904.

Haggerty, P. 1981. Women's work and child nutrition in Haiti. Master's thesis. Massachusetts Institute of Technology, Cambridge, MA.

Hernandez-Pena, P., M. D. L. Kageyama, I. Coria, B. Hernandez, and S. Harlow. 1999. Working conditions, labor fatigue and low birth weight among female street vendors. *Salud Publica de Mexico* 41(2): 101–9.

Himes, J., C. Landers, and J. Leslie. 1992. *Women, work, and child care.* Innocenti Global Seminar Report. Florence: UNICEF/ICDC.

Hoddinott, J., and L. Haddad. 1994. Women's income and boy–girl anthropometric status in the Côte d'Ivoire. *World Development* 22(4): 543–53.

Hoffman, L. W. 1989. Effects of maternal employment in the two-parent family. *American Psychologist* 44: 283–92.

Holmboe-Ottsen, G., O. Mascarenhas, and W. Wandel. 1988. Women's role in food production and nutrition: Implications for their quality of life. *Food and Nutrition Bulletin* 10(3): 8–15.

Horton, S. 1999. Marginalization revisited: Women's work and pay, and economic development. *World Development* 27(3): 571–82.

International Labor Organization/United Nations Center on Transnational Corporations (ILO/UNTC). 1988. *Economic and social effects of multinational enterprises in export processing zones.* Geneva: ILO/UNTC.

International Labor Organization (ILO). 1996. *Decent work for women: An ILO proposal to accelerate the implementation of the Beijing Platform for Action.* Geneva: ILO.

Ishii-Kuntz, M. 1995. *Paternal involvement and perception toward father's roles: A comparison between Japan and United States.* In *Fatherhood: Contemporary theory, research and social policy,* edited by W. Marsiglio. Thousand Oaks, CA.: Sage.

Joekes, S. 1989. Women's work and social support for childcare in the third world. In *Women, work, and child welfare in the third world,* edited by J. Leslie and M. Paolisso. Boulder, CO: Westview Press.

Joekes, S. 1995. Trade-related employment for women in industry and services in developing countries. Occasional paper no. 9. Geneva: United Nations Research Institute for Social Development.

Katzman, R. 1992. Why are men so irresponsible? *Cepal Review* 26: 45–87.

Kumar, S. 1978. Role of the household economy in determining child nutrition at low income levels: A case study in Kerala. Occasional paper no. 95. Ithaca, NY: Department of Agricultural Economics, Cornell University.

Lamontagne, J. F., P. L. Engle, and M. F. Zeitlin. 1998. Maternal employment, child care, and nutritional status of 12- to 18-month-old children in Managua, Nicaragua. *Social Science and Medicine* 46(3): 403–14.

Lee, E. 1997. Globalization and labour standards: A review of issues. *International Labour Review* 136(2): 173–89.

Leslie, J. 1989. Women's work and child nutrition in the third world. In *Women, work, and child welfare in the third world,* edited by J. Leslie and M. Paolisso. Boulder, CO: Westview Press.

Leslie, J., and M. Buvinic. 1989. Introduction. In *Women, work, and child welfare in the third world,* edited by J. Leslie and M. Paolisso. Boulder, CO: Westview Press.

Lokshin, M., E. Glinskaya, and M. Garcia. 2000. The effect of early childhood development programs on women's labor force participation and older children's schooling in Kenya. Gender and Development working paper series no. 15. Washington, D.C.: World Bank.

Martorell, R. 1996. Undernutrition during pregnancy and early childhood and its consequences for behavioral development. Paper prepared for World Bank conference, Early Child Development: Investing in the Future, April 8–9, Washington, D.C.

Mehra, R., and S. Gammage. 1999. Trends, countertrends, and gaps in women's employment. *World Development* 27(3): 533–50.

Munachonga, M. 1988. Income allocation and marriage options in urban Zambia. In *A home divided: Women and income in the third world,* edited by D. Dwyer and J. Bruce. Stanford, CA: Stanford University Press.

Myers, R. 1995. *The twelve who survive: Strengthening programmes of early childhood development in the third world.* London: Routledge.

Myers, R. 2000. Thoughts on the role of the "private sector" in early childhood. Paper prepared for the Year 2000 Conference on Early Childhood Development, Investing in Our Children's Future—from Science to Public Policy. Washington, D.C.: World Bank.

Nieves, I. 1981. A balancing act: Strategies to cope with work and motherhood in developing countries. Paper presented at the ICRW policy round table, The Interface between Poor Women's Nurturing Roles and Productive Responsibilities, International Center for Research on Women, December, Washington, D.C.

Olmsted, P. P., and D. P. Weikart, eds. 1995. *Families speak. Early childhood care and education in eleven countries.* Ypsilanti, MI: High/Scope Press.

Overseas Education Fund. 1979. *Child care needs of low income mothers in less developed countries: A summary report of research in six countries in Asia and Latin America (Korea, Malaysia, Sri Lanka, Brazil, Dominican Republic, Perú).* Washington, D.C.: Overseas Education Fund, League of Women Voters.

Palmer, I. 1991. *Gender and population in the adjustment of African economies.* Geneva: International Labor Organization.

Pearson, R. 1995. Male bias and women's work in Mexico's border industries. In *Male bias in the development process,* edited by D. Elson. Manchester, UK: Manchester University Press.

Popkin, B. 1980. Time allocation of the mother and child nutrition. *Ecology of Food and Nutrition* 9: 1–14.

Popkin, B. 1983. Rural women, work, and child welfare in the Philippines. In *Women and poverty in the third world,* edited by M. Buvinic, M. A. Lycette, and W. P. McGreevey. Baltimore, MD: Johns Hopkins University Press.

Rabiee, F., and C. Geissler. 1992. The impact of maternal workload on child nutrition in rural Iran. *Food and Nutrition Bulletin* 14(1): 43–48.

Rahmanidfar, A., A. Kirksey, T. D. Wachs, G. McCabe, Z. Bishry, O. M. Galal, G. G. Harrison, and N. W. Jerome. 1992. Diet during lactation associated with infant behavior and caregiver interaction in a semi-rural Egyptian village. *Journal of Nutrition* 123(21): 164–75.

Romero, A. T. 1995. Labour standards and export processing zones: Situation and pressures for change. *Development Policy Review* 13(3): 247–76.

Ross, C., and J. Mirowsky. 1995. Does employment affect health? *Journal of Health and Social Behavior* 36(3): 320–343.

Rossi, A. S. 1983. Gender and parenthood. *American Sociological Review* 49: 1–18.

Ruel, M. T., L. Haddad, and J. L. Garrett. 1999. Some urban facts of life: Implications for research and policy. *World Development* 27(11): 1917–38.

Salaf, J. 1990. Women, the family, and the state: Hong Kong, Taiwan, Singapore—newly industrialized countries in Asia. In *Women, employment and the family in the international division of labour,* edited by S. Stichter and J. L. Papart. Philadelphia: Temple University Press.

Seguino, S. 1997. Export-led growth and the persistence of gender inequality in the newly industrialized economies. In *Economic dimensions of gender inequality,* edited by J. Rives and M. Youseif. Westport, CT: Prager.

Shah, P. M., S. R. Walimbe, and V. S. Dhole. 1979. Wage-earning mothers, mother-substitutes, and care of the young children in rural Maharashtra. *Indian Pediatrics* 16(2): 167–73.

Smith, M., S. Paulsen, W. Fougere, and S. J. Ritchkey. 1980. Socioeconomics, education, and health factors influencing growth of rural Haitian children. *Ecology of Food and Nutrition* 13: 99–108.

Soekirman, 1985. Women's work and its effect on infants' nutritional status in Central Java, Indonesia. Paper presented at the Colloquium on Adequacy of Breast-feeding and Maternal Nutrition Status, 13th International Congress of Nutrition, August 18–23, Brighton, United Kingdom.

Standing, G. 1989. Global feminization through flexible labor. *World Development* 17(7): 1077–95.

Standing, G. 1999. Global feminization through flexible labor: A theme revisited. *World Development* 27(2): 583–602.

Standing, H. 1991. *Dependency and autonomy: Women's employment and the family in Calcutta.* London: Routledge.

Strauss, J., and D. Thomas. 1995. *Human resources: Empirical modeling of household and family decisions.* In *Handbook of development economics,* vol. 3, edited by T. N. Srinivasan and J. Behrman. Amsterdam: North-Holland.

Tanzi, V., and K. Chu. 2000. Social protection in a globalizing world: The role of the international community. Paper presented at the Rockefeller and Russell Sage Foundations Conference on Welfare State Policies in Emerging Market Economies, March, New York.

Tucker, K., and D. Sanjur. 1988. Maternal employment and child nutrition in Panama. *Social Science and Medicine* 26: 605–12.

Tzannatos, Z. 1999. Women and labor market changes in the global economy: Growth helps, inequalities hurt and public policy matters. *World Development* 27(3): 551–69.

United Nations (UN). 1995. *World's women 1995: Trends and statistics.* New York: UN.

United Nations Development Programme (UNDP). 1995. *Human development report.* New York: Oxford University Press.

Verbrugge, L. M. 1983. Multiple roles and physical health of women and men. *Journal of Health and Social Behavior* 24(1): 16–30.

Vial, L., and E. Muchnik. 1989. Women's market work, infant feeding practices, and infant nutrition among low-income women in Santiago, Chile. In *Women, work, and child welfare in the third world,* edited by J. Leslie and M. Paolisso. Boulder, CO: Westview Press.

Waiser, M. 1998. Early childhood care and development programs on Latin America: How much do they cost? LCSHD paper series no. 19, Latin America and the Caribbean Regional Office, Human Development Department, World Bank, Washington, D.C.

Wandel, M., and G. Holmboe-Ottesen. 1992. Maternal work, child feeding, and nutrition in rural Tanzania. *Food and Nutrition Bulletin* 14(1): 49–54.

Wolfe, B., and J. Behrman. 1982. Determinants of child mortality, health, and nutrition in a developing country. *Journal of Development Economics* 11: 163–94.

Wolfe, B., and R. Haveman. 1983. Time allocation, market work, and changes in female health. *American Economic Review* 73(2): 134–39.

Young, M. E. 1996. *Early child development: Investing in the future.* Washington, D.C.: World Bank.

Zohir, S. C., and P. Paul-Majumder. 1996. *Garment workers in Bangladesh: Economic, social and health conditions.* Research monograph no. 18, Bangladesh Institute of Development, Dhaka, Bangladesh.

Part III

The Relationship between Work and Population Health

7

Wage Poverty, Earned Income Inequality, and Health

S. V. SUBRAMANIAN AND ICHIRO KAWACHI

Economic disparity, defined primarily in terms of income and earnings inequalities, has been a persistent worldwide problem and a potential threat to the growth of nations. This problem has become of increasing concern to policy makers and others for various reasons. Most importantly, there has been growing evidence that the process of globalization—which gained force throughout the 1980s and 1990s—is increasing income inequalities both between and within countries (Galbraith, 2002). While economic disparity has implications for economic growth and development, what has been shown in recent years is the plausible role that economic disparity plays in shaping population health patterns and inequalities.

In this chapter, we review the evidence on international trends in income and earnings inequalities, their causes, and their potential consequences for population health. We first discuss the concept of income inequality and argue for the need to adopt a global perspective on this issue. We then describe trends in the world income distribution and review the different explanations that have been advanced to account for growing earnings differentials, focusing on the United States as a case example. We conclude by discussing the evidence that has linked income inequality to population health, the research on the social costs of economic disparities, and the implications of the available evidence regarding the world's rising income inequality, especially as it relates to health issues.

The Nature of Income Inequality

In the 1950s, Kuznets (1955) famously advanced the "*U-curve hypothesis*" of the relationship between economic growth and income inequality. Kuznets focused on the shifts in population in different sectors of the economy (e.g., agricultural/primary to manufacturing/secondary to service/tertiary) as a defining characteristic of the development process. The assumptions were, first, that the rural population's average per capita income is typically lower than the urban population's and, second, that income inequality is somewhat less pronounced in the rural population than in the urban one. Based on these assumptions, Kuznets postulated that, all other conditions being equal, a rise in the urban population means an increasing share for the more unequal of the two distributions, and that the distribution of per capita income tends to widen when per capita productivity in urban areas increases more rapidly than in the rural (agricultural) sector. Kuznets also postulated that a turning point would be reached at which inequality would eventually start decreasing with further development. Kuznets's analysis of longitudinal data for England, Germany, and the United States suggested eventual declining inequality with increasing per capita income.

Contrary to Kuznets's predictions, however, high levels of income disparity have persisted in many economically developed countries, and in many cases they have actually widened in the past 30 years. Increasing inequality in the most developed countries during the 1980s and the explosion of inequality in transition economies (such as those of Eastern and Central Europe) during the 1990s have pushed the issue of economic inequality to the center stage of the macroeconomic agenda (Galbraith, 1998b, 2002). Recent research has begun to cast doubt on the so-called equality–growth trade-off. Indeed, a burgeoning economic literature has revealed a *negative* correlation between income inequality and economic growth in cross-national data (Alesina and Rodrik, 1992; Benabou, 1996; Glyn and Miliband, 1994; Li, Squire, and Zou, 1998). For example, Alesina and Rodrik (1992) found that national income growth rates in 65 countries were negatively related to the share of national income going to the top 20% of earners. By contrast, larger shares going to low- and middle-income groups were associated with higher rates of growth. Increasingly, therefore, distributional concerns have become essential aspects of the overall assessment of economic performance rather than simply add-on considerations once efficiency has been established (as have been characteristic of traditional macroeconomics).

Alongside the concern about inequalities for economic growth and development is the concern about poverty. While inequality and poverty may be related, it is important to appreciate the uniqueness of the two concepts. *Poverty* refers to a standard of living below some benchmark (typically referred to as the *poverty line*), whether defined in absolute or relative terms. The *absolute* poverty definition draws on Rowntree's classic concept of a *socially acceptable* amount of money required to achieve minimum physical efficiency (Rowntree, 1910). The absolute poverty approach has been adopted by a number of countries, including the United States (Citro and Michael, 1995). In contrast to the absolute approach to poverty assessment, the *relative* approach defines poverty in terms of relation to the standards that exist elsewhere in a society. For example, in the Luxembourg Income Study, poverty is measured as a proportion (less than 50%) of the average disposable income per capita (Smeeding, O'Higgins, and Rainwater, 1990). Examples of countries whose governments adopt a relative approach to assess poverty are Armenia and Nigeria. *Inequality*, on the other hand, is a broader term and is defined over the entire distribution, not just the distribution of individuals or households below the poverty line, regardless of whether such a line is defined in absolute or relative terms. The distinction between poverty and inequality is important because, first, evidence suggests that each is independently associated with levels of population health (Subramanian, Belli, and Kawachi, 2002) and, second, policies that reduce one may not necessarily reduce the other. For example, a policy of reducing the taxation of the rich may stimulate economic growth (at least according to supply-side arguments) and reduce the number of people below the poverty threshold, but the same policy may increase disparity in the distribution of income. Conversely, because the degree of equality of the income distribution does not indicate the likelihood that any particular group in the population can achieve a minimally acceptable standard of living, policies that redistribute income may have no effect on the poverty rate, especially the relative one. Our focus in this chapter is on income inequality as observed across the entire distribution.

The renewed interest in income inequality, however, should be placed within a broader perspective. As Sen (1992) points out, the relevance of income (in its aggregate and distributive dimensions) lies in its instrumental value in shaping, among other things, population health—again in its aggregate and distributive dimensions. There has been a rapid increase in the number of empirical studies on the impact of income inequality—independent of poverty levels—on health outcomes, such as morbidity or mortality or as a cause of violence. Thus, the social, political, and academic relevance of the study of income inequality cannot be emphasized enough, both in its own right and crucially in its impact on population well-being and health. It is with this motivation that we present the existing evidence on income inequality.

Income inequality can be studied at all levels—local, regional, national, and international. Most economic analyses of inequality have been located primarily *within* national boundaries. Nonetheless, as more national economies become integrated into the global economic framework, there is a compelling reason to understand income inequalities in their global dimension. The global dimension is particularly important, since much of the observed income inequality, both within and between countries, is driven by wage and pay disparities (Galbraith, Jiaqing, and Darity, 1999). Thus, underlying the income inequality issue is the concern with the distribution of pay: the economic, social, and political relationship between the well paid and poorly paid. Since determination of pay and wages is based on labor market dynamics, which in turn is open to global economic compulsions and fluctuations, the study of income distribution (at any level) needs to include the global determinants in its analytical framework. In the following section, we present some recent studies that have considered earned income distribution and overall income distribution at the international level. While the former focuses mainly on industrial earnings, the latter includes income from other sources. Overall income data have wider coverage, while earned income data are largely absent for very poor, developing, and politically unstable countries.

Earned and Overall Income Inequality: An International Perspective

According to data compiled by the United Nations Development Program, the richest country in the world in 1820 was Great Britain, with a gross domestic product (GDP) per capita of $1750 in 1990 dollars. At that time, the poorest country in the world was China (GDP per capita of $523). By 1997, the richest country in the world, Luxembourg, reported a per capita GDP of $30,863, while the poorest country in the world, Sierra Leone, had a *lower* level of GDP in real terms ($410) than the poorest country, China, had in 1820. Put another way, the income ratio between the richest and poorest countries increased from a three-fold difference in 1820 to a more than seventy-five-fold one a century and a half later (UNDP, 1999).

Drawing on Milanovic's work (1998), we offer a few examples to illustrate the extent of global inequalities between 1988 and 1993. An American earning the average income in the lowest U.S. decile was still better off than two-thirds of the rest of the world's population. The ratio between the average income of the world's top 5% and the bottom 5% had increased from 78:1 in 1988, to 114:1 in 1993. Sixteen percent of the world's population received 84% of the world's income in unadjusted dollar terms. The richest 1% of people in the world received as much income as the bottom 57%.

Such striking snapshots of global inequalities have been supplemented and extended through the approaches of other researchers. In their pioneering work, for instance, Deninger and Squire (1996) established a basis for examining world inequality trends. Essentially, they mined the economic development literature starting from 1950 for surveys of income inequality and evaluated each available data point across countries on three criteria: (*1*) that the focus was on households, (*2*) all forms of income, including in-kind income, were considered, and (*3*) rural as well as urban areas were covered. Since the data were published in 1996, they have been a standard reference for a comprehensive set of inequality estimates for the distribution of household income across countries and through time. However, other researchers have improved on Deninger and Squire's original work and have identified different patterns. For instance, Galbraith, Jiaqing, and Darity (1999) argued that most work on world income inequality, including Deninger and Squire's, had failed to take into account the globalization of wage inequality. Specifically, they argued that Gini coefficients,[1] a standard measure for evaluating income inequality (see Kakwani, Wagstaff, and Doorslaer, 1997, for more discussion), are typically based on household income (which may include nonearned sources of income), not on annual earnings or hourly wages. However, it is wages and earnings that bear the direct effects of economic globalization. Thus, a measure of inequality restricted to the income sources of wages and earnings is, arguably, better suited to yielding an understanding of international income inequalities from a global perspective. The measurement of inequality that they present is a chain-linked index of earnings updated annually for changes in the structure of employment as well as changes in relative per capita earnings (for details on this index see Galbraith, Jiaqing, and Darity, 1999).

Galbraith and colleagues (1999) analyzed industrial earnings data from 17 Asian, 14 South American and Caribbean, 6 European, and 9 African countries, as well as 21 member nations of the Organization for Economic Cooperation and Development (OECD). Industrial earning data are essentially data that provide information on the industrial classification of manufacturing establishments along with their total employment and total payroll. Sources that provide such data, among others, include the Annual Survey of Manufacturers for the United States, the OECD Structural Analysis Database, the Economic Commission for Latin America and the Caribbean (ECLAC) data on industrial structure, and the United Nations International Development Organization (UNIDO) Industrial Statistics Dataset. On that basis and through various reports, they summarized the following trends:

1. Many countries compressed their wage structure in the 1970s, but most experienced rising inequality in the 1980s. Only a few reduced inequality during the 1990s. The United States experienced consistently rising inequality in annual earnings throughout the entire period, though with hourly wage rates it appears that the rise in inequality peaked in the early 1980s (Galbraith, 1998b).
2. Countries that are rich and strongly social democratic generally succeeded in controlling their wage structure from the 1970s to the 1990s, irrespective of their trade patterns. Germany, the Scandinavian countries, the Netherlands, Austria, and Denmark were notable examples of countries that had experienced stable or declining wage inequality, or increases that were modest by historical and international standards.
3. Large developing economies that were not fully integrated into the global capital markets (such as India) also managed to check the rise in inequality during the 1980s and early 1990s.
4. Developing countries that liberalized and globalized (such as Argentina and the Philippines) were subjected to larger swings in inequality than countries that did not (such as India).
5. Trends in inequality were linked to the patterns of political change in Latin America between 1970 and 1995. Inequality surged following military coups in Chile, Argentina, and Uruguay; inequality also rose following the establishment of postmilitary "liberal" regimes (Peru). Stabilization plans tended to arrest the rise in inequality in Brazil and Mexico, but not enough to offset earlier increases (Galbraith and Garza-Cantu, 1998).
6. Following the collapse of the Soviet Union, inequality in Russia skyrocketed. The stable patterns of income distribution observed in Eastern and Central Europe during the 1970s and 1980s also rose sharply in the 1990s.
7. In Africa, inequality trends in Nigeria and Algeria followed oil prices, while in South Africa inequality rose sharply in the early 1970s and again following the

end of the apartheid regime in the early 1990s, possibly due to postapartheid political, social, and economic instability.

Kanbur and Lustig (2000), using standard inequality measures based on overall household income and covering 66 countries (based on the count in Table 7-1), evaluated countries on the basis of whether inequality had increased, decreased, or remained unchanged during the 1980s and 1990s. They also observed sharp upward movements in a number of countries, as indicated in Table 7–1. In 11 countries in which inequality had increased (see column 1), the Gini coefficient increased by 9 points in five countries, between 10 and 19 points in seven countries, and by more than 20 points in two countries.

As Kanbur and Lustig (2000) observed, large increases in inequality were found in countries with very different structural characteristics. For instance, inequality rose in countries that were traditionally egalitarian (Thailand), as well as in ones that were marked by high inequality (Mexico); in developed nations (the United States, the United Kingdom) and in poor countries (Panama, Ethiopia); in long-standing market economies (Hong Kong) and in countries in transition (Russia, China). It is important to note, however, that for a substantial number of equally diverse countries, inequality remained practically unchanged (Colombia, India, Japan, Morocco, and Sweden) and that it fell in a few (Bangladesh, Canada, Honduras, and Tunisia). What accounts for these differences?

The above studies, while international in their coverage, are not necessarily focused on the notion of world income inequality. What these studies show is how, in different countries, income inequality has changed over time. They do not evaluate the extent to which different countries play a role in shaping world income inequality. Few studies have looked at income inequality in this manner, and we now turn to a discussion of such studies. Milanovic (1998), in an extensive and novel study of world income inequality covering 84% of the world's population and 93% of the world's GDP, makes the following observations:

1. World income inequality is not simply very high (a Gini coefficient of 66 based on income adjusted for differences in countries' purchasing power and almost 80 if one uses the current dollar incomes) but it has increased. The increase between 1988 and 1993 has been at the rate of 0.6 Gini points per year. To put this in perspective, this is a rather rapid increase for the period considered, faster than the increase experienced by the United States and the United Kingdom in the entire decade of the 1980s.
2. Because of the great disparity in average income from nation to nation, it is intercountry—not intracountry—inequality that is the major component of total income inequality in the world today. Korzeniewicz and Moran (1997) estimate that inequality across countries accounts for over 90% of current world income inequality as measured by the Gini index. The apportioned percentage varies

Table 7–1. Comparing the Average Gini Coefficient for the 1980s and 1990s

Inequality increased	Inequality decreased	Inequality did not change
Australia	Bahamas	Belgium
Belarus	Bangladesh	Chile
Brazil	Canada	Colombia
Bulgaria	Finland	Costa Rica
China	Ghana	India
Czech Republic	Honduras	Israel
Czechoslovakia	Indonesia	Japan
Denmark	Italy	Lesotho
Dominican Republic	Jamaica	Luxembourg
Estonia	Mauritius	Morocco
Ethiopia	Philippines	Netherlands
Finland	Slovakia	Portugal
Hong Kong	Spain	Sweden
Hungary	Tunisia	Venezuela
Jordan		Yugoslavia
Kazakhstan		
Kyrgyz Republic		
Latvia		
Lithuania		
Mexico		
Moldova		
New Zealand		
Nigeria		
Norway		
Panama		
Peru		
Poland		
Romania		
Russia		
Slovenia		
Taiwan		
Thailand		
Turkmenistan		
UK		
Ukraine		
USA		
Uzbekistan		

Source: Adapted from Kanbur and Lustig (2000).

across studies, but it is clear that the level of world inequality is due primarily to difference in average income across countries rather than to intracountry inequality (Berry, Bourguignon, and Morrisson, 1983). Crucially, an increase in intracountry inequality does not necessarily suggest an increase in world income inequality.

3. Increases in world income inequality between 1988 and 1993 occurred as both intercountry and intracountry inequality increased. However, since the relative proportions remained the same, it was the intercountry inequality that, being much larger, drove overall inequality up. More specifically, slow growth of rural per capita incomes in populous Asian countries (China, India, and Bangladesh) compared to income growth of large and rich OECD countries, plus fast growth of urban China compared to rural China and rural India, were the main reasons world income inequality increased.
4. The world inequality level depends to a large extent on what happens to the relative positions of China and India on one end of the spectrum and the United States, Japan, France, and Germany on the other end.

Now that we have outlined the income inequality patterns across countries and their unique contribution to world distributions, the key question is, what accounts for these differences? Atkinson (1998) addresses this question for the case of advanced industrialized countries. Noting that these countries experienced a divergent pattern in income inequality during the 1980s and early 1990s, he posits that in addition to differences in government policies, social norms may have played a role. While the Gini coefficient rose by more than 40% in the United Kingdom, over 10% in Japan and Germany (in the early 1990s), and close to 10% in the United States, it fell slightly in Canada and more dramatically in Italy and France. Put simply, all countries for which the Gini coefficient fell were governed by center-left social democratic governments. However, as Kanbur and Lustig (2000) observe, the question that remains largely unanswered concerns the causal direction of the link between government policies and income inequality. For instance, did countries with more egalitarian social norms vote for more leftist governments? Or, once the more right-wing governments were voted in, did inequality increase as a result of the influence on social norms by nonegalitarian leaders?

In the case of the transition economies of Eastern Europe and the former Soviet Union, the difference that government policies made on income inequality was probably more obvious. For instance, in Hungary, Poland, and Slovenia—where income inequality remained practically unchanged between the period right before and the years immediately after the dismantling of the Communist regime—the governments pursued what Milanovic (1998) called *populist* policies. While wage inequality contributed to increasing inequality, the cash social transfers had an equalizing and thus an offsetting effect. On the other hand, the countries such as Russia and Ukraine—which saw the sharpest increases in inequality—had governments that Milanovic called *noncompensators*.

The fact of rising income inequality within many countries is also being linked to issues of globalization (Richardson, 1995; Williamson, 1999; Wood, 1995). Mainstream economics advocates the *skill-based hypothesis*, which states that the rise in inequality is a matter of the relative gains for workers who possess higher levels of skill. The skill-based hypothesis of pay differentials, in turn, has been linked to (*1*) global trade patterns (specifically, the increase in the effective supply of less skilled workers) and (*2*) technological change (specifically, the increase in the effective demand for highly skilled workers). In recent years, the focus has been on the latter, that is, on the divide between *users* and *nonusers* of new technology and the extent to which they account for perceived differences in their relative pay as a function of differences in their relative productivity. However, Galbraith (1998b) strongly argues for a shift in the existing macroeconomic framework of *producers of technology* to *consumers of technology.*

According to dependency theorists, the affluence of rich countries today stems directly from the long-term economic exploitation of poor countries, originally through colonialism and more recently through globalization (Bradshaw and Wallace, 1996). Dependency theory has focused attention particularly on multinational corporate investment's role in slowing the economic development of poor countries, exacerbating the exploitation of women in poor countries, and increasing the political instability in some developing regions (Bradshaw and Wallace, 1996). Obviously, several other factors besides the activities of multinational corporations account for inequalities *between* countries, and no single factor is likely to explain everything. Furthermore, while dependency theorists have studied how globalization impoverishes the countries at the periphery of the world economy, relatively less attention has been paid to how the same processes affect inequality in the core countries (Morris and Western, 1999).

As our review has revealed so far, monitoring inequality (even within a decade) is more dynamic than was once thought. However, seeking explanations for increasing inequalities at a global level has limitations as well as strengths. We will accordingly discuss the underlying explanations for increased income inequality by using the case of the United States, a key country in shaping world income inequality. The United States is a useful case study of earnings inequality for two additional reasons: First, the size of the U.S. economy and the nation's population shifts during the past 50 years provide an informative setting to explore generic lines of reasoning about what produces wage disparities. Second, the evidence on the effects of income inequality on health in the United States is extensive.

Evolution of Earnings Inequality in the United States

Earnings inequality data (drawn from U.S. income tax data) suggest the occurrence of two peaks during the twentieth century: the first just before World War I and the second before the Great Depression (Williamson and Lindbert, 1980). From the 1930s to the 1950s, a general secular decline in earnings inequality occurred, as first documented by Kuznets (1953). The 1950s through 1970s saw the annual income of the median worker double, and, importantly, those at the bottom of the earnings scale made relatively greater progress during this period (Danzinger and Gottschalk, 1995). These trends underwent dramatic reversals in the early 1970s, with median earnings stagnating and then declining. Since the 1980s, the United States has witnessed a significant and steady increase in earnings inequality (Bernstein and Mishel, 1997).

The decline in the real earnings of low-paid Americans means that their living standards are markedly lower than those of low-paid workers in other industrialized countries. OECD estimates of hourly U.S. pay have shown that a male worker in the bottom decile of the earnings distribution earns 38% of the median income in the United States compared with 68% of the median income in Western Europe and 63% of the median income in Japan (Freeman, 1998). Low-paid German workers earn roughly twice as much per hour as low-paid Americans. Nor is it just at the bottom decile of the earnings distribution that American workers compare unfavorably with their counterparts in other countries. About one-third of American workers are paid less in purchasing-power units than comparable workers overseas. Not until the thirtieth to fortieth decile of earnings do Americans start to do better than Europeans (Freeman, 1998).

If the facts about the rising earnings disparity in the United States are beyond dispute, there is little consensus about what has caused it. The following discussion draws largely on the excellent overview of evidence provided by Morris and Western (1999). Briefly, four potential explanations for the rise in U.S. income inequality have been debated: the changing demographics of the labor force, the impact of economic restructuring, the role of political contexts and institutions, and the dynamics of globalization.

Changes in Supply: Demographic Shifts

Between 1950 and 1980 the U.S. labor force increased by 70%, with more than half of that expansion occurring during the 1970s. This trend coincided with four dramatic changes in the composition of the labor supply, all of which have been the subject of intense investigation regarding explanations for increasing wage inequalities in the United States. The first relates to the labor force entry of the baby boom generation, which is the cohort born between 1946 and 1964. Thus, the baby boomers reached age 18 between 1964 and 1980, and those years roughly mark their transition into the labor force (Bloom, Freeman, and Korenman, 1987; Easterlin, 1980). The share of the labor force comprising young workers (aged 20 to 24) grew by more than 40% during this period (Freeman, 1980). Some theorists (namely, those with a neoclassical view who advocate growth, concentration of resources based on comparative advantage, exports, and the fostering of technological change) would describe this increase in the labor supply as a factor that depresses the relative wages of new workers and, by extension, widens the overall wage distribution by lowering the bottom-tier wages.

However, the consensus is that the process described by this line of reasoning, while contributory, cannot be the major reason for the growth of earnings inequality (Dooley and Gootschalk, 1985; Schrammel, 1998). Among other things, the peak entry of baby boomers into the labor market—in the 1960s and early 1970s—occurred well before the surge in earnings inequality.

The second demographic change in the labor force involves the rise in women's labor force participation (Spain and Bianchi, 1996). The percentage of women aged 25 to 54 working for pay increased from 37% to 75% between 1950 and 1994. Such a rapid influx of workers with low levels of labor market experience might have accounted for the rise in earnings inequality. However, the fact that earnings inequality rose among both sexes suggests that other factors were at work (Blau, 1998; Blau and Kahn, 1994; Spain and Bianchi, 1996; Wellington, 1993).

A third shift in the labor force relates to the change in ethnic composition. While not as large as the age- and sex-specific changes, the 1965 amendments to the Immigration and Nationality Act brought about a rapid influx of Asians and Latin Americans into the labor market. Empirically, a majority of immigrants have less schooling on average than do U.S. natives (Borjas, 1994). If immigrants substituted for native workers, an increase in the number of immigrants would push wages down for less educated workers. Two main approaches have been adopted for testing the contribution of immigration to earnings disparities: spatial studies comparing earnings across localities (Borjas, Freeman and Katz, 1997; Card, 1997; LaLonde and Topel, 1991) and aggregate analyses linking immigration rates to earnings for different education groups (Borjas, Freeman, and Katz, 1992, 1997). Studies based on either of these approaches have not, however, implicated immigration as a major factor explaining the observed earnings disparities.

The fourth and final factor related to the change in labor force composition is the role of education. The growing wage gap between high school–educated workers and college-educated ones has been well established and has led to use of the term *education premium* (Blackburn, Bloom, and Freeman, 1990; Dooley and Gootschalk, 1985; Murphy and Welch, 1993). In contrast to the other compositional changes in the labor force, this rising education premium appears to be one of the few features in earnings trends that have clearly contributed to the growth in overall wage inequality. The rise in the college premium has been driven almost entirely by the collapse in the earnings of high school graduates and dropouts. From 1979 to 1994, the real weekly earnings of college graduates rose by 5%, while the earnings of high school graduates fell by 20% (Gottschalk, 1997), thus doubling the college premium. In turn, skills-biased technological change has been blamed for the college premium. The empirical evidence for a technology-driven increase in demand for skills, however, is weak (Berman, Bound, and Griliches, 1994; Howell and Wolff, 1991; Kozicki, 1997; Morris and Western, 1999; Pischke and DiNardo, 1997).

In summary, there is little doubt that the changes in a wage premium associated with a worker's having a college degree are more strongly implicated in the growth in earnings disparity compared to other demographic changes. However, there is continuing debate about the reasons for the changes in the education premium, and the microeconomic evidence regarding skills-based technological change is weak.

Changes in Demand: Macroeconomic Factors

It is important to look beyond the microeconomic evidence discussed thus far and consider as well macroeconomic factors that emphasize the role of economic restructuring (deindustrialization, changing employment relations), institutional and political factors (the minimum wage, unionization), and globalization (trade and capital flows).

Economic restructuring. The United States has witnessed a four-decade process of declining employment in the manufacturing sector coupled with the emergence of a service economy. Between 1950 and 1970, the share of employment in the manufacturing industry declined to 15%. The gap in the annual earnings between workers in so-called expanding industries (specifically, those in the service sector) and those in so-called contracting industries (those in the manufacturing sector) reached $10,000 in the 1980s—a post–World War II high (Costrell, 1988). The service sector was not only the major sector for employment (80% of all jobs were in this sector), but the sector also became fairly diverse. As a result, the dispersion of wages in the service sector turned out to be higher than that in the manufacturing sector. However, the evidence of sector changes' effects on income differentials has been inconclusive, especially since inequality has grown within sectors, not simply between them (Blackburn, 1990; Lawrence, 1984).

The rise in market-mediated employment relations—that is, ones involving and encompassing such practices as internal promotions; outsourcing; subcontracting; and temporary, contingent, and part-time contracts—is another aspect of economic restructuring that has been examined as a possible cause of rising earnings differentials. Although various researchers have studied outsourcing, temporary workers, and so on, most of the studies have been case oriented, rather than based on national surveys.[2] While market-mediated employment remains a crucial field for further research in developing explanations for income differentials, the current evidence related to it has not been systematic enough to ensure generalizability (Belous, 1989).

Institutional changes. In studies of income inequality, most researchers have overemphasized market-based explanations and have tended to neglect political and institutional factors. The evidence related to the minimum wage has fairly consistently supported the notion that the minimum wage plays a causal role in income inequality. This is especially true given the freeze in the minimum wage, at $3.35 per hour, from 1980 to 1990 (Blackburn, Bloom, and Freeman, 1990; Card, 1997). Importantly, researchers have repeatedly pointed out that the typical minimum-wage earners have not been teenagers but adults—predominantly women and minorities (Card, 1997).

Studies have shown the equalizing effect of labor unions on the earnings distribution, so the decline in unionization also provides a reasonable account for the rise in earnings inequality (Freeman and Medoff, 1984). In 1970, unions represented about 27% of all wage and salary earners in the United States; by 1993, only 15% of workers were unionized (Visser, 1996). Overall, these findings suggest that the decline in union density may account for about 20% of the overall rise in male wage inequality and as much as 50% of the rise for male blue-collar workers. As with other potential factors, however, there has also been evidence of increasing earning inequality among union members (Bratsberg and Ragan, 1997; Dinardo and Lemieux, 1996; Freeman, 1993).

Globalization. Finally, globalization and its associated processes, such as trade and capital flows, provide plausible mechanisms that may explain trends in earnings disparity. The consequences of trade for inequality are often considered alongside the effects of immigration, that is, the supply of less-skilled workers from less-developed countries (Abowd and Freeman, 1991; Borjas, Freeman, and Katz, 1997). The dramatic increase in international trade that occurred between 1978 and 1990 superficially supports the notion that trade has accentuated inequality (Sachs and Shatz, 1994), and various researchers (see, for example, Leamer, 1993, 1994; Wood, 1994, 1995) have argued for large trade effects and have cited evidence of downward pressure on less skilled workers' wages because of imports from less developed countries. However, others have been relatively conservative in assigning a role for trade in raising inequality (Krugman, 1995; Krugman and Lawrence, 1994; Lawrence and Slaughter, 1993). Krugman (1995), for example, has argued that trade makes up a minor share of total U.S. output and that its effects are concentrated in the manufacturing sector (which, in turn, makes up a small share of total employment).

Few researchers have examined the link between capital flows and earnings inequality. Capital flows can be divided into the foreign direct investments by U.S. multinationals and outsourcing (that is, delegating production to external suppliers). Foreign direct investments are unlikely to be the source of increasing earnings inequality, as recent trends have run in the wrong direction and the size of investment has been small. Krugman (1994) has suggested a net earnings loss in developed countries of 0.15% due to capital exports. On the other hand, Feenstra and Hanson (1996) have suggested that the impact of outsourcing may be larger than the direct investment effects. As Rodrik (1997) has argued, globalization and outsourcing make the demand for many types of labor more elastic—that is, the services of large segments of the working population can be more easily substituted for by the services of people across national boundaries. Moreover, the fact that workers can be substituted for each other more easily contributes to the undermining of the essential social bargain between workers and employers. As a result, workers now pay a larger share of the cost of improvements in work conditions and benefits; they incur greater volatility and job insecurity; and their bargaining power erodes, so they receive lower wages and benefits (Rodrik, 1997).

In summary, several factors have contributed to the trends in earnings disparity within the United States. Most analysts reject the notion that there is a single culprit, but they disagree about the relative contribution of individual causes. While recognizing the complex interactions between the different factors that we have discussed, some analysts assign more weight to macroeconomic factors, such as globalization or the decline in union density, while others emphasize microeconomic factors such as skills-biased technological change. There is also little consensus about the social significance of the rising earnings disparity. As Freeman (1998, 20–21) noted, "Some believe that increased inequality is not worth getting overly excited about. Perhaps increased disparity reflects increased mobility. Perhaps the market will cure the problem relatively quickly. Perhaps inequality is the price America must pay for its good employment record." Freeman's response to his own conjectures—a response we agree with emphatically—is that the United States, and indeed the rest of the world, ought to be deeply concerned about rising disparity

Income Inequality and Population Health

Why should the world care about rising income disparity? One reason is the growing body of literature that asserts that income inequality, over and above the effects of poverty, which has been extensively studied, harms population health (Subramanian, Belli, and Kawachi, 2002). While not all of the evidence has been consistent, a series of studies examining the issue through a variety of methods and in a variety of countries have suggested that income inequality is associated with population health. Cross-sectional ecological studies have suggested that increased income inequality is associated with lower life expectancy, higher infant mortality, and a poorer average health status in both developing and developed countries (for a survey of this evidence, see Kawachi, Kennedy, and Wilkinson, 1999). An inverse relationship between greater economic inequality and lower health achievement has been reported *within* countries as diverse as the United States (Kaplan et al., 1996; Kennedy, Kawachi, and Prothrow-Stith, 1996), the United Kingdom (Ben-Shlomo, White, and Marmot, 1996), Taiwan (Chiang, 1999), and Brazil (Landman et al., 1999), as well as *between* different countries (Waldman, 1992; Wennomo, 1993; Wilkinson, 1992). There are also compelling theoretical grounds for arguing that the health of a society depends not only on the average income of its members but also on the inequality of income within a society. The explanation is straightforward, as illustrated in Figure 7–1.

The relationship between individual income and life expectancy is concave, such that each additional dollar of income raises individual health by a decreasing amount (Fig. 7–1). In a hypothetical society consisting of only two individuals—a rich one (with income $x4$) and a poor one (with income $x1$)—transferring a given amount of money (amount $x4$ minus $x3$) from the rich individual to the poor will result in an improvement in the average life expectancy (from $y1$ to $y2$), because the improvement in the

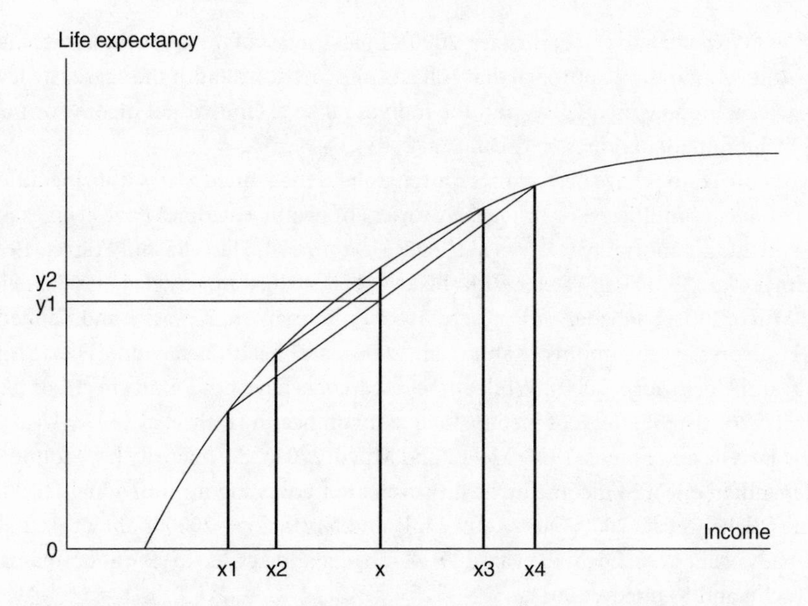

Figure 7–1. The concave relationship between income and life expectancy.

health of the poor person will more than offset the loss in health of the rich person. By extending this argument, one can see that given two societies with the same level of economic development, the society with the narrower distribution of income will have a better average health status, all other things being equal (Kawachi, 2000).

The basic reasoning behind this argument applies equally to the distribution of income *within* a country as to that *between* countries. In other words, a more equal world would be a healthier world. For example, the United Nations Development Program has estimated that the richest 200 individuals in the world own assets equal to the combined incomes of 41% of the world's people. A 1% annual contribution from the wealth of these 200 individuals would be sufficient to pay for basic education for every child in the world (at a cost of $7 to $8 billion annually), thereby vastly improving the life prospects of the world's poor citizens (UNDP, 1999).

What researchers have been trying to examine empirically is whether there is an additional effect of income inequality on population health over and above the effect just described. In other words, if all that matters about income inequality is the poor health of people near the bottom of the distribution, then policy makers could simply focus on reducing the number of poor people, by whatever means, without necessarily altering the distribution of income (such as would be accomplished by a trickle-down policy that focused exclusively on stimulating economic growth). However, many researchers have also asserted that income inequality per se may be damaging to population health. In order to tease out the potential health-damaging effects of income inequality from the known effects of individual poverty, research designs need to go beyond ecological studies (Wagstaff and van Doorslaer, 2000). In fact, a test of this hypothesis demands a multilevel analytical approach that collects information at both the aggregate level (area-level income inequality) and the individual level (individual income or poverty) (Subramanian, Jones, and Duncan, 2003).

The core studies have been carried out mainly in the United States utilizing different variants of multilevel techniques. A variety of health outcomes have been examined, including mortality (Daly et al., 1998; Deaton, 2001; Fiscella and Franks, 1997; Lochner et al., 2001), self-rated health (Blakely et al., 2000; Kennedy et al., 1998; Mellor and Milyo, 2001; Soobader and LeClere, 1999; Subramanian, Kawachi, and Kennedy, 2001), depressive symptoms (Kahn et al., 2000), and health behaviors (Diez-Roux, Link, and Northridge, 2000). While some researchers have not found effects, or have found inconsistent effects of income inequality on health (Daly et al., 1998; Deaton, 2001; Fiscella and Franks, 1997; Mellor and Milyo, 2001), the majority have found an independent effect of income inequality even after adjusting for individual-level income (Blakely et al., 2000; Diez-Roux, Link, and Northridge, 2000; Kahn et al., 2000; Kennedy et al., 1998; Lochner et al., 2001; Soobader and LeClere, 1999; Subramanian, Kawachi, and Kennedy, 2001).

Moreover, a close examination of these multilevel studies reveals a clearly emerging pattern of findings. The null studies have often lacked statistical power to detect the effects of income inequality on health outcomes. For example, the null studies by Daly and colleagues (1998) and Fiscella and Franks (1997) were based on comparatively small samples (6500 and 14,407, respectively). Positive studies, however, have tended to involve larger numbers. For example, Kennedy and colleagues (1998), studied 205,245 subjects, and Lochner and colleagues (2001) studied 546,888 subjects. In addition, some researchers have examined larger units of geographic aggregation, such as states (rather than smaller units such as counties, metropolitan areas, or neighborhoods), because states represent politically meaningful units and differentiate between levels of social spending that make a difference to health. It is noteworthy that few investigators have attempted to dissect the cross-level interactions between area-level inequality and the health of particular sociodemographic groups. That is, for whom is inequality most harmful and why? Some studies suggest that affluent individuals experience health benefits when they live in an area with high inequality (Kahn et al., 2000; Subramanian, Kawachi, and Kennedy, 2001). Other studies suggest that income inequality is particularly detrimental to the health of poor or near-poor individuals (Kennedy et al., 1998; Lochner et al., 2001).

The Social Costs of Economic Disparities

Even skeptics of the hypothesis linking income inequality and health appear to concede that rising economic disparity is associated with other social problems, including higher crime rates (Deaton, 2001). As Freeman (1998) noted, however, there is still no indisputable evidence that links homicide, violence, or crime to falling real wages and widening disparities. But the economic logic is clear:

> Whatever makes legitimate work less attractive makes crime more attractive. . . . It is clear that the real earnings of low skilled young men most prone to crime fell in the 1980s and 1990s, and that most of these men recognize they can do better on the street than in legitimate work. (225)

The relationship between crime and the thwarted American Dream, originally hypothesized by Merton (1968), has been confirmed in countless ethnographic studies (Anderson, 1990; Venkatesh, 1997). A spillover cost to American society of maintaining massive economic disparities has been the staggering rise in the prison and jail populations. Nationwide, the United States incarcerated 1.8 million offenders in 1999, up from 330,000 in 1972 (Butterfield, 1999). As of 1999, someone in America was arrested for a drug violation every 20 seconds; and every week, on average, a new jail or prison was built to lock up more people in the world's largest penal system (Egan, 1999). The State of California alone spent nearly $4 billion a year to operate the nation's largest prison system—more than the gross national product of such countries as Cambodia ($3.2 billion), Haiti ($2.9 billion), and Namibia ($3.4 billion). Between 1984 and 1999, California alone added 21 prisons to its penal system, compared with only one university campus added to the educational system during the same period. Even the vaunted low U.S. unemployment figures begin to look less attractive after data on the prison population are factored in. Including the incarcerated population as unemployed raises the U.S. male unemployment rate by about 2 points, largely erasing the U.S.–European difference in joblessness (Morris and Western, 1999).

Additional costs of a widening income gap are eroded social cohesion, reduced stability, and increased social tension (Kawachi and Kennedy, 1997). As Freeman (1998, 227) speculated: "Animus against CEOs, Wall Street, free trade and the like is one logical consequence of rising inequality. Animus against immigrants and ethnic groups other than one's own may grow."

The erosion of social cohesion that accompanies widening disparities may also hamper state efforts to invest in public goods. As Galbraith (1998a) has pointed out:

> More equal societies will tend to have lower private transfer burdens—less private capital, less debt, less conspicuous consumption and pecuniary emulation. People are willing to pay higher taxes for social insurance if they face a lower burden of private debts. Moreover, in a middle-class society, public services come to be seen as collective assets—something from which the population at large benefits directly. (16)

We have argued elsewhere that the erosion of social solidarity—as measured by declining levels of interpersonal trust and civic disengagement—is itself a threat to society

(Kawachi et al., 1997; Subramanian, Kawachi, and Kennedy, 2001). We concur with Freeman (1998) that what should worry Americans most about economic disparity is not so much the social pathologies exhibited by people on the lower rungs of the income distribution ladder but the acceptance of the new inequality by the better-off in society.

Conclusion

The facts about growing economic disparities across the globe and within U.S. society are beyond dispute, and in this chapter we have tried to show that such disparities are more than a benign side effect of globalization and American-style capitalism. Instead, rising disparities are threats to the well-being and health of societies around the world. While not all results have been consistent, studies from a range of countries, using a variety of methods and examining outcomes ranging from mortality to depressive symptoms, have found an association between income equality and health. The majority of studies have found an independent effect of income inequality even after adjusting for individual-level income (Blakely et al., 2000; Diez-Roux, Link, and Northridge, 2000; Kahn et al., 2000; Kennedy et al., 1998; Lochner et al., 2001; Soobader and LeClere, 1999; Subramanian, Kawachi, and Kennedy, 2001).

While a detailed discussion of the policy prescriptions to reduce inequalities is beyond the scope of this chapter, the experience of egalitarian nations (for example, Sweden and Canada) clearly demonstrates that market-based inequalities can be successfully addressed by social and economic policies that range from the radical down to the more incremental. These include implementing a more progressive taxation system, pursuing collective wage bargaining, maintaining a sustained full-employment policy, expanding earned income tax credits, increasing the child-care credit, and raising the minimum wage. Thus far, policy solutions have not been lacking, but the collective will and political leadership to carry them out have been missing. The mounting evidence on the social and health costs of economic disparities should, however, dispel the notion that continued apathy is a sustainable solution.

Note

1. The Gini coefficient is a formal numerical measure of inequality, with 0 signifying complete equality and 1 complete inequality.

References

Abowd, J., and R. B. Freeman, eds. 1991. *Immigration, trade and the labor markets.* Chicago: University of Chicago Press.

Alesina, A., and D. Rodrik. 1992. Distribution, political conflict, and economic growth: A simple theory and some empirical evidence. In *Political economy, growth and the business cycle,* edited by A. Cuckierman, Z. Hercowitz, and L. Leiderman. Cambridge, MA: MIT Press.

Anderson, E. 1990. *Street wise.* Chicago: University of Chicago Press.

Atkinson, A. B. 1998. Equity issues in a globalizing world: The experience of OECD countries. Conference on Economic Policy and Equity, International Monetary Fund, Washington, D.C.

Belous, R. S. 1989. *The contingent economy.* Washington, D.C: National Planning Association.

Benabou, R. 1996. *Unequal societies.* Cambridge, MA: National Bureau of Economic Research.

Ben-Shlomo, Y., I. R. White, and M. Marmot. 1996. Does the variation in socioeconomic characteristics of an area affect mortality? *British Medical Journal* 312: 1013–1014.

Berman, E., J. Bound, and Z. Griliches. 1994. Changes in the demand for skilled labor within U.S. manufacturing industries: Evidence from the annual survey of manufacturing. *Quarterly Journal of Economics* 109: 367–97.

Bernstein, J., and L. Mishel, 1997. Has wage inequality stopped growing? *Monthly Labor Review* 120(12): 3–16.

Berry, A., F. Bourguignon, and C. Morrisson. 1983. Changes in the world income distribution of income between 1950 and 1977. *Economic Journal* 93(37): 331–50.

Blackburn, M. L. 1990. What can explain the increase in earnings inequality among males? *Industrial Relations* 29(3): 441–56.

Blackburn, M. L., D. E. Bloom, and R. B. Freeman. 1990. The declining economic position of less skilled American men. In *A future of lousy jobs,* edited by G. Burtless. Washington, D.C.: Brookings Institution.

Blakely, T. A., B. P. Kennedy, R. Glass, and I. Kawachi. 2000. What is the lag time between income inequality and health status? *Journal of Epidemiology and Community Health* 54: 318–19.

Blau, F. D. 1998. Trends in overall well-being of American women, 1970–1995. *Journal of Economic Literature* 36(1): 112.

Blau, F. D., and L. M. Kahn. 1994. Rising wage inequality and the U.S. gender gap. *American Economic Review* 84(2): 23–28.

Bloom, D. E., R. B. Freeman, and S. D. Korenman. 1987. The labor-market consequences of generational crowding. *European Journal of Population* 3: 131–76.

Borjas, G. J. 1994. The economics of immigration. *Journal of Economic Literature* 32: 1667–717.

Borjas, G. J., R. B. Freeman, and L. F. Katz. 1992. On the labor market effects of immigration and trade. In *Immigration and the workforce: Economic consequences for the United States and source areas,* edited by G. J. Borjas. Chicago: University of Chicago Press.

Borjas, G. J., R. B. Freeman, and L. F. Katz. 1997. How much do immigration and trade affect labor market outcomes? Brookings Papers on Economic Activity 1.

Bradshaw, Y. W., and M. Wallace. 1996. *Global inequalities.* Thousand Oaks, CA: Pine Forge Press.

Bratsberg, B., and J. F. Ragan. 1997. Have unions impeded growing wage dispersion among workers? *Journal of Labor Research* 18(4): 593–612.

Butterfield, F. March 15, 1999. Number of inmates reaches record 1.8 million. *New York Times.* Section A, p. 14.

Capelli, P. 1992. Examining managerial displacement. *Journal of Academic Management* 35: 203–17.

Card, D. 1997. *Immigrant inflows, native outflows and the local labor market impacts of higher immigration.* Cambridge, MA: National Bureau of Economic Research.

Chiang, T.-L. 1999. Economic transition and changing relation between income inequality and mortality in Taiwan: regression analysis. *British Medical Journal* 319: 1162–65.

Citro, C. F., and R. T. Michael, eds. 1995. *Measuring poverty*. Washington, D.C.: National Academic Press.

Costrell, R. M. 1988. *The effects of industry employment shifts on wage growth 1947–1987*. Washington, D.C.: U.S. Congress, Joint Economic Committee, USGPO.

Daly, M., G. J. Duncan, G. A. Kaplan, and J. W. Lynch. 1998. Macro-to-micro links in the relation between income inequality and mortality. *The Millbank Quarterly* 76(3): 315–39.

Danzinger, S., and P. Gottschalk. 1995. *America unequal*. Cambridge, MA: Harvard University Press.

Deaton, A. 2001. Relative deprivation, inequality, and mortality. Princeton, NJ: Center for Health and Well-being, Princeton University.

Deninger, K., and L. Squire. 1996. A new data set measuring income inequality. *World Bank Economic Review* 10: 565–91.

Diez-Roux, A. V., B. G. Link, and M. E. Northridge. 2000. A multilevel analysis of income inequality and cardiovascular disease risk factors. *Social Science and Medicine* 50(5): 673–87.

Dinardo, J., and T. Lemieux. 1996. Diverging male wage inequality in the U.S. and Canada, 1981–88: Do institutions explain the difference? *Industrial and Labor Relations Review* 50(4): 629–51.

Dooley, M., and P. Gootschalk. 1985. The increasing proportion of men with low earnings in the United States. *Demography* 22: 25–34.

Easterlin, R. 1980. *Birth and fortune*. New York: Basic Books.

Egan, T. February 28, 1999. War on crack retreats, still taking prisoners. *New York Times*. Section 1, p. 1.

Feenstra, R. C., and G. H. Hanson. 1996. Globalization, outsourcing and wage inequality. Cambridge, MA: National Bureau of Economic Research.

Fiscella, K., and P. Franks. 1997. Poverty or income inequality as predictors of mortality: Longitudinal cohort study. *British Medical Journal* 314: 1724–28.

Freeman, R. B. 1980. The effect of demographic factors on age-earnings profiles. *Journal of Human Resources* 14: 289–318.

Freeman, R. B. 1993. How much has deunionization contributed to the rise in male earnings inequality? In *Uneven tides: Rising inequality in America*, edited by S. Danzinger and P. Gottschalk. New York: Russell Sage Foundation.

Freeman, R. B. 1998. The facts about rising economic disparity. In *The inequality paradox: Growth of income disparity*, edited by J. A. Auerbach and R. S. Belous. Washington, D.C.: National Policy Association.

Freeman, R. B., and J. L. Medoff. 1984. *What do unions do?* New York: Basic Books.

Galbraith, J. K. 1998a. *Created unequal: The crisis in American pay*. New York: Free Press.

Galbraith, J. K. 1998b. Globalization and pay. Remarks to the American Philosophical Society, November 14, Philadelphia, PA.

Galbraith, J. K. 2002. A perfect crime: Inequality in the age of globalization. *Daedalus* Winter: 11–25.

Galbraith, J. K., and V. Garza-Cantu. 1998. *Grading the performance of Latin American regimes*. Austin, TX: Lyndon B. Johnson School of Public Affairs.

Galbraith, J. K., L. Jiaqing, and W. A. Darity, Jr. 1999. *Measuring the evolution of inequality in the global economy*. Austin, TX: University of Texas.

Glyn, A., and D. Miliband, eds. 1994. *Paying for inequality: The economic cost of social injustice*. London: Rivers Oram.

Gottschalk, P. 1997. Inequality, income growth and mobility: The basic facts. *Journal of Economic Perspectives* 11(2): 21–40.

Howell, D. R., and E. N. Wolff. 1991. Trends in growth and distribution of skills in the US workplace, 1960–1985. *Industrial Labor Relations Review* 44: 486–502.

Hunter, L. W., and J. L. Lafkas. 1998. *Firm evidence of the information age? Information technology, work practices, and wages.* Philadelphia: Financial Institutions Center, The Wharton School, University of Pennsylvania.

Kahn, R. S., P. H. Wise, B. P. Kennedy, and I. Kawachi. 2000. State income inequality, household income and maternal mental and physical health: Cross sectional national survey. *British Medical Journal* 321: 1311–15.

Kakwani, N., A. Wagstaff, and E. V. Doorslaer. 1997. Socioeconomic inequalities in health: Measurement, computation, and statistical inference. *Journal of Econometrics* 77(1): 87–103.

Kanbur, R., and N. Lustig. 2000. *Why is inequality back on the agenda?* Washington, D.C.: World Bank.

Kaplan, G. A., E. Pamuk, J. W. Lynch, R. D. Cohen, and J. L. Balfour. 1996. Income inequality and mortality in the United States: Analysis of mortality and potential pathways. *British Medical Journal* 312: 999–1003.

Kawachi, I. 2000. Income inequality and health. In *Social epidemiology*, edited by L. F. Berkman and I. Kawachi. New York: Oxford University Press.

Kawachi, I., and B. P. Kennedy. 1997. Health and social cohesion: Why care about income inequality? *British Medical Journal* 314: 1037–40.

Kawachi, I., B. P. Kennedy, K. Lochner, and D. Prothrow-Stith. 1997. Social capital, income inequality and mortality. *American Journal of Public Health* 87: 1491–98.

Kawachi, I., B. P. Kennedy, and R. G. Wilkinson, eds. 1999. *Income inequality and health: A reader.* New York: New Press.

Kennedy, B. P., I. Kawachi, R. Glass, and D. Prothrow-Stith. 1998. Income distribution, socioeconomic status and self-rated health: A U.S. multilevel analysis. *British Medical Journal* 317: 917–21.

Kennedy, B. P., I. Kawachi, and D. Prothrow-Stith. 1996. Income distribution and mortality: Cross-sectional ecological study of the Robin Hood index in the United States. *British Medical Journal* 312: 1004–07.

Korzeniewicz, R. P., and T. P. Moran. 1997. World economic trends in the distribution of income, 1965–1992. *American Journal of Sociology* 102: 1000–39.

Kozicki, S. 1997. The productivity growth slowdown: Diverging trends in the manufacturing and service sectors. *Economic Review* 82(Q1): 31–46.

Krugman, P. 1994. Does third world growth hurt first world prosperity? *Harvard Business Review* 72(4): 113–21.

Krugman, P. 1995. Growing world trade: Causes and consequences (with discussion). *Brookings Papers on Economic Activity* 1: 327–77.

Krugman, P., and R. Z. Lawrence. 1994. Trade, jobs, and wages. *Scientific American* 270: 44–49.

Kuznets, S. 1953. *Shares of upper income groups in income and savings.* New York: National Bureau of Economic Research.

Kuznets, S. 1955. Economic growth and income inequality. *American Economic Review* 45(1): 1–28.

LaLonde, R. J., and R. H. Topel. 1991. Labor market adjustments to increased immigration. In *Immigration, trade and the labor market*, edited by J. M. Abowd and R. B. Freeman. Chicago: University of Chicago Press.

Landman, S. C., F. I. Bastos, F. Viavaca, and C. L. T. Andrade. 1999. Income inequality and homicide rates in Rio de Janeiro, Brazil. *American Journal of Public Health* 89: 845–50.

Lawrence, R. Z. 1984. Sectoral shifts and size of the middle class. *Brookings Review*, Fall: 3–11.

Lawrence, R. Z., and M. Slaughter. 1993. International trade and American wages in the 1980s: Great sucking sound or small hiccup? *Brookings Economic Micro* 2: 161–226.

Leamer, E. E. 1993. Wage effects of a U.S.–Mexican free trade agreement. In *The Mexico–I.S. Free Trade Agreement*, edited by P. M. Garber. Cambridge, MA: MIT Press.

Leamer, E. E. 1994. *Trade, wages and revolving door ideas.* Cambridge, MA: National Bureau of Economic Research.

Li, H., L. Squire, and H. Zou. 1998. Explaining international and intertemporal variations in income inequality. *Economic Journal* 108: 26–43.

Lochner, K., E. R. Pamuk, D. Makuc, B. P. Kennedy, and I. Kawachi. 2001. State-level income inequality and individual mortality risk: A prospective multilevel study. *American Journal of Public Health* 91(3): 385–91.

Mellor, J. M., and J. Milyo. 2001. Reexamining the evidence of an ecological association between income inequality and health. *Journal of Health Politics, Policy and Law* 26(3): 487–522.

Merton, R. K. 1968. *Social theory and social structure.* New York: Free Press.

Milanovic, B. 1998. *Income, inequality and poverty during the transition from planned to market economy.* Washington, D.C.: World Bank.

Morris, M., and B. Western. 1999. Inequality in earnings at the close of the 20th century. *Annual Review of Sociology* 25: 623--57.

Murphy, K. M., and F. Welch. 1993. Industrial change and the rising importance of skill. In *Uneven tides: The rising inequality in America*, edited by S. Danzinger and P. Gottschalk. New York: Russell Sage Foundation.

Pischke, J.-S., and J. E. DiNardo. 1997. The returns to computer use revisited: Have pencils changed the wage structure too? *Quarterly Journal of Economics* 112: 291.

Richardson, D. J. 1995. Income inequality and trade: How to think, what to conclude. *Journal of Economic Perspectives* 9(3): 33–56.

Rodrik, D. 1997. *Has globalization gone too far?* Washington, D.C.: Institute for International Economics.

Rowntree, B. S. 1910. *Poverty: A study of town life.* London: Macmillan.

Sachs, J. D., and H. J. Shatz. 1994. Trade and jobs in U.S. manufacturing (with discussion). *Brookings Papers on Economic Activity* 1: 1–84.

Schrammel, K. 1998. Comparing the labor market success of young adults from two generations. *Monthly Labor Review* 121(2): 3–48.

Sen, A. K. 1992. *Inequality reexamined.* Cambridge, MA: Harvard University Press.

Smeeding, T., M. O'Higgins, and L. Rainwater, eds. 1990. *Poverty, inequality and income distribution in comparative perspective.* New York: Harvester Wheatsheaf.

Soobader, M.-J., and F. LeClere. 1999. Aggregation and the measurement of income inequality: Effects on morbidity. *Social Science and Medicine* 48: 733–44.

Spain, D., and S. M. Bianchi. 1996. *Balancing act: Motherhood, marriage and employment among American women.* New York: Russell Sage Foundation.

Subramanian, S. V., P. Belli, and I. Kawachi. 2002. The macroeconomic determinants of health. *Annual Review of Public Health* 23: 287–302.

Subramanian, S. V., K. Jones, and C. Duncan. 2003. Multilevel methods for public health research. In *Neighborhoods and health*, edited by I. Kawachi and L. F. Berkman. New York: Oxford University Press.

Subramanian, S. V., I. Kawachi, and B. P. Kennedy. 2001. Does the state you live in make a difference? Multilevel analysis of self-rated health in the U.S. *Social Science and Medicine* 53: 9–19.

UNDP. 1999. *Human development report.* New York: Oxford University Press.

Venkatesh, S. 1997. The social organization of street gang activity in an urban ghetto. *American Journal of Sociology* 103(1): 82–111.

Visser, J. 1996. *Unionisation trends revisited.* Amsterdam: Centre for European Social Industrial Relations.

Wagstaff, A., and E. van Doorslaer. 2000. Income inequality and health: What does the literature tell us? *American Journal of Public Health* 21: 543–67.

Waldman, R. J. 1992. Income distribution and infant mortality. *The Quarterly Journal of Economics* 107(4): 1283–1302.

Wellington, A. J. 1993. Changes in the male/female wage gap, 1976–85. *Journal of Human Resources* 28(2): 83–141.

Wennemo, I. 1993. Infant mortality, public policy, and inequality—a comparison of 18 industrialised countries 1950–85. *Sociology of Health and Illness* 15: 429–46.

Wilkinson, R. G. 1992. Income distribution and life expectancy. *British Medical Journal* 304: 165–68.

Williamson, J. G. 1999. *Globalization and inequality then and now: The late 19th and late 20th centuries compared.* Cambridge, MA: National Bureau of Economic Research.

Williamson, J. G., and P. H. Lindbert. 1980. *American inequality: A macroeconomic history.* New York: Academic Press.

Wood, A. 1994. *North–South trade, employment and inequality: Changing fortunes in a skill-driven world.* New York: Oxford University Press.

Wood, A. 1995. How trade hurt unskilled workers. *Journal of Economic Perspectives* 9(3): 15–32.

8

Gender Inequality in Work, Health, and Income

MAYRA BUVINIC, ANTONIO GIUFFRIDA,
AND AMANDA GLASSMAN

In Latin America and the Caribbean, more women than men have entered the labor force since the 1980s. By choice or need, women have assumed increasingly indispensable roles in the economy, and their contribution to family income has enabled poor families to cope with financial hardship. This region's countries, each with its own peculiarities, have replicated a trend that has been occurring worldwide since the last decades of the twentieth century—the rapid incorporation of women into paid employment.[1] The feminization of the workforce is a consequence of, first, reduced fertility and more female schooling—both of which have expanded the supply of female workers—and, second, the globalization of labor markets, which has increased the demand for female labor. In addition, the growing social acceptance of women in the workplace, evident in much of the world, has helped reduce cultural barriers against their participation in economic activities.

What are the implications of these trends for women's health status? This chapter reviews the empirical evidence about the effects of women's paid work on their health in Latin America. We begin with a brief description of the changing nature of labor markets and women's labor force participation. We then explore women's occupational health risks and mention some initiatives that seek to respond to these risks. Next, we look at the existing evidence for the positive effects of paid work on women's health and child health. Finally, we provide policy recommendations.

The Context

Changing Labor Markets

Globalization, or the global integration of production and trade, has had marked effects on labor markets around the world. In Latin America, as elsewhere in the world, there has been substantial growth in the number of workers employed in the service sector, including financial activities, at the expense of those working in the agricultural sector. Technological advances, global competition, and labor market deregulation have changed employment processes and conditions. There has been a move away from formal sector, nine-to-five jobs with labor contracts, tenure, and employment benefits toward less permanent arrangements with employers, including subcontracting, part-time work, and short-term contracts with few employment benefits (Lora and Marquez, 1998).

The growth of the service sector and the "informalization" of working conditions have increased the demand for female labor for two reasons. First, women are disproportionately found in service jobs. Second, women often work in labor markets that continue to be segmented by sex, forcing them to accept work under more precarious, less than ideal employment contract conditions in the informal sector (Beneria, 2001; Standing, 1999). This willingness to work in less desirable settings has also increased workers' exposure to occupational hazards. Informal sector work, by definition, takes place outside formal legal standards and regulation and, therefore, outside monitoring by the government or by formal sector workers' associations (unions). In addition, Latin American and Caribbean unions are comparatively weak and largely male-dominated member organizations that generally fail to represent the interests of female workers (Greenhouse, 2001).

The last characteristic of the Latin American and Caribbean labor market is its high level of unemployment and underemployment, along with the lack of unemployment and social security insurance for informal sector workers. Many of the region's workers, therefore, may be willing to tolerate hazardous working conditions rather than lose their main source of income (Giuffrida, Iunes, and Savedoff, 2001).

The Feminization of the Workforce

The past three decades have witnessed a progressive feminization of the Latin American workforce. The percentage of women in the labor market is still below that of industrial economies, but the upward trend is consistent and unambiguous. Table 8–1 shows, in a majority of the 26 countries listed, a rise in the proportion of women in the paid labor force from 1990 to 1997. In this period, women's labor force participation increased by about 5%, and the gap between male and female economic activity rates in Latin America and the Caribbean as a whole decreased by 4%. Still, on average, women's economic activity rate is about 10% lower in Latin American countries than in Canada, the United States, and the United Kingdom, and women represent 38% of the total labor force compared to approximately 45% in more developed countries. Just as globalization has increased the demand for female labor, decreased fertility rates, lower infant mortality rates, and women's educational gains have increased the supply of women available for labor force participation. The region's demographic transition, characterized by such trends, has affected the supply of female workers and

Table 8–1. Indicator of Economic Activity of Women in Latin America and the Caribbean (LAC) (%)

	Adult (aged 15+) economic activity rate			
	1990		1995/1997	
Country	Women	Men	Women	Men
Argentina	29	79	41	76
Bahamas	65	81	67	81
Barbados	60	76	62	73
Belize	24	86	34	79
Bolivia[a]	46	84	56	74
Brazil[b]	44	85	51	82
Chile	32	75	35	75
Colombia[b]	46	80	52	78
Costa Rica[b]	33	83	36	81
Dominican Republic	34	86	38	86
Ecuador[a]	28	85	49	81
El Salvador	51	80	41	79
Guatemala	28	90	32	88
Guyana	37	84	40	85
Haiti	58	82	57	82
Honduras[b]	34	87	41	88
Jamaica	62	77	69	81
Mexico	34	84	39	84
Nicaragua	40	87	44	86
Panama[b]	39	79	43	80
Paraguay	51	83	35	87
Peru[a]	29	80	55	78
Suriname[c]	30	74	33	64
Trinidad and Tobago	38	74	47	74
Uruguay[a]	44	75	47	74
Venezuela	38	82	41	81
LAC	41	81	46	80
Stage 2	39	84	41	81
Stage 3a	35	83	43	81
Stage 3b	42	79	49	79
Stage 4	52	77	56	76
Canada	59	76	57	73
United States	53	75	54	72
United Kingdom	58	76	60	75

[a]The data relate to the urban survey conducted in the main departmental capitals of the country.

[b]Data are estimated to correspond to standard age groups.

[c]The data relate to the districts of Wanica and Paramaribo.

Source: United Nations (2000).

in part explains the rise in women's labor force participation (Duryea and Székely, 2000).

The transition to lower fertility and infant mortality rates reduces the time women need to spend in household (versus market) production, and in bearing and caring for children. Household income mediates women's time allocation between market and nonmarket work. Children, particularly the young, can be cared for by the mother, by friends or relatives (including older daughters, elderly people, or kin or friends outside the household who may provide this type of support on a reciprocal basis), or by paid caregivers. In countries where the government does not subsidize child care, the use of day-care centers and paid child-care services is an option available only to middle- and upper-income households.

Women's education and labor force participation. Another key determinant of women's labor supply is the level and distribution of education. Duryea and Székely (2000) used an instrumental variable technique to decompose the determinants of female labor market participation in Latin America, based on panel data from 22 countries from 1980 to 1996. This study showed that while participation rates in Latin America increased by approximately 35% during the 1980s, approximately 10% of that increase was associated with reductions in fertility and another 3% was linked to the gains in women's schooling.

In the past four decades, the region has shown impressive gains in female education. Historically, male cohorts completed on average more years of education than their female counterparts. However, these gender differences disappeared in the cohort of men and women born in 1970, and women today complete, on average more years of education than men. And women with more schooling participate more in the labor market, as Figure 8–1 shows for women aged 30 to 45. This figure, however, also shows that in the late 1990s female economic activity rates increased because less educated women were working at higher rates than at the beginning of the decade (Duryea, Cox Edwards, and Ureta, 2001). It is quite possible that these women increased their participation rates to help families handle economic crises, as they had done when faced with economic contraction in prior decades—in the 1970s and the early 1980s (Leslie, Lycette, and Buvinic, 1988). In fact, recent evidence from Colombia supports this assertion (Székely, Hilgert, and Glassman, 2000).

Converging trends. The feminization of the region's workforce, therefore, can be explained by a number of converging trends. On the demand side, globalization, with its preference not only for service sector and manufacturing work but also for informal job arrangements, has expanded opportunities for female labor—most often, however, in jobs that pay lower wages than men's jobs (as documented below). On the supply side, as noted earlier, the reduction in fertility and mortality rates and the gains in women's schooling have increased the supply of women workers. Economic

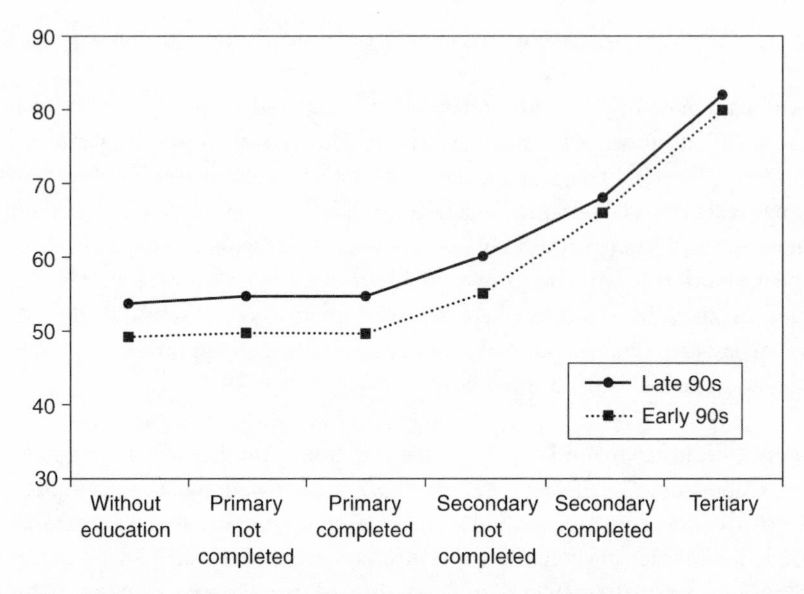

Figure 8–1. Percent of women economically active in Latin America, by educational level (ages 30–45). Averages of 18 Latin American and Caribbean household surveys. Source: Duryea, Cox Edwards, and Ureta (2001).

crises, another result of globalization, seem to have further buttressed this supply by drawing low-income women into the labor force in order to help families weather these crises.

Segregated Occupations

While more women are working, Latin American women are still segregated into specific job categories. In fact, women face a more segmented-by-gender labor market in Latin America than in other world regions (Horton, 1999). Table 8–2 shows this segmentation by gender in economic activities in various countries. A labor market segmented by gender has implications both for women's economic opportunities and for occupational health and safety. Segregated markets restrict mobility and opportunity. With regard to economic opportunities, women are effectively barred from generally better-paid male-dominated occupations. With regard to occupational health and safety, occupational health risks are not distributed proportionately across the genders, so the gains of predominantly male labor unions will likely leave female workers' occupational health and safety concerns unaddressed. Women will need to join workers' unions or will need to form their own. Anecdotal evidence suggests that women are becoming somewhat more visible in the regional union movement, although as they seek broader representation, they may encounter the same barriers that women trying to unionize historically faced in the United States and other industrial countries (Greenhouse, 2001; Kaufman and Gonzalez, 2001).

The female workforce is overrepresented in the service sector (wholesale and retail trade; restaurants and hotels; and community, social, and personal services) and underrepresented in agriculture, and this employment structure has changed relatively little since 1970. Much of the growth in women's employment from 1990 to 1998, as shown in Table 8–3, took place in the service sector, which accounted for 60% of new jobs created. Wholesale and retail trade made up another 34% of new jobs, while manufacturing, transport, communication, and finance represented only 6% of the new jobs for women. On the other hand, new jobs for men were more equally distributed among the economic activities considered.

Official statistics estimate that the female workforce represents approximately 20% of the economically active population in the agricultural sector (see Table 8–2; ILO, 2000). It is important to emphasize, however, that the female share of the officially counted agricultural labor force, in Latin America as elsewhere in the developing world, is subject to substantial underestimation. More accurate estimates produced by the Instituto Interamericano de Cooperación para la Agricultura (Chiriboga, Grynspan, and Pérez, 1995; Grynspan, 1999) have shown that women make up at least 37% of the agricultural labor force in the region. They work as unpaid workers on family farms, as well as seasonal wage laborers in commercial agriculture; they are involved in small-scale agricultural processing, and they sell agricultural products in local markets. This means that at least 7 million women are invisible in the official counts and that occupational health risks of women in this sector are likely to be grossly underestimated.

Women's share in manufacturing is affected by the presence of the *maquila,* the export-oriented manufacturing companies that are set up offshore to take advantage of the reduced costs of labor. While in many countries (including Argentina, Brazil, and Chile) men predominate in manufacturing, and while the average representation of women in the sector declined in the 1990s, in countries like El Salvador, Mexico, and the Dominican Republic this share is large (over 60% of the workforce) and has expanded. Globalization has given increased visibility to *maquila* operations and their health risks (Greenhouse, 2001).

The Quality of Female Employment

What is the quality of the largely segregated jobs women get? Women are disproportionately represented in low-paid employment and underrepresented as administrators and managers, although for some this situation has improved in the past two decades (Gammage and Schmitt, 2001). Most of women's low-paid jobs are in the informal sector. In 1999, 50% of all women's jobs were in the informal sector, many

Table 8–2. Distribution of Labor Force by Economic Activity in Latin America and the Caribbean (LAC) (%)

Country	Sex	Agriculture, hunting, forestry, and fishing	Mining and quarrying	Manufacturing	Electricity, gas, and water	Construction	Wholesale and retail trade, and restaurants and hotels	Transport, storage, and communication	Financing, insurance, real estate, and business services	Community, social, and personal services	Activities not adequately defined
Argentina[a]	Men	1.1	0.4	19.1	0.9	13.6	23.8	11.1	9.4	19.5	1.1
	Women	0.2	0.0	9.7	0.3	0.4	21.5	2.3	9.3	37.8	18.5
Brazil	Men	26.0	1.68[b]	14.0	—	11.3	13.3	5.9	2.0	25.8	—
	Women	19.3	0.5	8.4	—	0.7	13.7	1.0	1.7	54.7	—
Chile[c]	Men	19.4	2.1	16.3	0.9	12.0	15.0	10.3	7.0	17.0	—
	Women	4.6	0.3	12.6	0.2	0.8	25.5	3.3	8.5	44.4	—
Colombia[a]	Men	1.6	0.4	18.4	0.9	7.8	25.1	12.4	9.8	23.4	0.3
	Women	0.5	0.1	18.5	0.3	1.0	27.7	2.2	7.7	41.7	0.2
Costa Rica[c]	Men	26.9	0.2	15.2	1.4	9.3	17.8	7.6	1.9	18.3	1.5
	Women	4.7	0.1	16.8	0.3	0.3	26.7	1.8	2.2	28.3	18.9
Ecuador[a]	Men	10.5	0.5	15.8	0.7	9.4	25.5	9.4	5.9	22.1	0.1
	Women	2.3	0.0	13.0	0.2	0.4	37.6	1.4	4.1	40.9	0.1
El Salvador	Men	37.3	0.1	14.8	0.6	8.8	17.0	6.3	3.7	11.4	—
	Women	6.3	0.0	24.5	0.1	0.4	37.1	0.6	3.7	27.2	—

Honduras[c]	Men	49.8	0.2	12.2	0.5	7.8	12.4	3.5	2.1	11.6	—
	Women	8.9	0.2	23.8	0.2	0.4	37.1	0.5	2.3	26.6	—
Jamaica[c]	Men	29.0	0.8	10.1	0.7	13.7	13.9	8.4	5.0	18.2	0.2
	Women	9.9	0.2	7.3	0.4	0.7	31.8	2.8	7.6	39.3	0.1
Mexico	Men	26.9	0.5	18.0	0.7	8.1	16.6	5.9	3.5	18.6	1.2
	Women	9.2	0.1	20.5	0.2	0.3	31.2	1.5	4.2	20.9	12.0
Panama	Men	25.3	0.1	10.1	0.9	11.0	20.7	9.8	5.6	15.4	1.2
	Women	1.9	0.0	9.2	0.4	0.8	28.0	3.4	8.5	33.6	14.3
Peru[a]	Men	7.9	0.7	14.0	0.9	9.3	26.8	14.3	7.9	18.0	0.3
	Women	3.3	0.1	10.6	0.2	0.3	45.8	1.5	5.3	22.3	10.6
Trinidad	Men	10.8	5.2	12.2	1.7	17.6	12.6	9.6	6.2	24.0	0.1
& Tobago	Women	3.4	1.4	8.2	0.7	2.8	25.8	3.6	11.5	42.5	0.1
Uruguay[d]	Men	5.8	0.2	18.0	1.2	14.2	19.3	8.7	6.4	26.2	—
	Women	1.2	—	12.8	0.7	0.5	20.4	2.7	6.9	54.8	—
Venezuela[c]	Men	15.6	1.5	14.5	1.0	12.3	20.7	9.0	5.2	20.0	0.3
	Women	1.5	0.4	11.7	0.4	0.9	30.2	1.6	6.5	46.5	0.3

[a]Urban agglomerations.

[b]Includes electricity, gas, water, and sanitary services.

[c]Civilian population that is employed.

[d]Includes those in the professional army; excludes those performing compulsory military service.

Source: Calculations based on data from ILO (1999b).

Table 8–3. New Jobs by Economic Activities in Latin America and the Caribbean, 1990–1998 (%)

Economic activity	Men	Women
Manufacturing	14	3
Wholesale and retail trade	24	34
Transport, communication, and finance	25	3
Services	37	60

Source: ILO (1999a).

of them in domestic service, the segment of the informal sector with the lowest pay and the least social protection. This category of female employment increased by 1.3% during the 1990s, as indicated in Table 8–4.

Women's unemployment rates tend to be higher than men's, as noted in Table 8–5. The recent economic recessions linked to global and domestic financial crises have led to a disproportionate increase in the level of female unemployment, which grew from 6.1% in 1990 to 11.2% in 1998. There is also evidence that discrimination against women tends to increase as unemployment levels go up. Such discrimination is rationalized on the grounds that employing women pushes up the male unemployment rate and that men need jobs more than women (Lim, 1996). The problem of women's unemployment tends to be especially serious at both ends of the age range—that is, for young, first-time workers and for older women. Female unemployment rates are higher than male rates at all levels of household income and education, but the highest rate (and gender gap) is observed among the poor, with about 19.2% unemployment in 1998. As a result, approximately one of every five poor women is unemployed, even if she is actively seeking a job (Lim, 1996).

Reducing Wage Differentials by Gender

Women's wages, relative to men's, have been rising slowly but steadily for the past two decades. Although there is still a gender gap in wages, by the late 1990s women in Latin America earned wages that compared quite favorably to men's. Of the 15 countries with available data, the wage ratio was below 80% (of male wages) for only two countries (Honduras and Guatemala). In two others (Colombia and Costa Rica), by the end of the decade the wage gap had reversed in favor of women (Duryea, Cox Edwards, and Ureta, 2001). These advances in the reduction of the wage gap by gender have not, however, benefited all women equally. A most unfortunate feature of women's progress in Latin America is that it has not been shared by all. As a result, while the wage gap between the sexes has narrowed, there is evidence that the wage gap *among* women has grown (Buvinic, 2001). Poor women have been left behind. A majority of women work for low wages because of economic need in informal sector occupations where they have no social security coverage and are exposed to occupational health hazards.

Some labor force surveys that record informal sector work more reliably have shown, for instance, that women earn, on average, 25% less than men in the formal sector but 48% less in the informal sector. Within the informal sector, the largest gender inequality is observed among self-employed workers. Self-employed men earn about 39% less than those employed in the formal sector; self-employed women earn less than 70% of the salary of their formal sector counterparts. Domestic workers, who represent 15.8% of all female workers in Latin America, earn only 23% of the salary of the average male in the formal sector (ILO, 1999a).

Women Left Behind

Evidence that disaggregates social and economic indicators by gender, as well as ethnicity or race, has shown that among the poor, indigenous women, women of African descent and female heads of households with young children exhibit the lowest levels of well-being. For instance, indigenous girls in Guatemala are least likely to attend school. In Bolivia and Guatemala, indigenous women are most likely to work in informal occupations, and they show the lowest earnings in the labor market given the same level of schooling compared to nonindigenous women (Duryea, Cox Edwards, and Ureta, 2001). Female-headed families, especially those with younger children, are more numerous in the lowest income (destitute) category in 9 out of 13 countries studied (ECLAC, 1997). Female household heads work in the market more than other women, and their low earnings help explain the link between female-headed households and poverty (Buvinic and Gupta, 1997). In Brazil, women of African descent are disproportionately represented among poor female heads of households with young children (Barros, Fox, and Mendonca, 1997). A study in Chile showed that a period of fast economic growth (from 1987 to 1994) left behind poor female-headed households. Poverty was more intense for female household heads than for their male counterparts, and these women also suffered the highest unemployment rates (Anríquez and Buvinic, 1997).

Health measures compound concerns about the well-being of poor women. Like economic indicators, health indicators disaggregated by income show widening disparities between better-off and poor women. In absolute terms, poor women are most vulnerable. In six countries studied, females in the bottom 20% of the income distribution reported the highest burden of health problems relative to both men and women in other income quintiles. And although a greater proportion of these women had a health problem, they were least likely to have sought treatment. Inequality is concentrated in this group: at the same levels of need, poor women do not receive similar levels of care (Henderson, Montes, and Glassman, 2000). Further, poorer women spend more money on health care as a percentage of their income and are least likely to be covered by health insurance plans.

Table 8–4. Structure of Urban Employment in Latin America and the Caribbean, 1990–1999

	Women					Men				
	Formal	Informal				Formal	Informal			
	Total	Total	Self-employed	Domestic service	Small business	Total	Total	Self-employed	Domestic service	Small business
Latin America										
1990	**52.6**	**47.4**	23.2	13.8	10.4	**60.6**	**39.4**	21.6	0.5	17.3
1999	**50.1**	**49.9**	23.4	15.1	11.4	**56.1**	**43.9**	24.3	0.8	18.8
Argentina										
1991	**44.5**	**55.5**	26.5	14.3	14.7	**50.1**	**49.9**	28.2	0.5	21.2
1998	**48.6**	**51.4**	20.4	15.8	15.2	**52.0**	**48.0**	24.1	0.3	23.6
Brazil										
1990	**52.4**	**47.6**	21.3	16.7	9.6	**63.9**	**36.1**	19.6	0.5	16.0
1999	**48.3**	**51.7**	20.7	20.9	10.1	**56.3**	**43.7**	26.4	0.9	16.4
Chile										
1990	**54.1**	**45.9**	20.1	14.7	11.1	**66.5**	**33.5**	21.3	0.2	12.0
1998	**55.2**	**44.8**	17.4	13.1	14.3	**67.1**	**32.9**	19.2	0.1	13.6
Colombia										
1990	**53.5**	**46.5**	26.3	5.0	15.2	**55.0**	**45.0**	22.6	0.1	22.3
1998	**51.2**	**48.8**	27.7	4.7	16.4	**50.7**	**49.3**	28.4	0.2	20.7
Costa Rica										
1990	**52.5**	**47.5**	18.6	15.8	13.1	**62.3**	**37.7**	19.1	0.3	18.3

1999	**47.5**	**52.5**	19.6	16.6	16.3	**56.8**	**43.2**	17.7	0.6	24.9
Ecuador										
1990	**37.9**	**62.1**	39.9	12.1	10.1	**48.3**	**51.7**	32.6	0.7	18.4
1998	**35.9**	**64.1**	46.7	9.4	8.0	**45.5**	**54.5**	28.9	1.0	24.6
Honduras										
1990	**28.0**	**72.0**	50.5	14.6	6.9	**54.9**	**45.1**	25.7	0.5	18.9
1999	**32.4**	**67.6**	49.8	9.9	7.9	**46.8**	**53.2**	28.6	0.7	23.9
Mexico										
1990	**60.1**	**39.9**	18.7	12.0	9.2	**62.4**	**37.6**	19.1	0.7	17.8
1999	**58.8**	**41.2**	19.2	11.4	10.6	**60.4**	**39.6**	17.8	1.2	20.6
Panama										
1991	**61.9**	**38.1**	14.0	17.8	6.3	**65.5**	**34.5**	23.8	1.0	9.7
1999	**57.8**	**42.2**	19.9	14.6	7.7	**63.3**	**36.7**	24.4	1.2	11.1
Peru										
1991	**37.2**	**62.8**	40.4	11.6	10.8	**53.6**	**46.4**	28.9	0.6	16.9
1998	**35.4**	**64.6**	38.7	11.9	14.0	**54.7**	**45.3**	23.8	0.5	21.0
Uruguay										
1990	**53.5**	**46.5**	18.5	16.2	11.8	**66.2**	**33.8**	18.6	0.2	15.0
1999	**52.1**	**47.9**	19.8	17.0	11.1	**60.7**	**39.3**	24.5	0.2	14.6
Venezuela										
1990	**60.7**	**39.3**	22.8	10.4	6.1	**61.7**	**38.3**	22.0	0.4	15.9
1999	**48.6**	**51.4**	36.6	5.9	8.9	**52.4**	**47.6**	29.6	0.2	17.8

Source: ILO (2000).

Table 8–5. Unemployment Rates by Household Earnings and Years of Studies in Latin America and the Caribbean, 1990–1998 (%)

	Household earnings			Years of studies				
	Low	Medium	High	0–5	6–9	10–12	13 or more	**Total**
1990								
Women	11.8	4.7	2.2	4.4	7.6	6.9	4.1	**6.1**
Men	9.3	3.6	1.5	4.7	5.8	5.1	2.7	**5.1**
Difference	2.5	1.1	0.7	–0.3	1.8	1.8	1.4	**1.0**
1998								
Women	19.2	8.8	4.5	9.8	13.9	11.7	6.7	**11.2**
Men	13.0	5.5	2.9	8.1	8.9	7.3	4.6	**7.6**
Difference	6.2	3.3	1.6	1.7	5.0	4.4	2.1	**3.6**

Source: ILO (1999a).

Poor Women at High Risk

As was made clear in preceding sections, the question of how paid work affects health (both positively and negatively) is a pertinent one for most women in the region's workforce and a critical one for poor women. The latter have increased their labor force participation rates in recent years, often as a result of need (although many cannot find work); have faced higher health risks (both occupational and general ones) than better-off women; and have received very low wages. Women's wages, when they are adequate, are positively related to their own as well as their children's health (as discussed in the next section). When wages are too low, the opposite effect may occur: work, in combination with other factors that exacerbate disadvantages, may lead to stagnation or deterioration in women's and their children's health.

Occupational Health Hazards for Women

Gender Differences

Quantitative information on occupational hazards in Latin America and the Caribbean is scarce and has serious limitations. Official statistics, derived from disability compensation systems in Latin America, are available only for the relatively small proportion of the workforce who work in the formal sector and receive compensation for their injury or illness. However, even if workers are covered by a reporting system, the poor identification of occupational diseases and the legal and bureaucratic features of the systems raise questions about the estimates' validity and accuracy. Giuffrida, Iunes, and Savedoff (2001) applied the rates of the population covered by reporting systems to the whole workforce and estimated that around 27,000 fatal occupational accidents occurred in the region in 1998, which represents 0.135 fatal accidents per 1000 workers. Taking into account underreporting and the likely higher exposure to occupational hazards in the informal sector, the estimate was raised to 68,000 fatalities, representing 0.338 fatal accidents per 1000 workers. The same study also estimated between 27 and 51 million occupational accidents causing 3 or more days' absence from work (Table 8–6).

An examination of existing statistics on compensated occupational injuries and illnesses reveals that women and men have distinctive patterns. The 1999 figures on work accidents among workers affiliated with the Mexican Social Security Institute, a parastatal organization that provides medical insurance and services to formal sector workers, who represent about one-third of all the workers in the country, reveal that men have higher rates of reported work-related occupational accidents and illnesses at all age groups.[2] Similarly, Giuffrida, Iunes, and Macías (2001), analyzing data from a 1996 Mexican household survey, found that, after controlling for age and work characteristics, women were less likely than men to report work-related impairments.

Women and men are exposed to different types of work hazards, since they mostly work in different occupations. (As noted earlier, the region exhibits the highest degree of occupational segregation by gender). For instance, men predominate in mining, while women constitute the majority of the workers in the flower export business. The former suffer accidents and respiratory diseases, while the latter suffer the negative health effects of exposure to pesticides. While men reported more physical work-related impairments, women reported higher proportions of mental or intellectual work-related impairments (discussed in the section on emotional and mental stress later on). One interpretation of this data is that women face fewer physical risks at work than men but greater risks from the psychosocial work environment, such as stress associated with lower pay, disapproval of women's employment, or sexual harassment. While still at the level of conjecture, it may be that women in the region, in comparison to men, are in occupations that elevate the risk of chronic diseases (cardiovascular diseases, cancers) but decrease the risk of injuries or accidents. This hypothesis requires further study.

Table 8–6. Estimated Annual Occupational Fatalities in Latin America and the Caribbean (1998)

Work-related accidents	Estimates
Estimated number of fatal accidents	27,270–68,147
Fatality rate (per 1000 workers)	0.135–0.338
Fatal accidents reported in official statistics	7443
Fatal accidents unreported	19,827–60,704
Nonfatal accidents with 3 or more days out of work (millions)	27–51

Source: Giuffrida, Iunes, and Savedoff (2001).

Women's illness and injury rates may be artificially lowered by technical factors. If working women spend less time at the workplace than their male counterparts, then female accident rates, which are usually calculated per worker rather than per hour worked, may appear lower for this reason. Another element that may have important implications for epidemiological research is the difficulty in accounting for the existence of male–female task segregation. Since women and men with the same job titles often perform different tasks, they may have different amounts and types of exposure to work-related hazards (Messing et al., 1994).

When comparisons are made within the same industry, the results of studies comparing gender exposure to occupational hazards are variable. Sometimes women report more accidents than men and sometimes fewer. One example from the Latin American and Caribbean region involves a study that documented the occupational health problems among a sample of 497 workers in the *maquiladora* industry, the export processing and manufacturing firms in Mexico's northern free trade zone, in Nogales (Sonora, Mexico). According to that study, female workers had a greater probability of suffering work-related diseases and illnesses than male workers (Balcazar, Denman, and Lara, 1995). Another study that looked at the prevalence of byssinosis (an occupational lung disease) among workers in a cotton mill in Managua found that female workers had a much higher rate of the disease than did male workers (Velazquez et al., 1991). This result was attributed to different exposures of the sexes in both workplace and nonworkplace settings (for example, exposure to household wood stove smoke). Female health-care workers showed a higher prevalence of tuberculosis than their male counterparts in a tertiary care center in Mexico City (Ostrosky-Zeichner et al., 2000). The prevalence of tuberculosis was particularly high among nurses, most of whom were women; thus, gender differences were attributed to job segregation in the workplace.

Reproductive Health

Various researchers have shown that during pregnancy, women's respiration and metabolism are more active, and health hazards from exposure to chemicals in the workplace increase (Mattison, 1999). Moreover, exposure to some types of occupational hazards may produce negative consequences for the fetus and newborn. For example, it has been shown that a pregnant woman's exposure to chemicals such as pesticides may also affect the fetus (Waliszewski et al., 2000), and links have been established between maternal exposure to pesticides and higher child mortality rates due to congenital malformations (Jasso and García, 2000).

Physical stresses and hazards have been associated with an increased risk of miscarriage, low birth weight, and prematurity. Evidence of an association between labor fatigue and low birth weight was found in one study of a group of Mexico City women who worked as street vendors during pregnancy (Hernandez-Pena et al., 1999). A statistical relationship between low birth weight, maternal working conditions (such as a work week longer than 50 hours), and problems at work was found in a study that analyzed data from 2623 workers who gave birth in Mexico City hospitals in 1992 (Cerón-Mireles et al., 1997).

Maternity protection laws in the region are quite comprehensive and, on average, entitle women to 3 months of maternity leave and to full or nearly full wages during this period (see Table 8–7). However, these protections apply only to workers in the formal sector of the economy covered by social security. For example, under Mexican labor law, women are entitled to take a 12-week maternity leave and to receive their full wages during this period from the Mexican Social Security Institute. However, to be eligible for the social security–funded maternity leave wage subsidy, workers must have contributed to the social security fund for 30 weeks in the 12-month period prior to the maternity leave; otherwise, the employer must pay 100% of the maternity leave wage benefit. Thus, even though all working women are legally entitled to 12 weeks of paid maternity leave, the majority of the female workforce, being employed in the informal sector, would not receive any subsidy from the Social Security Institute. In both the formal and the informal sectors there are many cases of employers who have refused to hire pregnant women in order to avoid paying maternity wages, have forced women to resign before they could claim maternity leave, or have allowed women to take maternity leave but have refused to pay them while on leave (Human Rights Watch, 1998).

Emotional and Mental Stress

Women in both developed and developing countries report higher rates of psychological distress, consult more health practitioners, and take more medication for mental health concerns than do men (WHO, 2001). Work-related stress has been suggested as an explanatory factor related to the higher incidence of mental health problems among women (Pérez et al., 2000; Wollersheim, 1993), which in turn are associated with many chronic diseases. A major factor potentially affecting women's mental health status is the difficulty of reconciling work with family duties. If women's and men's work differs in the workplace, their situations diverge even more outside the workplace. Most women combine paid work and domestic activities such as cleaning, cooking, and child care. The result is that a woman's workday is, on average, longer than that of a man. Data from a recent national household survey in Nicaragua showed that if time spent both in the workplace and in the household is considered, employed women work, on average, 1 hour and 10 minutes more than men do each day.

A study of university teachers in Caracas, Venezuela, found that women with greater workloads in home tasks were more likely to complain of anxiety and depression (Blanco and Feldman, 2000). Another study, based on interviews with poor rural women in Mexico, found strong evidence of increasing emotional and psychological disorders as a result of the increased intensity in these women's use of time (Roldán, 1985).

Table 8–7. Maternity Leave Benefits in Latin America and the Caribbean (1998)

Country	Length of maternity leave	Percentage of wage paid in covered period	Provider of coverage
Antigua and Barbuda	13 weeks	60%	S.S. + possible employer supplement
Argentina	90 days	100%	Social security
Bahamas	8 weeks	100%	40% employer / 60% S.S.
Barbados	12 weeks	100%	Social security
Belize	12 weeks	80%	Social security
Bolivia	60 days	100% of national min wage + 70% of wages above min wage	Social security
Brazil	120 days	100%	Social security
Chile	18 weeks	100%	Social security
Colombia	12 weeks	100%	Social security
Costa Rica	4 months	100%	50% employer / 50% S.S.
Cuba	18 weeks	100%	Social security
Dominica	12 weeks	60%	S.S./employer
Dominican Republic	12 weeks	100%	50% employer / 50% S.S.
Ecuador	12 weeks	100%	25% employer / 75% S.S.
El Salvador	12 weeks	75%	Social security
Grenada	3 months	100% (2 months), 60% for third month	S.S./employer
Guatemala	12 weeks	100%	33% employer / 67% S.S.
Guyana	13 weeks	70%	Social security
Haiti	12 weeks	100% for 6 weeks	Employer
Honduras	10 weeks	100% for 84 days	33% employer / 67% S.S.
Jamaica	12 weeks	100% for 8 weeks	Employer
Mexico	12 weeks	100%	Social security
Nicaragua	12 weeks	60%	Social security
Panama	14 weeks	100%	Social security
Paraguay	12 weeks	50% for 9 weeks	Social security
Peru	90 days	100%	Social security
Saint Lucia	13 weeks	65%	Social security
Trinidad and Tobago	13 weeks	60%–100%	S.S./employer
Uruguay	12 weeks	100%	Social security
Venezuela	18 weeks	100%	Social security

Source: United Nations (2000).

Stress at work is also likely to be related to the degree of control over duties to be carried out and over the organization of work (Hall, 1989). Jobs assigned to women are characterized by a limited latitude for decision making, and they are more likely to be stressful (Cerón and Pimentel, 2000). A study based on cross-sectional data from a poor community in the city of Salvador in northeast Brazil also found that informal work—where women are overrepresented—was associated with a number of physiological symptoms (Santana et al., 1997). However, the study did not determine whether the statistical association was a casual relationship, and the researchers failed to control adequately for differences in socioeconomic status that could be associated both with physiological symptoms and with informal work.

Musculoskeletal Disorders

A major research area in occupational health is musculoskeletal problems, which include arthritis, carpal tunnel syndrome, and inflammation of various joints. Musculoskeletal disorders of the upper limbs are now among the most frequent work-related diseases in many Latin American and Caribbean countries (Reis et al., 2000). Musculoskeletal problems are a major occupational risk factor for women because of the nature of the tasks assigned to many women in factories and offices that require high levels of repetitive work and involve repetitive strain. For example, the prevalence of carpal tunnel syndrome, a work-related ailment characterized by wrist pain and loss of manual sensitivity, is 2 to 10 times more frequent in women than in men (De Krom et al., 1990). In Latin America and the Caribbean, high prevalence rates of musculoskeletal disorders have been recorded among female workers involved in the assembly operations in *maquiladora* plants and in secretarial jobs (Meservy et al., 1997; Ribeiro, 1997).

Mechanical equipment injuries account for a high proportion of all work-related injuries in all occupations (Gardner et al., 1999). Poorly designed and improperly used machinery and equipment are major causes of injury, particularly in the manufacturing sector. In the design of equipment and tools, the anthropometric data (standard or average height and weight measurements) used do not always reflect the characteristics of the working population who will use them. Most of the personal protective equipment and tools used worldwide are designed for men from Germany or the United States (Gardner et al., 1999). This means that many female workers are therefore not properly equipped for their protection.

Sexual Harassment

Sexual harassment at work is a health and safety matter as well as an issue of human rights. The influx of women into the workforce over the past 30 years has both magnified the problem and enabled women to be more vocal about their own defense. *Sexual harassment* may be defined as any non-work-related behavior having a sexual component (Gutek, 1985). Many behaviors constitute sexual harassment, but the two main categories are (*1*) quid pro quo harassment, in which economic penalties are placed on employees who refuse sexual advances, and (*2*) hostile work environment claims involving a hostile, offensive workplace atmosphere caused by sexual harassment, without threat of economic loss. Harassment in a general sense is one example of discrimination: a group or individual with more power or confidence picks on a weaker group or individual. Those responsible are often men in a position of authority over the person they are harassing. More generalized workplace harassment that is not tied to group membership and is known by many names, including *bullying*, *mobbing*, and *emotional abuse*, has recently become the focus of more research and policy attention (Keashly, 1998; Rayner, 1997; Sheehan, Barker, and Rayner, 1999). Among examples of these behaviors are excluding someone from key work activities, giving someone the silent treatment, demeaning someone in front of others, yelling and screaming at someone, flaunting status differences, and taking credit for another's work.

Sexual harassment in the workplace, especially in its more extreme forms, may have serious physical and emotional consequences for the targets. These include physical injury, depression, fatigue, headaches, sleeplessness, hostility, inability to concentrate, lower job satisfaction and organizational commitment, and deterioration of interpersonal relationships at work (Gutek and Koss, 1993; Vaux, 1993). Women are far more likely to experience sexual harassment than men because of women's status and role in society and in the workplace. Sexual harassment has been described as one of the most common and least discussed occupational health hazards for women. Studies in developed countries have shown that about 45% to 50% of women have experienced sexual harassment at some time during their working lives (Labour Research Department, 1999; Sheffey and Scott, 1992).

However, not much is known about the incidence of sexual harassment in Latin America. In Argentina, a survey of 302 women revealed that 47.4% had been the object of sexual harassment (Unión del Personal Civil de la Nación, 1997). In Uruguay, a survey of 1295 individuals found that 15% knew of a female colleague who had experienced sexual harassment (Raga, 1999). Certain groups of women are particularly vulnerable: live-in domestic workers and women who work in nontraditional occupations such as those in the *maquiladoras*. For example, in her study of the *maquiladoras*, La Botz (1994) described sexual harassment as endemic.

The Health Benefits of Women's Paid Work

The Impact of Work on Health

As noted earlier, a positive correlation is often found between health and participation in the labor market. Thus, despite the argument that exposure to hazards in the working environment may damage health, women who work in paid jobs report, on average, better physical well-being than others, most of whom are unemployed, retired, or keeping house. Table 8–8 shows the self-reported health status of Brazilian

Table 8–8. Health Status of Women Aged 15 Years and Older by Work Status (%)

	Brazil: employed*		Jamaica: economically active†	
Self-assessed health	Yes	No	Yes	No
Excellent	14.91	9.33	28.7	27.0
Very good	24.01	19.05	28.9	22.5
Good	39.87	35.57	28.2	24.1
Fair	19.07	28.59	11.4	14.8
Bad	2.14	7.46	2.9	11.6

Sources: * *Pesquisa sobre padrões de vida* (IBGE, Brazil, 1995–96); † *Jamaican Survey of Living Conditions* (Statistical Institute of Jamaica, 1989).

women aged 15 years and older, by occupational status. A higher proportion of working women, compared to nonworking women, assessed their health as excellent, very good, or good. Similar patterns emerge in other countries of the region, such as Jamaica. The positive correlation between employment and health generally remains significant and substantial, with adjustment for age, education, marriage, and race (Bird and Fremont, 1991; Ross and Mirowsky, 1995).

A plausible mechanism or process is needed to support the hypothesis of a causal relationship. Some researchers have argued that labor market participation may improve women's health status because of increased self-esteem, social contacts, and support (Ross and Mirowsky, 1995). Conversely, specific forms of nonemployment may be unhealthy. In particular, those who were laid off or fired, or who cannot find work, have a low sense of control and low levels of social support, and consequently suffer distress. Failure to get or keep a job may result in demoralization and neglect, and thus in poor health. Thus, involuntary unemployment may diminish health, whereas voluntary nonemployment, which includes being in school, being retired, or homemaking, may not (Pearlin et al., 1981).

A positive indirect effect of employment is related to the fact that paid jobs increase household income and decrease economic hardship, and both of these effects improve physical well-being. The seminal model developed by Grossman (1972) posits that individuals choose to allocate their available time and money so as to achieve the combination of health and other goals they value most, given their available resources (such as income). Women in paid employment bring additional income and augment the total amount of resources available in the household.

Researchers have repeatedly demonstrated the positive empirical relationship between income and health at the individual and national levels (Fiscella and Franks, 1997; Preston, 1975; Pritchett and Summers, 1996). These findings support the hypothesis that individuals and households maximize their utility (including health) according to their budget constraints. Thus, work has a positive effect on health because women in paid jobs are more likely to be able to afford medical care, higher-quality diets, and better housing for themselves and their children (Parker and Wong, 1997).

The Impact of Health on Work

Despite the facts and arguments supporting a causal interpretation, other researchers have argued that much or most of the correlation between health and employment results from a selection of healthy people into employment and of unhealthy ones out of it (Repetti, Matthews, and Waldron, 1989; Waldron, 1991). Evidence of various sorts supports this view. Physical impairments can limit both the physical demands of employers on their employees and the tasks that can be accomplished by employees. Even in the absence of a specific disease, many common or chronic diseases erode energy and concentration, and thus reduce both the labor supply and wage rates (Luft, 1975; Schultz and Tansel, 1997). A recent edited volume (Savedoff and Schultz, 2000) contains numerous studies carried out in Latin America to examine the empirical relationship between health and labor income. In one study, researchers analyzed data from Mexico that suggested an association between a decline of 1 year in age at menarche—an indicator that is closely linked with adult health—and a wage increase in adulthood of 23% to 26% (Knaul, 2000). A study in Colombia found that 1 more day of disability is associated with a decrease in annual earnings by rural women of about 13% (Ribero and Nuñez, 2000). In Peru, 1 less day of reported illness in a month increased the wage rate of urban and rural women by 3.4% and 6.2%, respectively (Cortez, 2000). A similar effect was estimated among Jamaican women (Neitzert and Handa, 2000).

Joint Examination of Health and Work

Clearly, women's work decisions, labor income, and health are jointly determined and linked in a complex relationship. The linkages are represented in Figure 8–2, based on the models suggested by Wolfe and Haveman (1983) and Haveman and colleagues (1994).

Women's Work and Children's Health

For women, work is also linked with the well-being of their offspring. Figure 8–3 shows the complexity of the relationship between mothers' work and their children's health. Women's work can negatively affect children's health because of reductions in the amount of time devoted to child care and breast-feeding. Negative associations have been found in the case of pregnant women. Work during pregnancy may produce negative effects on the development of the fetus, which may affect the child's health. As noted in the previous section, some evidence has shown a relationship between low birth weight and extremely poor maternal working conditions in Mexico.

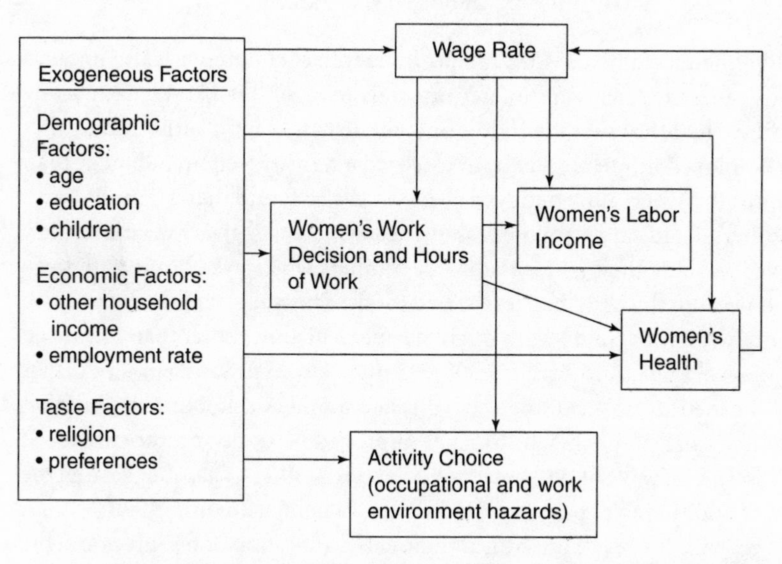

Figure 8–2. A model of the linkages between women's work and health.

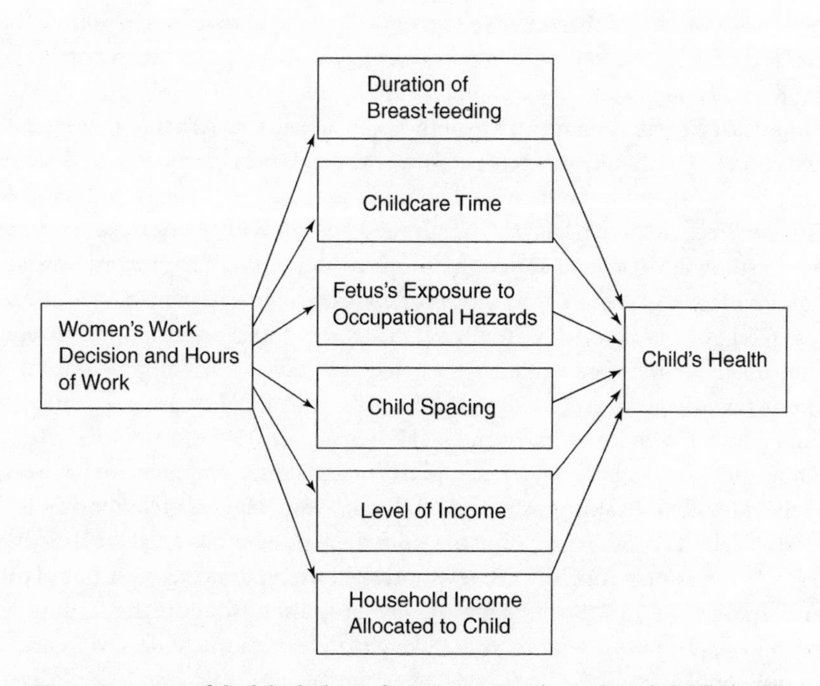

Figure 8–3. A model of the linkages between women's work and child's health.

On the other hand, women's work can positively affect children's health because of the positive income effect and longer intervals between births. A recent study based on Nicaraguan households in low-income urban communities found that children of employed mothers were both closer to a healthy weight and taller than those whose mothers were not employed. This study also found that in families with working mothers, child care was poorer, both because the caregivers were less likely to be observed washing their hands than were mothers who stayed home with their children and because the child had less varied foods. This suggests that the positive associations of work with child health might be due to income rather than improved care (Lamontagne, Engle, and Zeitlin, 1998). Another study, in Santiago, Chile, that controlled for genetic factors (mothers' height) and mothers' schooling showed that children's nutritional status (height for age) improved when poor mothers earned incomes. This finding was not replicated for nonpoor mothers, again suggesting the importance of additional income for children's well-being (Buvinic, 1998).

There is a growing literature on the intrahousehold allocation of resources and the role of individual preferences in household decision making. According to this literature, a household member's control over resources outside the family—such as unearned income, wage rate, or employability—affects the intrafamily distribution of resources. This happens because the person has greater bargaining power and, hence, can influence decision making (Alderman et al., 1995; Handa, 1996; Manser and Brown, 1980; McElroy, 1990). Preferences may differ within the household, and several studies have shown that, relative to men, women tend to favor children in their resource allocation behavior, with implications for their own health (Dwyer and Bruce, 1988; Kennedy and Peter, 1992; Thomas, 1990).

Empirical evidence supports this hypothesis. In Jamaica, maternal work was related to the reduction of family budgets because of expenditures on tobacco and alcohol (usually for consumption by men) and increases in the demand for goods that would positively affect children's health, such as food and preventive health care (Handa, 1994). A study in Guatemala found that women who earned a higher proportion of the family income gained significantly more control over decision making in all areas except food purchases, which were already primarily women's decisions. Controlling for potentially confounding variables, the percentage of the total family income earned by women was highly associated with children's nutritional status, suggesting that income control by mothers may benefit children (Engle, 1993).

Altogether, the available evidence suggests that maternal employment has a positive effect on child health (Leslie and Paolisso, 1989), and this relationship is reflected in Table 8–9. Summary statistics from the Demographic and Health Surveys (DHS), a series of nationally representative household surveys on population characteristics and health status and service utilization, support the finding that women in paid employment are more likely to give birth to children who are not underweight.

Table 8–9. Proportion of Children Smaller Than Average or Very Small at Birth, by Mother's Occupational Status (%)

	Guatemala (1998–1999)	Nicaragua (1998)
Paid employee	26.43	29.84
Did not work	32.47	31.36
Self-employed	28.54	25.25
Unpaid worker	25.00	34.78
Average	31.36	30.29

Source: Authors' calculations based on DHS.

Discussion and Policy Implications

It is a fact that all women work: they perform multiple roles of market production, home production, and reproduction. Although women work, on average, longer hours than men and contribute substantially to family income, the work of many women goes unrecognized. The findings presented in this chapter suggest that the following short-term policy actions would go a long way toward improving the health and well-being of women in the labor market.

Reduce Discrimination in the Labor Market

In relation to the disadvantages and discrimination that Latin American and Caribbean women face in the labor market, one can distinguish between situations where employers do not hire women or pay them less than men (*1*) because of cost and productivity concerns and (*2*) because of prejudices and gender biases. These considerations may help policy makers identify crucial points of intervention and the appropriate actions to take. In relation to the first point, women may display lower levels of productivity as expressed through wages than men because they are disadvantaged in terms of having lower levels of education, training, and previous work experience—factors that directly affect worker productivity. Interruptions in work experience because of childbearing or family responsibilities may compound their disadvantages in the labor market. However, these differences between male and female workers may also reflect earlier discrimination that prevented women from obtaining education, training, and experience in the first place.

To protect working women, many countries have adopted special measures, including the prohibition of night work, underground work, and other activities considered dangerous for women, and especially their reproductive health. Other measures have limited the weekly number of hours of work and overtime work, and have been oriented to the protection of women's traditional role as mother and wife.

In recent years, however, such measures have been increasingly questioned because protective legislation has sometimes led to discriminatory consequences, reducing women's access to employment. Moreover, employers may exclude women, as a working group, from hazardous occupations instead of removing the workplace risks for the protection of all workers' health. Thus, legislation and regulation in the countries of the region need to be reviewed in order to eliminate direct and indirect discrimination.

Because the majority of poor women in the Latin American and Caribbean region work in the informal sector and in agriculture, their status in these sectors is key to the improvement of their well-being. The income—and thus the ability—to promote the health of a substantial fraction of the lowest-income women can be improved by increasing productivity in these sectors. Improved productivity and its effect on wages, along with efficiency gains, may also free up time and thereby reduce women's time conflicts with their family responsibilities, while higher wages may allow for paid child care. Women may significantly improve their productivity if they are given technical assistance and training to improve the management of their activities, as well as better access to credit and other factors of production.

Reduce Underlying Inequalities in Education and Health

The link between women's education and improved health is well established. Women's education is also clearly related to access to paid occupations, with higher-quality jobs and better wages. Schooling and knowledge may also improve efficiency in the production of health. Studies have consistently found that mothers' education is positively correlated with their children's health and nutrition in developing countries (Cochrane, Leslie, and O'Hara, 1982). Women's educational attainment and health status have improved significantly in the past three decades. Unlike women in other developing regions of the world, young Latin American and Caribbean women attain, on average, higher educational levels than the region's men. (In the health arena, women live longer than men but are reported to suffer more often from morbidity and disability.) Nevertheless, increasing inequality in the distribution of education among women in different income, ethnic, and racial groups has translated into higher inequality of work opportunities and wages. This underlying inequality in human capital investment presents serious challenges to the promotion of women's health and well-being.

A disproportionate number of women will accumulate disadvantages (such as uneducated, unskilled, poor, single working mothers) and will be among the most vulnerable in the labor market. To deal with women's disadvantaged position, governments should pursue targeted programs to improve women's health, education, and training, as well as to provide support services and improve employment opportunities. Finally, it is important to ensure that interventions are introduced as early as possible to avoid a process of cumulative disadvantage.

Work Toward Comprehensive Social Insurance for the Poor

As noted earlier, the informal sector—casual employment, subcontracting, part-time work, home-based work, short-term employment, and self-employment—provides the bulk of opportunities for women in the region, particularly poor women. It provides alternatives to the traditional standard employment model, which typically restricts women's options. More flexible management of working hours and flexibility in the place of work could also benefit women. However, many women go into the informal sector because they have no other choice. In the informal sector, occupational health safety standards are not normally observed, and enforcement by the labor inspectors is difficult. Given that women's employment in the informal sector represents more than half of the total jobs, it is essential to find ways to protect women and other vulnerable groups from the more negative aspects of such work.

In addition to facing occupational health hazards, women in the informal sector have little access to health or unemployment insurance benefits. In six countries studied (Brazil, Dominican Republic, Jamaica, Mexico, Paraguay, Peru), only 5% of women in the poorest 20% of the income distribution have public or private health insurance, and this low coverage is not compensated for by public health services, in which the same inequitable patterns of access and utilization hold (Henderson, Montes, and Glassman, 2000). Lack of health insurance means that out-of-pocket payments represent a large proportion of total health spending, and adverse health episodes may have extreme impoverishing effects, moving the whole household into poverty (Wagstaff, 2000). Like general health insurance, occupational accident insurance is limited to the formal sector.

Few countries in the region are able to afford universal unemployment insurance, and few programs aimed at smoothing consumption during periods of unemployment are available for informal sector workers. Recently, several countries in the region have begun to finance workfare programs, which essentially function as unemployment insurance for the informal sector on a limited scale.[3] This lack of protection against income drops due to unemployment or catastrophic illness has important consequences for general health status, as well as food consumption levels and their impact on health.

How can formal sector protection be extended to the informal sector? Increasing formalization is one option. Formalized work relations would promote better labor conditions and allow for enforceable labor rights and access to formal social risk management instruments, such as health, accident, sickness, pension, and unemployment protection. Further, since informal sector businesses and individuals are unlikely to self-insure, governments may need to correct market failure (Holzmann and Jorgensen, 1999). However, the very factors that created the extensive informal sector in Latin America make greater formalization difficult to implement. High nonwage costs in the form of direct and indirect taxes, regulation, and licensing (in many cases, with weak links between contributions and benefits) create strong incentives for informality. In 1999, for example, mandatory contributions to social security[4] as a percentage of the region's gross wages varied between 11% in Honduras and

48% in Argentina, leading to a high regional average, only slightly lower than the rates in the Organization for Economic Cooperation and Development member countries (IDB, 2001). Argentina, Uruguay, Colombia, Brazil, and Peru have contribution rates relative to gross domestic product that are higher than the Organization for Economic Cooperation and Development average.

Many studies have suggested that the costs of labor market regulations are borne both by workers in the form of lower take-home wages or reduced employment and by employers in the form of increasing costs and lower profits. Also, the effectiveness of payroll taxes is low; rates are high, and so is tax evasion in the formal sector.[5] Nonwage labor costs are not the only barrier to formality. Limited access to credit in financial markets, burdensome administrative requirements for property ownership, and business creation and lack of credible legal protections also create substantial disincentives and are the subject of a growing literature. Thus, to increase formalization in the short term, governments may have to pursue two possibly contradictory courses. First, they must consider the reduction of social security–related and other taxes that neither workers nor employers perceive as providing sufficient benefits. Second, they should improve the organization and quality of tax-financed services and regulations in order first to strengthen the link between contributions and benefits and second to create incentives for formality.

Another feasible short-term option is to provide a larger safety net for the poor. While governments in the region face resource constraints and the need to maintain low nonwage labor costs, they may be able to reallocate, at least temporarily, existing spending so that it is shifted from inefficient public social programs to targeted social insurance programs for the poorest, especially poor women.

Empower Female Workers

The process of empowering people in the workplace has been a successful means of improving the work environment. However, the particular needs of women have thus far received very little attention in the establishment of health promotion policies, since women are underrepresented in decision-making bodies such as national safety councils, occupational health services, trade unions, and firm-level safety and health committees. Action to empower women in the formal sector needs to improve their representation in labor market institutions and in collective bargaining structures, especially at leadership levels. For those working in the informal sector, group or collective representation is crucial, and the rights to associate freely and to organize are fundamental to women's empowerment.

El Salvador's duty free, export-oriented apparel factories employ mostly women (80% of the total workforce). According to the *New York Times* (April 24, 2001, A1) a recent report by the government found unhealthy air and water conditions, large amounts of forced overtime, and frequent dismissal of workers who supported labor unions. But some factories have taken proactive measures to improve conditions through the creation of a group of independent monitors made up of local union, religious, and academic leaders who meet regularly with workers to hear complaints, investigate problems, make spot checks, and look over books. All agree that human rights violations in the factory are down in comparison to other factories. Nevertheless, lack of freedom to organize remains.

A good sign in the region is the professionalization of nongovernmental organizations that look after women's concerns. They have fought hard to improve women's sexual and reproductive health, and have focused increasingly on improving their occupational health. Examples include Coverco, a nongovernmental organization in Guatemala set up to monitor labor conditions in the *maquila* industry and in agriculture. Governments and international agencies need to nurture and strengthen nongovernmental organizations such as Coverco, as well as women's associations and groups in civil society, by, among other things, providing training and funding and creating conditions that encourage local philanthropy.

Occupational Safety Research and Information Gathering

Occupational health and safety in Latin America and the Caribbean is still in its infancy, and the region has fewer experts, less safety and monitoring equipment, and less enforcement than do developed nations (Delclos et al., 1999). Occupational safety and health research in the region is underfunded. Estimates show that only about 5% of occupational health research in the world takes place in developing countries, which clearly demonstrates a severe imbalance between the share of the population, the severity of the problem, and the resources available in these countries (Partanen et al., 1999). Moreover, women are studied less often than men, and in many studies involving both women and men, differences between the sexes often are not investigated (Niedhammer et al., 2000). Thus, scientific research oriented toward the well-being of female workers is needed to yield a better understanding of women's conditions (Dumais, 1992).

Information about women's work and health at work is particularly scarce, since standard occupational classifications frequently omit the types of work undertaken by women, especially those related to "invisible" occupations in the informal sector and in agriculture. Thus, it is important to enhance the efforts of data collection agencies, including those that collect information on employment, in order to have a reliable basis for policies related to women in the workplace. In particular, it is important to have this information disaggregated by income, as well as by ethnic and racial groupings.

ACKNOWLEDGMENT

The views and interpretations presented in this chapter are those of the authors and should not be attributed to the Inter-American Development Bank or to any individual acting on its behalf.

Notes

1. The region of Latin America and the Caribbean is made up of the following countries: Argentina, the Bahamas, Barbados, Belize, Bolivia, Brazil, Chile, Colombia, Costa Rica, the Dominican Republic, the eastern Caribbean, Ecuador, El Salvador, Guatemala, Guyana, Haiti, Honduras, Jamaica, Mexico, Nicaragua, Panama, Paraguay, Peru, Suriname, Trinidad and Tobago, Uruguay, and Venezuela.

2. Examination of IMSS data from the 1995–1999 period reveals that the number of occupational accidents reported by male workers diminished by more that 7%, while women's work-related accidents increased by 12%. Considering rates, occupational accidents among male workers decreased about 10% more than those among women, suggesting that improvements in occupational safety were concentrated in occupations with a predominantly male workforce.

3. Workfare programs, such as Trabajar in Argentina and Empleo en Acción in Colombia, generally finance construction or infrastructure rehabilitation activities and provide temporary workfare jobs to unskilled workers. Given this emphasis, they tend to employ men rather than women.

4. Social security programs include pensions, disability and death pensions, health insurance, maternity benefits, unemployment insurance, workers' compensation, and family allowances.

5. In Guatemala, for example, only 5% of taxes are actually collected. Chile leads the region, with a 20% collection rate (IDB, 2001).

References

Alderman, H., P. A. Chiappori, L. Haddad, J. Hoddinott, and R. Kanbur. 1995. Unitary versus collective models of the household: Is it time to shift the burden of proof? *World Bank Research Observer* 10(1): 1–19.

Anríquez, G., and M. Buvinic. 1997. Poverty alleviation for male-headed and female-headed households in a fast growing economy: A case study for Chile. Washington, D.C.: Inter-American Development Bank. Mimeographed.

Balcazar, H., C. Denman, and F. Lara. 1995. Factors associated with work-related accidents and sickness among maquiladora workers: The case of Nogales, Sonora, Mexico. *International Journal of Health Services* 25(3): 489–502.

Barros, R., L. Fox, and R. Mendonca. 1997. Female-headed households, poverty, and the welfare of children in urban Brazil. *Economic Development and Cultural Change* 45(2): 231–57.

Beneria, L. 2001. Changing employment patterns and the informalization of jobs: General trends and gender dimensions. Paper presented at the workshop Women at Work: A Challenge for Development, March 17, Santiago, Chile.

Bird, C. E., and A. M. Fremont. 1991. Gender, time use, and health. *Journal of Health and Social Behavior* 32: 114–29.

Blanco, G., and L. Feldman. 2000. Home-making responsibilities and health in working woman. *Salud Pública de México* 42(3): 217–25.

Buvinic, M. 1998. Costs of adolescent childbearing. *Studies in Family Planning* 29(2): 201–9.

Buvinic, M. 2001. La mujer en el mundo del trabajo: progresos y desafios. Paper presented at workshop, Women at Work: A Challenge for Development, March 17, Santiago, Chile.

Buvinic, M., and G. R. Gupta. 1997. Female-headed households and female-maintained families: Are they worth targeting to reduce poverty in developing countries? *Economic Development and Cultural Change* 45(2): 259–80.

Cerón, F. E., and P. B. M. Pimentel. 2000. Flexibilidad y salud mental: el caso de las trabajadoras industriales. Paper presented at the fourth Reunión Nacional de Investigación en Salud en el Trabajo. January 20–21, México, D.F.

Cerón-Mireles, P., C. Sánchez-Carrillo, S. D. Harlow, and R. Nuñez-Urquiza. 1997. Maternal working conditions and low birth weight in Mexico City. *Salud Pública de México* 39(1): 2–10.

Chiriboga, M., R. Grynspan, and L. E. Pérez. 1995. *Mujeres de maíz: Programa de análisis de la política del sector agropecuario frente a la mujer productora de alimentos en centroamérica y panamá.* San José, Costa Rica: Inter-American Development Bank and Instituto Interamericano de Cooperación para la Agricultura (IICA).

Cochrane, S., J. Leslei, and D. J. O'Hara. 1982. Parental education and child health: Intracountry evidence. *Health, Policy and Education* 2: 213–50.

Cortez, R. 2000. Health and productivity in Peru: Estimates by gender and region. In *Wealth from health: Linking social investments to earnings in Latin America,* edited by W. D. Savedoff and T. P. Schultz. Washington, D.C.: Inter-American Development Bank.

Deininger, K., and L. Squire. 1996. A new data set measuring income inequality. *World Bank Economic Review* 10(3): 565–91.

De Krom, M., A. Kester, P. Knipschild, and F. Spaans. 1990. Risk factors for carpal tunnel syndrome. *American Journal of Epidemiology* 132(6): 1102–10.

Delclos, G. L., S. A. Felknor, M. T. Morandi, L. J. Schulze, L. S. Tovar, and L. Yanes. 1999. The role of information dissemination in sustainability of international partnership. *International Journal of Occupational and Environmental Health* 5: 203–8.

Dumais, L. 1992. Impact of the participation of women in science: On rethinking the place of women especially in occupational-health. *Women and Health* 18(3): 11–25.

Duryea, S., A. Cox Edwards, and M. Ureta. 2001. *A survey of women in the labor market.* Washington, D.C.: Inter-American Development Bank. Mimeographed.

Duryea, S., and M. Székely. 2000. Labor markets in Latin America: A look at the supply-side. *Emerging Markets Review* 1(3): 199–228.

Dwyer, D., and J. Bruce, eds. 1988. *A home divided: Women and income in the third world.* Stanford, CA: Stanford University Press.

Economic Commission on Latin America and the Caribbean (ECLAC). 1997. *Las mujeres en América Latina y el Caribe en los años noventa: Elementos de diagnóstico y propuestas.* Serie Mujer y Desarrollo no. 18. Santiago, Chile: ECLAC.

Engle, P. L. 1993. Influences of mothers' and fathers' income on children's nutritional status in Guatemala. *Social Science and Medicine* 37(11): 1303–12.

Fiscella, K., and P. Franks. 1997. Poverty or income inequality as predictor of mortality: Longitudinal cohort study. *British Medical Journal* 314 (7096): 1724–27.

Gammage, S., and J. Schmitt. 2001. Statistical appendix of women's status in Latin America and the Caribbean, 1970–2000. Paper presented at the workshop Women at Work: A Challenge for Development, March 17, Santiago, Chile.

Gardner, D., J. A. Cross, P. N. Fonteyn, J. Carlopio, and A. Shikdar. 1999. Mechanical equipment injuries in small manufacturing business. *Safety Science Journal* 33: 1–12.

Giuffrida, A., R. Iunes, and H. Macías. 2001. *Workers' health in Latin America: An econometric analysis of work-related injuries.* Health Note Report No. 5. Washington, D.C.: IDB.

Giuffrida, A., R. Iunes, and W. Savedoff. 2001. *Occupational safety in Latin America and the Caribbean: Economic and health dimensions of the problem.* Sustainable Development Department Technical Study Series No. 121. Washington, D.C.: Inter-American Development Bank.

Greenhouse, S. May 10, 2001. Labor abuses in El Salvador are detailed in document. *New York Times*, Section A, p. 12.

Grossman, M. 1972. On the concept of health capital and the demand for health. *Journal of Political Economy* 80: 223–55.

Grynspan, R. 1999. *Perspectiva de género y nueva ruralidad.* San José, Costa Rica: Instituto Interamericano de Cooperación para la Agricultura (IICA).

Gutek, B. A. 1985. *Sex and the workplace: Impact of sexual behavior and harassment on women, men and organizations.* San Francisco: Jossey-Bass.

Gutek, B. A., and M. P. Koss. 1993. Changed women and changed organizations: Consequences of and coping with sexual harassment. *Journal of Vocational Behavior* 42: 28–48.

Hall, E. M. 1989. Gender, work control and stress: A theoretical discussion and an empirical test. *International Journal of Health Services* 19: 725–45.

Handa, S. 1994. Gender headship and intra-household resource allocation. *World Development* 22: 1535–47.

Handa, S. 1996. Maternal education and child attainment in Jamaica: Testing the bargaining power hypothesis. *Oxford Bulletin of Economics and Statistics* 58(1): 119–37.

Haveman, R., B. Wolfe, B. Kreider, and M. Stone. 1994. Market work, wages, and men's health. *Journal of Health Economics* 13(2): 163–82.

Henderson, P., J. L. Montes, and A. Glassman. 2000. Access, utilization and household spending on women's health: An analysis of household surveys in six countries. Background paper prepared for *The health of women in Latin America and the Caribbean: A convergence of interests*, edited by R. Levine, A. Glassman, and M. Schneidman. Washington, D.C.: Inter-American Development Bank, World Bank and Pan American Health Organization, 2002.

Hernandez-Pena, P., M. D. L. Kageyama, I. Coria, B. Hernandez, and S. Harlow. 1999. Working conditions, labor fatigue and low birth weight among female street vendors. *Salud Pública de México* 41(2): 101–9.

Holzmann, R., and S. Jorgensen. 1999. Social protection as social risk management: Conceptual underpinnings for the social protection sector strategy paper. Social Protection Discussion Paper no. 9904. Washington, D.C.: World Bank.

Horton, S. 1999. Marginalization revisited: Women's work and pay, and economic development. *World Development* 27(3): 571–82.

Human Rights Watch. 1998. *A job or your rights: Continued sex discrimination in Mexico's maquiladora sector.* Report vol. 10 (1B). New York: Human Rights Watch.

Instituto Brasileiro de Geografia e Estadistica (IBGE). *Pesquisa sobre padrões de vida.* 1995–96. Brasilia, Brazil: IBGE.

Instituto Mexicano del Seguro Social (IMSS). 1999. *Memoria Estadística 1999.* México, D.F.: IMSS.

Inter-American Development Bank (IDB). 2001. *Report on social and economic progress in Latin America and the Carribean.* Washington, D.C.: IDB.

International Labor Organization (ILO). 1999a. *Latin America and Caribbean 1999 labour overview.* Geneva: ILO.

International Labor Organization (ILO). 1999b. *Yearbook of labour statistics.* Geneva: ILO.

International Labor Organization (ILO). 2000. *Latin America and Caribbean 1999 labour overview.* Geneva: ILO.

Jasso, B., and J. Garcķa. 2000. Plaguicidas y malformaciones congénitas en México. Paper presented at the fourth Reunión Nacional de Investigación en Salud en el Trabajo, January 20–21, Mexico, D.F.

Kaufman, L., and D. Gonzalez. 2001. Labor standards clash with global reality. *The New York Times.* Late Edition—Final, Section A, Page 1, Column 1, April 24.

Keashly, L. 1998. Emotional abuse in the workplace: Conceptual and empirical issues. *Journal of Emotional Abuse* 1: 85–117.

Kennedy, E., and P. Peter. 1992. Household food security and child nutrition: The interaction of income and gender household head. *World Development* 20: 1077–85.

Knaul, F. M. 2000. Health, nutrition and wages: Age at menarche and earnings in Mexico. In *Wealth from health: Linking social investments to earnings in Latin America,* edited by W. D. Savedoff and T. P. Schultz. Washington, D.C.: Inter-American Development Bank.

La Botz, D. 1994. Manufacturing poverty: The maquiladorization of Mexico. *International Journal of Health Services* 24(3): 403–8.

Labour Research Department. 1999. *Women's health and safety: A trade union guide.* Labour Research, no. 21. London: Labour Research Department.

Lamontagne, J. F, P. L. Engle, and M. F. Zeitlin. 1998. Maternal employment, child care, and nutritional status of 12- to 18-month-old children in Managua, Nicaragua. *Social Science and Medicine* 46(3): 403–14.

Leslie, J., M. Lycette, and M. Buvinic. 1988. Weathering economic crises: The crucial role of women in health. In *Health, nutrition, and economic crises: Approaches to policy in the third world,* edited by D. E. Bell and M. R Reich. Dover, MA: Auburn House.

Leslie, J., and M. Paolisso. 1989. *Women, work, and child welfare in the third world.* Washington, D.C.: American Association for the Advancement of Science.

Lim, L. L. 1996. *More and better jobs for women: An action guide.* Geneva: ILO.

Lora, E., and G. Marquez. 1998. The employment problem in Latin America: Perceptions and stylized facts. Working paper no. 371, Office of the Chief Economist, Inter-American Development Bank, Washington, D.C.

Luft, H. 1975. The impact of poor health on earnings. *Review of Economics and Statistics* 57: 43–57.

Manser, M., and M. Brown. 1980. Marriage and household decision making: A bargaining analysis. *International Economic Review* 21: 31–44.

Mattison, D. R. 1999. Differences between males and females and the consequences for risk assessment and regulation. In *Risk assessment strategies in relation to population subgroups,* report of a workshop held in Leicester on 24–25 April 1997, edited by the Risk Assessment and Toxicology Steering Committee. University of Leicester, UK: Institute for Environmental and Health.

McElroy, M. 1990. The empirical content of Nash-bargained household behavior. *Journal of Human Resources* 25: 559–83.

Meservy, D., A. J. Suruda, D. Bloswick, J. Lee, and M. Dumas. 1997. Ergonomic risk exposure and upper-extremity cumulative trauma disorders in a maquiladora medical devices manufacturing plant. *Journal of Occupational and Environmental Medicine* 39(8): 767–73.

Messing, K., L. Dumais, J. Courville, A. M. Seifert, and M. Boucher. 1994. Evaluation of exposure data from men and women with the same job title. *Journal of Occupational Medicine* 36(8): 913–17

Neitzert, M., and S. Handa. 2000. Gender and the impact of health on labour force participation in Jamaica. Jamaica: University of the West Indies. Mimeographed.

Niedhammer, I., M. J. Saurel-Cubizolles, M. Piciotti, and S. Bonenfant. 2000. How is sex considered in recent epidemiological publications on occupational risks? *Occupational and Environmental Medicine* 57(8): 521–27.

Ostrosky-Zeichner, L., M. S. Rangel-Frausto, E. Garcia-Romero, A. Vazquez, M. J. Ibarra, and S. P. de Leon-Rosales. 2000. Tuberculosis in healthcare workers: Importance of surveillance and control programs. *Salud Pública de México* 42(1): 48–52.

Parker, S. W., and R. Wong. 1997. Household income and health care expenditures in Mexico. *Health Policy* 40(3): 237–55.

Partanen, T. J., C. Hogstedt, R. Ahasan, A. Aragón, M. E. Arroyave, J. Jeyaratnam, K. Kurppa, R. Loewenson, I. Lundberg, A. V. F. Ngowi, C. F. L. Mbakaya, L. Stayner, K. Steenland, E. Weiderpass, and C. Wesseling. 1999. Collaboration between developing and developed countries and between developing countries in occupational health research and surveillance. *Scandinavian Journal of Work, Environment, and Health* 25(3): 296–300.

Pearlin, L. I., M. A. Lieberman, E. G. Menaghan, and J. T. Mullan. 1981. The stress process. *Journal of Health and Social Behavior* 22: 337–56.

Pérez, P., B. Maribel, R. E. Gómez, and L. Enríquez. 2000. Mujer, trabajo industrial y salud mental en Naucalpan: dinámica de una población vulnerada. Paper presented at the fourth Reunión Nacional de Investigación en Salud en el Trabajo, January 20–21, Mexico, D.F.

Preston, S. H. 1975. The changing relation between mortality and level of economic development. *Population Studies* 29: 231–48.

Pritchett, L., and L. H. Summers. 1996. Wealthier is healthier. *Journal of Human Resources* 31: 841–68.

Raga, A. 1999. Problemas de Trabajo. El País, Montevideo, Uruguay. Available at www.cifra.com.uy/co 270699.htm

Rayner, C. 1997. The incidence of workplace bullying. *Journal of Community and Applied Social Psychology* 7(3): 199–208.

Reis, R. J., T. M. M. Pinheiro, A. Navarro, and M. Martin. 2000. Profile of occupational disease outpatients and the presence of repetitive strain injury. *Revista de Saude Pública* 34(3): 292–98.

Repetti, R. L., K. A. Matthews, and I. Waldron. 1989. Employment and women's health. Effects of paid employment on women's mental and physical health. *American Psychologist* 44(11): 1394–401.

Ribeiro, H. P. 1997. Lesões por Esforços Repetitivos (LER): Uma doença emblemática. *Cadernos de Saúde Pública* 13(2): 85–93.

Ribero, R., and J. Nuñez. 2000. Adult morbidity, height and earnings in Colombia. In *Wealth from health. Linking social investments to earnings in Latin America*, edited by W. D. Savedoff and T. P. Schultz. Washington, D.C.: Inter-American Development Bank.

Roldán, M. 1985. Industrial outworking: Struggles for the reproduction of working class families and gender subordination. In *Beyond employment: Household, gender and subsistence*, edited by N. Redclift and E. Mingione. Oxford: Basil Blackwell.

Ross, C. E., and J. Mirowsky. 1995. Does employment affect health? *Journal of Health and Social Behavior* 36: 230–43.

Santana, V. S., D. Loomis, B. Newman, and S. D. Harlow. 1997. Informal jobs: Another occupational hazard for women's mental health? *International Journal of Epidemiology* 26(6): 1236–42.

Savedoff, W. D., and T. P. Schultz. 2000. *Wealth from health. Linking social investments to earnings in Latin America.* Washington, D.C.: Inter-American Development Bank.

Schultz, T. P., and A. Tansel. 1997. Wage and labor supply effects of illness in Cote d'Ivoire and Ghana: Instrumental variable estimates for days disabled. *Journal of Development Economics* 53(2): 251–86.

Sheehan, M., M. Barker, and C. Rayner. 1999. Applying strategies for dealing with workplace bullying. *International Journal of Manpower* 20(1/2): 50–56.

Sheffey, S., and R. Scott. 1992. Perceptions of sexual harassment in the workplace. *Journal of Applied Social Psychology* 22: 1502–20.

Standing, G. 1999. Global feminization through flexible labor: A theme revisited. *World Development* 27(3): 583–602.

Statistical Institute of Jamaica in conjunction with the Planning Institute of Jamaica. 1989. *Jamaican survey of living conditions.* Kingston, Jamaica: Statistical Institute of Jamaica.

Székely, M., M. Hilgert, and A. Glassman. 2000. Criterios para estimar el valor de un subsidio condicionado en Colombia. Washington, D.C.: Inter-American Development Bank. Mimeographed.

Thomas, D. 1990. Intrahousehold resource-allocation: An inferential approach. *Journal of Human Resources* 25(4): 635–64.

Unión del Personal Civil de la Nación. 1997. *Estudio sobre acoso sexual: Violencia laboral.* Buenos Aires: Secretaría de la Mujer, Unión del Personal Civil de la Nación.

United Nations (UN). 2000. *Women 2000: Trends and statistics.* New York: UN.

Vaux, A. 1993. Paradigmatic assumptions in sexual harassment research: Being guided without being misled. *Journal of Vocational Behavior* 42: 116–35.

Velazquez, A. M., D. C. Christiani, R. McConnell, E. A. Eisen, and M. Wilcox. 1991. Respiratory disease in a textile factory in Nicaragua. *American Journal of Industrial Medicine* 20: 195–208.

Wagstaff, A. 2000. *Technical note A: Research on equity, poverty and health: Lesson for the developing world.* Washington, D.C., U.S.: World Bank.

Waldron, I. 1991. Effects of labor force participation on sex differences in mortality and morbidity. In *Women, work, and health: Stress and opportunities,* edited by M. Frankenhaeuser, U. Lundberg, and M. Chesney. New York: Plenum Press.

Waliszewski, S. M., A. A. Aguirre, R. M. Infanzon, and J. Siliceo. 2000. Carryover of persistent organochlorine pesticides through placenta to fetus. *Salud Pública de México* 42(5): 384–90.

Wasserman, E. 1999. Environment, health, and gender in Latin America: Trends and research issues. *Environmental Research Section A* 80(3): 253–78.

Wolfe, B. L., and R. Haveman. 1983. Time allocation, market work, and changes in female health. *American Economic Review* 73(2): 134–39.

Wollersheim, J. P. 1993. Depression, women and the workplace. *Occupational Medicine: State of the Art Reviews* 8(4): 787–94.

World Health Organization (WHO). 2001. *The world health report 2001. Mental health: New understanding, new hope.* Geneva: WHO.

9

Women, Labor, and Social Transitions

PARVIN GHORAYSHI

Over the past few decades, perhaps more than ever before, problems of work have been at the forefront of public consciousness and debate, as well as academic theorizing and research. Structural and technological changes at both the national and international levels have raised questions about the nature and place of work in various societies: What is work? Why and how is it divided up, organized, and rewarded? Could it be different? Considerable changes in both the real world of work and the academic analysis on the nature of work have occurred.

One of the most important additions, as well as challenges, to the study of work has come from the growing research on women and work (Armstrong and Armstrong, 1990; Boserup, 1970; Creighton and Omari, 2000; Dickinson and Schaeffer, 2001; Roos, 1985; United Nations, 2000). This literature spans many disciplines and draws attention to the ways in which the position of female workers is determined by the sexual division of labor and by women's role in reproductive, domestic, and productive work as a whole (Leacock and Safa, 1986; Stanley, 1987). The studies to date have analyzed, among other things, the interplay between gender and class, the impact of state policies and ideologies on women's participation in the labor market, the influence of globalization and the new technology on women's work, and the ways women themselves have been influential in changing their working lives. In general, this scholarship has revealed both the complexity and the centrality of women's work in various parts of the world (Bodman and Tohidi, 1998; Redclift and Sinclair, 1991; Smith, 1987).

Within women's studies, interest in the study of women in developing countries rose with the inauguration of the United Nations (UN) Decade for Women in 1975. Various UN agencies, the World Bank, national governments, many Western agencies for international development, and even multinational corporations identified with the field. As a result, during the past two decades, social scientists have compiled an impressive body of research on women's work and their position in society in Africa, Asia, Latin America, the Caribbean, and the Middle East (Davies, 1983; Ghorayshi, 1994; Mies, 1986; Moghadam, 2000).

Iranian women's position in the labor market is the detailed case example of this chapter. In Iran, especially after the Islamic revolution of 1979, issues related to women's work and position in society have received increasing attention, as has been true in other nations. Scholars have discussed the impact of the revolution on women (Afshar, 1998a; Millett, 1986; Neshat, 1980), analyzed women's rights and status under Islam (Mahdavi, 1983; Neshat, 1980), talked about the burden of Islamic ideology (Afshar, 1984), and focused on a range of other issues (Betteridge, 1980; Sanasarian, 1982). The writings on various aspects of women's lives continue to grow (Afshar, 1998b; Haeri, 1989; Nafisi, 1994; Paidar, 1995).

Iranian women's position in the labor market has attracted the attention of researchers (Afshar, 1981, 1997; Moghadam, 1988, 1991, 1995, 2000; Tabari and Yeganeh, 1982). However, this scholarship has tended to focus on urban women who are in the formal sector of the economy and are in the paid labor force. Moreover, these researchers did not discuss and analyze the multidimensional nature of women's work systematically. In addition, as I demonstrate in this chapter, much of what we know about women and work in Iran is based on official statistics that use the traditional structural approaches to employment. It focuses on whether a person works full-time or part-time, is self-employed or an employee, or is in a temporary or permanent position. Structural approaches to work prevent us from grasping the multilayered nature and complexity of women's work. Moreover, such approaches do not enable us to assess jobs from the perspective of workers themselves and how work affects their well-being.

In the first section of this chapter, using the research findings from various parts of the world, I emphasize the significance of gender as a category of analysis in our understanding of the nature of women's work. In the second section, I discuss how government policies and our method of large-scale data collection in Iran (as elsewhere) have contributed to our narrow conception of women's work. In the third section, I use examples from my original case studies in Iran[1] to discuss the varied nature of women's work: paid employment, work in the household, and family work. In the fourth section, I use women's own words to show the complex impact of women's multiple roles on their well-being. I conclude that women's work is complex and multidimensional, that it cannot be limited to paid work, and that narrow definitions of *work* do not allow us to understand the relationship between women's work and their well-being.

Understanding Gender Inequality

Social scientists have challenged the sex-blind analysis of work and have established that no consideration of the division of labor can ignore the significance of gender in explaining the experience and organization of work (Gannagé, 1986; Waring, 1999). They have questioned any explanation that attributes differences primarily to biologically determined factors and use the term *gender* to label socially constructed differences between women and men (Armstrong and Armstrong, 1990; Sydie, 1987). While these studies have drawn our attention to the nonbiological origins of women's position, the conditions under which women participate in the labor force remain a considerable problem (Basow, 1992; Joekes, 1987; Loutfi, 1985; Smith, 1987; Stacey, 1987).

These social scientists have discussed the distinct nature of women's work and their differing pattern of participation in the labor force. On the basis of empirical research, anthropologists and other social scientists have compiled massive evidence regarding the centrality of women's contributions in both industrialized and developing countries (Armstrong and Armstrong, 1990; Boserup, 1970; Leacock and Safa, 1986; Waring, 1999). In a classic study, Boserup (1970) showed that women are the key producers of food in Africa. Other researchers have stressed the importance of women's work in various types of production, both for sale and for subsistence (Kandiyoti, 1988; Suda, 1989). Women are producers, traders, migrant workers, and wage laborers, and they are divided on the basis of class and other factors (Kabeer, 1992; Radcliffe, 1990). Researchers have shown, again and again, that women have a subordinate position both in the household and in the labor market (Dickerscheid, 1990; Hirschberg and Hirschberg, 2001; Hopkins, 1992; Phillips, 1989; Seager, 1997). It has also been widely documented that women's paid employment is segregated and concentrated in a limited number of paid occupations, and that much of women's work remains invisible (Ghorayshi, 1994; hooks, 1989; Kandiyoti, 1988; Labrecque, 1996; Mies, 1986; Seager, 1997; Smith, 1987).

Moreover, scholars of women's studies have focused on the importance of women's work inside the home, as well as on the interplay between paid work and family life (Gannagé, 1986; Ghorayshi, 1996). They have rightly pointed out that we need to go beyond the traditional structural approaches to the study of work, where the focus is on paid employment, and recognize that theories of work must consider all types of labor, paid or unpaid. This broader view requires including the unpaid labor done in family enterprises and the volunteer work performed at every level of society (Waring, 1999). By stressing the importance of gender in current analyses of work, scholars have criticized research and theories on work for ignoring the experience of women as women and for downplaying women's experience as workers (Gannagé, 1986; Reeves, 1986; Smith, 1987; Waring, 1999).

With the growth of literature on women's contributions globally and in specific countries, it has become clear that a combination of extremely complex variables affect the definition of a *man* or a *woman* within a specific population (Dumont, 1992; Hirschberg and Hirschberg, 2001). While there are similarities in women's lives, there are also tremendous differences, and those require concepts that can detail the variations (Anderson, 1988; Barrett and McIntosh, 1985; hooks, 1988). The multidimensional nature of women's work cannot be grasped without developing knowledge of the links between gender and other social relations within a particular society (Dumont, 1992; Labrecque, 1996). Within such a perspective, the historical, social, and cultural specificity that affects women's working lives needs to be emphasized.

In Iran, as elsewhere, gender is a social construct. Moreover, when we talk about working women in Iran, we must not draw a picture that is monolithic and homogeneous. The most crucial fact is that Iranian women, like their counterparts elsewhere, do not constitute a unified group. In 1996, 29 million of Iran's more than 60 million people were women. Of these women, 61.3% lived in urban areas, 38.3% were in rural areas, and the rest were categorized as unsettled (Statistical Centre of Iran, 1998, 58). Apart from urban and rural divisions, there are differences among women based on education, type of work, language, age, income, and many other factors.[2] When all these factors are taken into account, we find that a narrow notion of work cannot detail the complexity of Iranian women's working lives.

In what follows, I discuss some of the major factors that have been crucial in determining women's work and women's participation in public life. The presence or absence of women in the paid labor market, women's expected role in society, how statistics define women's work, and so on have to be understood within the political, social, and cultural context of Iran.

Institutionalizing Gender Inequity

Women and State Policies

In both the industrialized and developing worlds, there is general agreement that the state has played and continues to play a central role in the formulation of social policies, development strategies, and legislation that shape opportunities for women (Baker, 1995; Flora, 1986; O'Connor, Orloff, and Shaver, 1999; Parpart and Staudt, 1988; Peterson, 1992). The state can act as a facilitator or as an obstacle to the integration of women in public life. In the Middle East, governments have been major determinants of women's legal and economic status, to the extent that some scholars differentiate governments in this region by the position they assign to women in the family and in society (Afkhami, 1995; Esposito, 1982; Mernissi, 1991). However, it is important to note that, in this region, there are variations in state policies regarding the mobilization of female labor and women's integration into the formal economy. As Moghadam (1993, 54) stated:

> In some cases, a regime's search for political legitimacy, a larger labor force, or an expanded social base has led it to construct health, education and welfare services conducive to greater work participation by women, and to encourage female activity in the public sphere. Examples are the Iraqi Baathists during the 1960s and 1970s, the Pahlavi state in Iran in the same period, Tunisia under the late President Habib Bourguiba, and Egypt under Nasser and afterward. In other cases, state managers remain wedded to the ideology of domesticity and refrain

from encouraging female participation in the paid labor force. Examples are Saudi Arabia, Algeria and Jordan.

Moreover, we cannot ignore the Islamist resurgence in this area, exemplified by movements as varied as Jamat'ti Islami in Pakistan, Ikhwan al-Muslimin in Egypt, the Islamic Republic of Iran, the Islamic Salvation Front (FIS) in Algeria, and the Taliban in Afghanistan. For the "Muslim fundamentalist every domestic issue is negotiable except women's rights and their position in society. . . . [They] insist on singling out women's relations to society as the supreme test of authenticity of the Islamic order" (Afkhami, 1995, 1).

In Iran, in the immediate aftermath of the Islamic Revolution, the public behavior of women became a central issue and gender inequality was institutionalized. The following discussion shows the overwhelming impact of state policies on women's position in the labor market and in the society at large.

Constructing Women as Wives and Mothers

When the Islamic government came to power, a reversal of the trend toward gender equity was central to the policies of the state and has been widely documented (Esfandiari, 1997; Keddie, 2000; Shahidian, 1991). After the revolution of 1979, Iranian women came under close scrutiny, and the government was set to change their role and status. The Shah's regime was denounced as decadent and was cited as having caused the corruption of womanhood.[3] At the heart of the revolutionary state's position regarding women was the belief in the biological and psychological differences between the sexes. Of course, using biology to determine the destiny of women in Iran cannot be attributed solely to the policies of the Islamic regime, since many of the policies reflected legacies of the past. Sexist attitudes, women's inferior position within the household and outside the home, limitations on women's mobility, and so on existed prior to the Islamic Revolution and were deeply rooted in the economic, social, political, and cultural structure of Iran. Overall, during the Islamic Revolution, both continuities and breaks within Iran's gender system became evident (Moghadam, 1991; Poya, 1999).

During its early years, 1979–1981, the Islamic state adopted policies that forcefully emphasized the distinctive roles of men and women, as well as the importance of family life and domestic responsibilities for women. The constitution of the Islamic republic was ratified, and under the heading "Women and the Constitution," it emphasized that the Islamic government viewed the family as the cornerstone of society and saw women as having the precious function of motherhood (Poya, 1999, 66). The Family Protection Act, the Shah's reform of women's rights, was suspended. Men were given the exclusive right to divorce and were allowed to take four wives (Haeri, 1989, 1994). The Council of the Islamic Revolution ratified the Islamic Family Legislation in

October 1979. As a result, a woman had to obtain the permission of her male kin to work, travel, study, and change her place of residence (Tabari and Yeganeh, 1982). The Islamic government used a variety of methods to discourage women from employment. On May 3, 1979, a decree forbade female judges to work: women were designated as unfit to judge, and the Ministry of Justice refused to issue decrees confirming female judges (Yadgar Azadi, 1992[4]). Many women lost their jobs in the legal profession, and many others were removed from top government posts. The age of retirement for women in the paid labor force was reduced from 50 to 45 (Poya, 1999, 67; Tabari and Yeganeh, 1982). Women were barred from sports on the grounds that coaches, judges, and spectators in such events included men. In the realm of education, women were excluded from studying in many technological fields, some engineering areas, veterinary sciences, and some arts programs (Ghorayshi, 1993; Shahidian, 1991). All coeducational schools were abolished, and female teachers were assigned to girls' schools while men were assigned to boys' schools. Either priority was given to men or courses were identified as unsuitable for women (Mojab, 1987). In general, women's biology was used to justify their segregation in public, as on buses (Tabari and Yeganeh, 1982), and their restriction to the home.

The Islamic government's position on women was reproduced and reinforced in the media, during Friday prayers, and in the schoolbooks. Among the most widely noted changes were the revisions in textbooks, most evidently in the illustrations. After the revolution, far fewer women appeared in textbook illustrations, and those who were included had domestic roles (Moghadam, 1991). The differing positions of men and women in the family and society were supported by the prominent Shii clergies, as Poya (1999) noted. Other prominent people besides the clergy supported such positions as well. An example is Zahra Rahnavardi, a female writer on women's issues, who argued that for women, motherhood and wifehood are the road to freedom and liberation (Poya, 1999, 65).

Drastic changes did take place, but soon it became clear that the Islamic government had underestimated the popularity of the prerevolutionary reforms. The gains that women had made in education, employment, and other areas before the revolution could not be reversed by redefining Islam and changing laws. A combination of factors contributed to the gradual comeback of women's rights. The revolutionary period ended in 1986, the war with Iraq ended in 1988, and the Ayatollah Khomeini died in 1989. By the end of the 1980s, a new phase had begun in the development of the Iranian state, referred to as the *period of reconstruction* and marked by a reversal in the state's economic, gender, and employment policies (Afshar, 1998b; Keddie, 2000; Poya, 1999). The government was in need of skilled professionals, including women. As noted in the later discussion of women in the paid labor market, the government began to override its earlier policies. In general, at present, the Islamic government is more tolerant toward women who work in the public sphere, but it continues to see the private sphere as the most suitable one for women.

The Power to Define

The construction of woman as wife and mother has left its impact on social scientists' concepts and methods of data collection. Census data, the major source of large-scale information on population in developing countries such as Iran, provide general, but limited and partial, information on working women. Since women are seen as mothers and wives, many of their contributions, as I will discuss later, go undocumented by census data.[5] It is also widely acknowledged that problems of definition and procedure plague the collection of data—and labor force statistics in particular—in almost all situations, in both industrialized and developing countries alike (Anker, 1983; Armstrong and Armstrong, 1983; Dixon, 1982; Ghorayshi, 1993; Moghadam, 1991; Poya, 1999; Safilios-Rothschild, 1985; UN, 1980; Waring, 1999). Census statistics—which follow the recommendations of either the Inter-American Statistical Institute (IASI) or the United Nations Statistical Commission—have been designed to capture a "type of activity whose underlying model is the activity of males in developed economies characterized by continuity, an eight-hour workday, and a five- or six-day workweek" (Recchini de Lattes and Wainerman, 1986, 74; Waring, 1999).

A large proportion of women's work in Iran, and in developing countries in general, however, is discontinuous, part-time, seasonal, frequently difficult to distinguish from domestic activities, and performed within the traditional sector of the economy, in family enterprises, or in what has been termed the *informal economy*. The problems with data gathering are usually reinforced by others, such as the personal biases of the census interviewers, who tend to view women, even when they work in the fields, primarily as housewives helping their husbands. For instance, in the village of Rostamkola, one of the case studies used in this research and described later in this chapter, women stated very clearly that officials had never asked them whether they worked and what kind of work they performed. The women of this village, like many other women who live in rural areas, do not appear in official reports as part of the economically active population of Iran, despite their central role in the households, on the farms, and in the villages (Ghorayshi, 1998, 2001). The invisibility of adult female workers in these statistics is related to women's gender roles and the assumptions about the labor force that shape the design of the statistical information.

The failure of the official statistics to provide accurate information is particularly obvious with regard to the documentation of women's work (United Nations, 1991). The definitions of *work*, *family income*, *family labor*, and *economically active* used in census statistics mask the multidimensional nature of women's contribution to households and national economies. Many of the household activities so prominent in women's lives do not fit or do not have a place in census categories, and many of women's activities such as family, community, and volunteer work are best described as invisible work. The key words in labor force definitions are *economic*, *pay*, *profit*, or *market exchange.* Only those activities that are part of the formal sector of the economy are considered labor force activities. The problem is particularly acute in developing countries, where women are frequently presented as economically inactive members of the society, even though their labor is essential for the survival of their families, production units such as farms and small businesses, and communities (Ghorayshi, 1997). These difficulties are particularly obvious in the agricultural sector, where women's unpaid labor is crucial for the survival of household production, where it is impossible to draw a line between domestic work and farmwork, where women tend animals and grow foodstuffs in their kitchen gardens, and where trades or small crafts are added to agricultural work in a seasonal mix of household activities. As a whole, the overwhelming majority of women perform tasks that are interlinked and do not fit the commonly used narrow definition of *work*.

The Iranian census, like its counterparts elsewhere, makes women's work invisible. In the 1996 census, there were more than 22 million women older than 10, of whom more than 20 million were categorized as being economically inactive. Slightly more than 13 million of these women were categorized as homemakers (Statistical Centre of Iran, 1998, 95). It is important to note that the category of homemaker does not accurately reflect what women do. For example, in the village of Rostamkola, women did not see themselves as housewives. In fact, there was not a single woman in this village whose work could be limited to what has been termed *housework* in the literature (Ghorayshi, 1998). This problem also exists when women work in other types of household production units (Friedl, 1989; Tohidi, 1991). For instance, the growing number of small family businesses that produce garments, referred to as *towlidi*, rely on the labor of family members, especially women. Moreover, a large number of women work in small or medium-sized private enterprises whose employers do not declare them as workers in order to avoid paying taxes and offering insurance (Poya, 1999). Statistics do not include these categories of women who effectively contribute to their household units, small enterprises, and the national and international economies.

The underestimation of what women do has affected women's perceptions of their own work, since women internalize society's view of their activities. Many women in Iran still feel that work outside the household is demeaning, and they have accepted their government's construction of women's acceptable roles as being wives and mothers (Friedl, 1989). In many cases, in my interviews, it was common to see women label many aspects of their work as unimportant and unproductive. Running errands, producing crafts to contribute to the family's income, caring for children, doing domestic work, and completing other types of work were not credited by many women. Women's self-perception is certainly an obstacle to gathering accurate data. Also, the multicultural nature of the population adds another layer of difficulty in collecting accurate data. For instance, the refugee population of Afghanis in Iran, estimated to be more than 2 million, many working illegally and in the informal sector, complicates enumeration, and the problems associated with the coverage of the tribal and unsettled population have been extensively documented in the literature. Compounding such problems is the fact that, in Iran, the low level of education, the lack of exposure to the formal process of data collection, and the sociopolitical climate have created an immense problem for the gathering of data through formal interviewing and survey methods. The reliance on written words markedly limited our ability to gather accurate data because, among women aged 6 years or older, one out of four in urban areas and one out of three in rural areas are illiterate, and the literate population often has an elementary-level education or less (Statistical Center of Iran, 1998). Moreover, many Iranian women live in small towns or villages—in fact, 38.3% of all Iranians live in rural areas (Statistical Centre of Iran, 1998)—and have had little contact with the world outside their families and communities, have not been exposed to the formal methods of data collection, and do not favor structured interviewing, in which formal interviewers use tape recorders—facts that became evident in my research. Another key issue is that, in Iran, "research is not supported and has not found its proper place" (Motiee and Sarhaddi, 1994, 164).

Women's Work Is Multilayered

As noted at the beginning of this chapter, the growing research on women in the past few decades has shown both the centrality and the complexity of women's work in various parts of the world. This literature has made it clear that women are simultaneously responsible for various types of activities and that the specific nature of their work has to be understood within the social, economic, political, and cultural contexts of each country. The focus in the following section is on Iran and, specifically, on women's work in the paid labor market, in household units, and in the family, as revealed through case studies I conducted from 1989 to 1998.

Paid Employment

Keeping in mind the shortcomings of the census statistics, I use labor force data to present a broad picture of women's position in the formal sector of the Iranian economy.

Despite difficulties, more women have joined the job market in recent years: 1,212,000 in 1976, 975,000 in 1986, and 1,765,000 in 1996 (Statistical Center of Iran, 1998, 95). While the proportion of women in the paid labor force declined from 12.9% in 1976 to 8.2% in 1986, it went up to 8.7% in 1991 and to 9.1% in 1996. The exigencies of modern life had to be reconciled with religious and cultural traditions. As Ramazani (1993) noted, the government began to override its earlier policies. For instance, bans or quotas on some educational fields were repealed, and the number of educated women increased. In recent years, a number of factors have been pushing women to work outside their homes. The rising level of women's education, the decreasing size of the family (Salehi-Isfahani, 2000), and the growing economic pressures on households have increased women's likelihood of seeking paid work. In addition, an increasing public validation of women's work has been emerging over the past decade.

It is important to note that women fought back and used various tactics and strategies to counteract the existing limitations, especially during the early years of the Islamic government. Dissatisfied Islamic and secular women campaigned in the press, the parliament, and elsewhere, and their efforts led to new discussions and reforms concerning the position of women. Female Majles (members of Parliament) deputies pushed for reforms in family matters, including policies pertaining to marriage, polygamy, divorce, child custody, and other issues. A new core group of Islamic women—including relatives of major male political figures—interpreted Islam in more gender-egalitarian ways. Women who lost jobs or were shut out after the revolution imaginatively carved out new working lives. For instance, female lawyers refused to accept the government's attempts to remove women from legal practice by firing all female judges and excluding women from the law faculty. Some continued to practice in the name of a male family member, while others worked as legal advisors to companies, and female deputies fought for them (Keddie, 2000, 9). Female authors who faced financial and political difficulties have been taking their books into the streets for sale (Sherkat, 2000b). Aside from the large number of working-class women, women made their mark in a great variety of middle-class professions. They set up small businesses and went in unprecedented numbers into professions including medicine, teaching, and law. Women more than ever before became active in literature and the arts. The number of female writers, dramatists, filmmakers, sculptors, and painters grew after the revolution of 1979 (Esfandiari, 1997; Keddie, 2000).

A growing number of Iranian women are entering the world of business. During the past decade, women's magazines, especially *Zanan* and *Zan-e-Rouz*, have been an important venue for the discussion of what women do. They have offered extensive profiles on women in certain occupations and have done a good job of presenting female entrepreneurs. Today, some women employ many workers and run successful businesses (Sherkat, 2000a). These female entrepreneurs operate large and small enterprises, some from their homes and others outside their homes. Women are involved in such wide-ranging paid activities as preaching in women's gatherings, designing clothes, having their own orchestra and entertainment services, catering food, traveling for business purposes to the free trade zone areas such as Kish and Qatar, and conducting various trade activities, such as selling crafts, household items, and other products.

Considering the difficulties women have faced, their current involvement in various activities in the paid labor force is impressive. However, according to census data, as of 1996 women still accounted for less than 10% of the total labor force. In the private sector, only 3% of the employers, 6.6% of the self-employed, and 7.6% of the wage and salary earners were women (Statistical Centre of Iran, 1996, 1998). In many sectors of the economy at that time, the percentages of women were still small: mining, 4%; construction, 0.9%; electricity, gas, and water supply, 0.3%; and hotels and restaurants, 2.3%. Nor were women equally represented in all government sectors. For instance, the percentages of women who worked in the government and were covered under the civil service code were as follows: the Ministry of Education, 46.2%; the Ministry of Health,

42%; the Ministry of Culture and Higher Education, 20.5%; the Ministry of Roads and Transportation, 16%; the Office of the President, 15.5%; the Ministry of Foreign Affairs, 7.2%; the Ministry of Defense, 6%; and the Islamic Consultative Assembly, 5%. In addition, only 5.6% of the government employees covered under the nation's labor law were women. In general, women in the paid labor force were concentrated in low-paid and low-status occupations. In the government sector, the overwhelming majority of women were employed in teaching, health services, and various types of low-paid office work. Similarly, large proportions of women in the private sector consisted of agricultural laborers, domestic servants, and those who worked in the garment, textile, leather, and food processing industries. A very small percentage of women in the private sector occupied specialized positions such as accountants, physicians, and top office managers (Ghorayshi, 1996). Based on the analysis of the census data, researchers have rightly argued that there is a marked gender asymmetry in the paid labor market in Iran and that it must be given serious attention. Women are concentrated in feminized job sectors and occupy the lower level of the occupational ladder (Afshar, 1997; Bagherian, 1991; Kousha and Mohseni, 1997; Moghadam, 1991).

Work in Household Units

Household commodity production units, based on the contributions of family members, are widespread in many parts of developing countries, including Iran. These units of production are particularly important in rural areas of Iran, where 38.3% of the population resides. In 1995, there were 11,421,321 women in the rural areas, of whom 8,362,526 were older than 10. By the census data definitions, only 893,980 women—that is, 10.7%—were considered economically active (Statistical Centre of Iran, 1996). Of course, as other researchers (Moghadam, 1991; Poya, 1999; Sarhaddi, 1992) have noted, even a superficial observation of rural Iran makes it clear that census information falsifies women's reality. In what follows, I use the example of my fieldwork in the village of Rostamkola between 1994 and 1998 to demonstrate the centrality of women's work for the survival of farms, households, and the village (Ghorayshi, 1997, 1998, 2001).

In the village of Rostamkola, the household (*Khanevar*) proved to be the basis of production. Households relied on three primary sources of income: agricultural production, orchard and garden produce, and service and wage work. They also depended on money earned through the sale of citrus fruits, tomatoes, and other garden vegetables. On the one hand, village households had many characteristics of small-scale subsistence enterprises in that they produced some of the agricultural products they needed. On the other hand, they depended on the market for selling their products and satisfying their increasing consumption needs. The labor contribution of all members of the family, including women, was central to the survival of the household. Women generally worked from dawn to dusk, and their working life in agricultural production started at a young age, continued after their marriage, and extended into old age. Women were active on the farm, in the household, and in the village. For the most part, farmwork was labor intensive, and modern technology was either unavailable or too expensive and beyond the financial reach of the majority of villagers. The overwhelming majority carried out their work in trying conditions. The scarcity of the means of transportation, the inaccessible roads, and the long distances between farms and the individual dwellings—coupled with the fact that "good women" did not drive cars or tractors or ride bicycles—made women's work very difficult.

Agricultural household activities were not limited to what is known in the literature as *domestic work* but also included many tasks essential for the reproduction of farm and village. For instance, households grew tomatoes for both consumption and sale, as well as for preparing the seeds for the next year's planting. The processing of the seeds and the cleaning of the products for sale took place within the household and was the responsibility of household members, especially women. In Rostamkola, even women who had paid employment were active in various aspects of farmwork. For instance, a teacher, a part-time nurse, and a superintendent of the school—all women—were involved in the community and in every aspect of farming. In fact, these civil servant women relied on the success of their farming, rather than their paid work, for their their contribution to the family income.

While women in Rostamkola played a critical role within and outside their households, men generally owned the land, the most important means of production—as was made clear by the life stories of women in this village. Likewise, marketing, especially wholesale marketing, was in the hands of men. Typically, husbands determined the allocation of financial resources, especially when large sums of money were involved, and wives made decisions about expenses related to day-to-day household finances. In the great majority of cases, the women of Rostamkola did not know the total cash income of their own households.

The expansion of the market and the need for cash income in this village had affected men and women differently in that it had forced many men to outmigrate in search of paid work. The dominant ideology, both patriarchal and religiously strict, did not approve of women's movement outside the village. As we have discussed earlier, the Islamic government forcefully emphasized the importance of family life for women (Haeri, 1994; Moghadam, 1991; Poya, 1999). Men moved freely within and outside the village, but they put restrictions on women's mobility. Making frequent journeys into town provoked suspicion and was regarded as inappropriate for proper women. Therefore, men, especially those in the younger generation, left the village in search of work. With the growing outmigration of men, more and more women had been left to take care of the farm households, so that Rostamkola had been experiencing the feminization of farms (Ghorayshi, 1998). The image of the household as a unit headed solely by a man represents a view of social relations incongruent with the realities experienced in this village. With few exceptions, men in Rostamkola could not afford to be the sole providers for their households.

The example of women's work in Rostamkola's agricultural households is not intended to be generalized to all rural areas in Iran, but it could be applicable to other types of commodity production units based on the labor of family members. As I found in Rostamkola, other case studies have shown that women are very active in both tribal and agricultural areas, as well as in a range of family enterprises (Friedl, 1989; Motiee and Sarhaddi, 1994; Poya, 1999; Sarhaddi et al., 1989; Sarhaddi, 1992). In general, we know very little about women's experiences when they work within their own household units.

Family Work

Defining *work* as that which is done for pay or profit limits our understanding of women's work at home. Family work is separate and distinct from market-oriented work. While most wage work takes place in factories and offices, reproductive work—that is, childbearing and child rearing, plus feeding, clothing, and caring for the household members—takes place at home. Whereas wage labor in the formal sector is paid, reproductive labor is not. While the wage laborer works under the direction of a boss, reproductive labor is done under a different form of authority relations—namely, the unequal relations of power within the household based on gender and generation. Housework is essential for the survival of the household, but it carries little prestige or reward, and as noted in the discussion of census data, it is not counted as work (Ghorayshi, 1998; Recchini de Lattes and Wainerman, 1986; Waring, 1999).

In this section, I examine women's family work by discussing the findings from two original case studies that were part of a larger project I conducted on women's work in Iran from 1989 to 1998. The methodology employed in this part of the study was based on semistructured interviews, participant observation, and focus group discussions. The first sample focused on 40 women who were working full-time in the paid labor force. In the private sector, one was a garment worker; another, a medical secretary; and still another, a nurse. In the government sector, 18 women were teachers, 5 were in health care services, 12 did administrative and office work, 1 was a research officer, and 1 was an engineer. These women were aged 24 to 50. Three were widows, three were divorced, and the rest were married. All, except for one divorced woman, had children. Over half of the women had a university education; of these, two had Ph.D.s, one was an engineer, and one was a physician. Four women had an elementary education, and the rest either had graduated from high school or had completed technical or nursing programs after high school. In terms of religion, four women were very religious, four indicated that they were agnostic, and the rest—that is, the majority—were not practicing Muslims but had taken part in religious ceremonies occasionally. Ten lived in low-income families, 23 were in middle-income families, and 7 were in upper-middle or upper-income families.

The second sample was composed of 30 women, aged from 20 to 54, who were full-time homemakers. All except four had children, and two-thirds had school-age children. Among these women, two were widows, four were single, and the rest were married. Two women were illiterate, six had finished elementary school, four had a university education, and the rest had a high school diploma. One-third of these women were from working-class families, half came from middle-class backgrounds, and five lived in high-income households.

The findings from both case studies showed that reproductive work—childbearing, child rearing, feeding, clothing, and caring for the household members—had stayed within the sphere of the family. Despite the variations in age, education, and family size, women were, with few exceptions, in charge of the basic domestic tasks (Ghorayshi, 1996; Sharifi, 1990). Women performed much of the work of social reproduction, such as food preparation, shopping, cleaning, socialization of children, care and support of adults, and nurturing of kin and community ties. Although men occasionally helped with these tasks, the rising level of inflation, widespread unemployment, the high cost of living, and migration related to the search for work, together with other factors, had created a situation such that women had to carry the burden of unpaid domestic work. As noted earlier, however, this pattern fit with the society's emphasis on the roles of mother and wife. Regardless of women's other types of work, Iranian women bear the responsibility for unpaid household work.

My research revealed that women played a central role in responding to the social and personal needs of the household members in that the women allocated resources and fulfilled family needs. Furthermore, the domestic role of women required them to act as intermediaries between various members of the household, especially between husbands and sons and between daughters and male family members. Although such efforts involved conflict and tension management, they were not classified as skilled work because these tasks, like many other tasks and activities traditionally undertaken by women, were considered a natural extension of their gender role (Baxandall and Gordon, 1995). Women's ability to manage social relations was rarely, if ever, acknowledged as a skill.

In considering women's family work in Iran, we have to note that drastic changes after the revolution of 1979, some of which we have discussed earlier, had added another layer to what women are expected to do at home. People's leisure time had been curbed both by the unavailability of leisure outlets and by the state's rigid restrictions on and perceptions of leisure. For instance, radio and television programs had been altered to cater to the needs of the revolutionary government, and Western public forms of entertainment had been canceled. Also, many of the public holidays had been assigned to religious ceremonies. For the majority of the people, the main channel of entertainment had been limited to getting together with friends and family. Women had to bear the brunt of the work for these activities. Preparing and serving food, keeping the house in a presentable condition, and washing and cleaning after visitors' departure were among the responsibilities of women during family gatherings.

In sum, my case studies have made it clear that family and work are neither separate nor fixed categories but intersect in complex ways. In general, within the household everyone turns to the wife, mother, or daughter for solutions to household problems. Combining family work and other types of work is a problem for all classes of women. The nature of each role can profoundly influence women's health, but this fact confounds the problem, since supportive policies for women are so lacking and since gender inequalities are extensive.

Women's Work and Health

The market-driven definition of *work* as employment has affected the nature of research. Studies of working women's health tend to concentrate on the relationship between women's paid employment and health rather than on the relationship between women's work as a whole and health. Even more recent theoretical models regarding women's work and well-being have continued to separate women's paid work from other types of work that women do (Nippert-Eng, 1996). Such an outlook, as I have already argued, does not accurately reflect the context, meaning, and multilayered nature of women's work.

Women's health research is rapidly evolving, but the relation between Iranian women's work and health remains unexplored. In what follows, I use women's words from my case studies to show the impact of their multilayered work activities on their well-being.

Injuries Resulting from Sexism

In the case studies, I asked women questions about their work requirements, work pace, conflicting demands, and overtime, as well as questions assessing their skill development, task variety, decision-making authority, and support systems. Their responses made it clear that work and health were intricately intertwined in their everyday lives. Women did not compartmentalize their work or their health to the degree that health care professionals and researchers would. As explored in this section, the research revealed that working women's health and their concerns varied with the type of work they did, the place of their work, their class position, their position within the multiple relations of power, both in the society and in the workplace, and other factors. It appeared that there were similarities, as well as major differences, between women who combined paid work with family work, those who did mainly family work, and those rural women who were commodity producers. In varying degrees, women's work had both positive and negative impacts on their health and well-being.

Women were simultaneously in charge of many tasks that affected the amount of time and resources they had left for themselves. For instance, Fati, one of the village women, had problems with her eyes, but she could not find the time to visit a doctor. "It is about two years that my eyes bother me. I plan to go to the doctor, but I have been either too busy, or I had to spend the money on other things. . . . I know I have to do something about my eyes." A cartographer in a large government institution stated, "My day starts at 6:00 A.M. and ends close to midnight. My husband works at two jobs, and he is hardly around. I feed the kids, take them to school, attend to my office work, [and] use my break to do grocery shopping. I pick [up] my kids from school and help them in their homework. I prepare food, clean, wash, etc. In the weekend I visit my sick parents and get them what they need. . . . Honestly, not much is left to do anything else. . . . I am often tired, and I know why, but, at this point, I do not have any other choice." Juggling multiple roles is a common problem and a major cause of fatigue, anxiety, and stress. Research has clearly shown that stress has both short- and long-term negative health impacts (Long and Kahn, 1993; Stark-Adamec and Andrew, 1995). Among the major sources of stress for women were the many forms of gender discrimination, such as occupational segregation by sex, the limiting of women to low-paid occupations, and lower pay than men. For instance, a female pharmacist with a high-status job in the government stated, "I am well paid, have a good position, and am in charge of this pharmaceutical lab. They need me and they know it, too. But, I face sexism. Often, both men and women in my place of work attempt to undermine what I do. What they do is subtle and hard to describe. . . . I can tell you, some days, I come home feeling I do not want to go back, even if I love what I do. . . . It is hard to be a working woman in this country." A village woman angrily questioned the sexual division of labor: "I work in the rice field in trying conditions, carry the goods on my head to the market, walk a number of kilometers daily. I do all this and more, but they tell me I cannot run that little tractor. The guy drives it and gets twice as much as I do. . . . You tell me, whose work is harder and needs more skill?" Similarly, a homemaker questioned her position within the household: "In my household the assumption is that I do not work outside the house and I am responsible for all the housework. . . . When my husband comes from office, he expects to be served, as if he is in a restaurant. . . . Oh, he makes me mad. . . . Is it written in my forehead that cooking, cleaning, etc. is for women?" Some women had internalized the dominant gender ideology, but most working women in my studies explicitly defied gender differences based on biological sex distinctions that govern the allocation of power and authority in the labor market and in the household. More broadly, the literature on women's work and health in general has provided strong evidence that workplace discrimination based on sex, affecting the division of labor, the type of work women do, and their pay, is associated with women's deteriorating health (Bird, 1999; Jackson and Palmer-Jones, 1998; Long and Kahn, 1993; McCall, 2001; Stark-Adamec and Andrew, 1995).

Gender inequality was experienced differently by women in various social classes. Wealthier women reduced the tension caused by their multiple layers of work by reassigning some of the work related to domestic activities and infant care to lower-class women of their own or different ethnic groups. These domestic workers, in turn, often were forced to leave their infants with relatives or friends. In the rural areas, women from well-off households hired poor women to do menial agricultural work. These helpers tended to be lower-class poor women who faced the combined stresses of poverty and menial labor.

In my study, domestic work and child care did not seem to create as great a problem for the women in the village as they did for urban women. In general, households in Rostamkola enjoyed an elaborate system of support involving relatives, friends, and neighbors (Ghorayshi, 2001). The major concern for women in the village seemed to relate to their lack of ability to control their means of production and the products of their labor. With few exceptions, the economic ownership of land was in the hands of men even when women had legal ownership. One woman angrily stated, "When my father died, I did inherit some land, but my older brother cultivates my land. . . . I continuously raise the question with my brother and the village head, but no one listens. . . . Where is the justice?" Another woman complained while pointing outdoors to a large rice field: "You see this rice field. . . . I am 35 years old and have developed rheumatism from working in this rice field, having my feet up to my knees in the water. . . . We have produced these bags of rice, but my husband takes them to the wholesale market. . . . I do not see the money." Another source of tension for women in this agricultural village was the growing crisis of the economy and the increasing amount of their work. As noted earlier, the outmigration of men in search of work meant that many women had become the guardians of their households (Ghorayshi, 1998).

Rewards of Work

As the literature on work shows, employment positively affects individuals' health in a variety of ways (MOW, 1987; Naylor, Willimon and Osterberg, 1996). Employment can bring women separate sources of income, autonomy, and social ties independent of familial relationships. Even though employed women are concentrated in female-dominated and low-paid jobs, for the most part the advantages of holding a job outweigh the disadvantages (Apter, 1993; Lee, 1998).

In my interviews, women indicated many reasons for their paid employment. For the overwhelming majority of them, money was the primary reason. Women of all ages, regardless of their marital status, worked to support themselves and their household members. Even though the women in my study faced negative attitudes toward their employment, they were very confident that without their income, their families would be unable to meet the rising costs of living. They also used their employment in the public sphere to open new spaces for themselves in the household and in the society. Employed women seemed to have increased their influence in their households' daily life by shaping household decisions more directly. In addition, the overwhelming majority of women in this study had expanded their social life through their paid work, since they had developed new friendships and contacts with nonrelatives. For many educated women, working in the public sphere also had boosted their self-image and self-worth, since they could use their skills and fulfill their career dreams.

It became evident in this case study that working in the household was different from pursuing employment in urban areas. For the women studied, agricultural work was part of their identity, even though they were unpaid. They, like their counterparts in the city, were well aware that their work was central to their households' survival. Despite the limitations that these women faced in their daily lives, they valued their work. In fact, these women's identity was based on their position as direct producers. They saw themselves as being *Za're* or *dehghan*, people who cultivate the land. For these women, working in the field was an indication of being healthy and economically useful and active. In addition, farmwork in this village was done in cooperative groups. Working on the farm not only put the women in direct contact with others but also included them in many economic and social circles associated with farmwork.

Conclusion

This study showed that the notions of men's work and women's work are not natural but are, instead, social and political constructs. In addition, the female population is clearly stratified, and women's experiences of gender inequality are greatly determined by their class position, the type of work they do, and the place of their work. My interviews with women also showed that work, in its varied forms, is a source of both satisfaction and stress. The overwhelming majority of women indicated that they work under strain, and they identified their major sources of dissatisfaction as being the juggling of various tasks, the lack of time and of control over their work, the gender gap in pay, occupational segregation, the sexual division of labor, and the general invisibility of their work.

The case studies provided strong evidence that women's work is multidimensional and is not synonymous with wage and salary work. We need to reconceptualize women's work to reflect the multiple contexts and dimensions of contributions by women, as well as the diversity and differences among them. The different types of work handled by women do affect each other and cannot be compartmentalized. In turn, what women do affects their health and well-being. Narrow definitions of *work* do not lend themselves to the study of the relationship between women's work and their well-being. In order to be able to interpret the relationship between women's work and health, we must better understand how various women conceptualize both their work and their health. One of the challenges in the study of women's work and health is the recognition that terms such as *work*, *job*, *employment*, and *health* have different meanings to different groups.

ACKNOWLEDGMENT

I would like to thank the anonymous reviewer who provided comments on an earlier version of this chapter.

Notes

1. In this study, I draw examples from three case studies, all of which are part of a larger project on the political economy of women in Iran. They are based on continuing original fieldwork research in Iran that I have been involved with since 1989.

2. Farsi is the official language of Iran, but the population is composed of a variety of ethnic groups that speak their own languages or dialects and have their own traditions and cus-

toms. Women come from diverse ethnic groups: Persian, Turkish, Mazandarani, Gilani, Luri, Baluchi, and so on. We do not have detailed information on all of these groups. (Statistical Centre of Iran, 1998). There are also differences among women in terms of their education. Of the over 25 million women older than 6, close to 6 million are illiterate (Statistical Centre of Iran, 1998).

3. Iran experienced rapid modernization in the twentieth century, especially during the Pahlavi regime. As part of his White Revolution, Mohammad Reza Shah, from 1962 on, introduced measures to improve women's status. We must note that the beneficiaries of modernization during the Pahlavi regime were middle- and upper-class women. However, changes in education, employment, and other areas were starting to affect all classes of women. At that time, there was a cultural division within the Iranian society. On the one hand, there was a new middle class, with a secular ideology and Western education and ways of life. On the other hand, the working classes and the traditional middle class continued to follow what they considered to be Islamic norms, including veiling for women and traditional marriage and family practices (see also Keddie, 2000; Poya, 1999, 53).

4. The calendar year commonly referred to in Iran is different from the calendar year generally referred to in Western countries. In general, the Western calendar year can be converted to the Iranian calendar year by subtracting 621 although this conversion is inexact because the Iranian calendar year starts on March 21. To assist readers interested in locating Iranian source documents, the references include both Western and Iranian calendar years.

5. This problem is compounded by the fact that assumptions underlying the construction of many definitions, scales, inventories, coding, editing, tabulations, and indexes are biased against women. There are sex-related biases in the process of design, collection, and analysis of census data. The data are not only conditioned by the questions asked or not asked, but also by the choices of response that are offered to respondents (Ghorayshi, 1993; United Nations, 1980, 1991; Waring, 1999).

References

Afkhami, M., ed. 1995. *Faith and freedom: Women's human rights in the Muslim world.* Syracuse, NY: Syracuse University Press.

Afshar, H. 1984. Muslim women and the burden of ideology. *Women's Studies International Forum* 7(4): 247–50.

Afshar, H. 1981. Women in the work and poverty trap in Iran. *Capital and Class* 37: 62–85.

Afshar, H. 1997. Women and work in Iran. *Political Studies* 14: 755–67.

Afshar, H. 1998a. Behind the veil: The public and private faces of Khomeini's policies on Iranian women. In *Structure of patriarchy: The state, the community and the household in modernizing Asia,* edited by B. Abrawal. London: Zed Books.

Afshar, H. 1998b. *Islam and feminists: An Iranian case study.* New York: St. Martin's Press.

Anderson, M. L. 1988. Moving our minds: Studying women of color and reconstructing sociology. *Teaching Sociology* 16(2): 123–32.

Anker, R. 1983. Female labor force participation in developing countries: A critique of current definitions and data collection methods. *International Labor Review* 122(6): 709–24.

Apter, T. 1993. *Working women don't have wives: Professional success in the 1990s.* New York: St. Martin's Press.

Armstrong, P., and H. Armstrong. 1983. Beyond numbers: Problems with quantitative data. *Alternate Routes* 6: 1–40.

Armstrong, P., and H. Armstrong. 1990. *Theorizing women's work.* Toronto: Garamond Press.
Bagherian, M. 1991. Eshteghal va bikari zanan as didgahe tows'eh (Women's employment and unemployment from development's standpoint). *Zanan* 1: 4–12.
Baker, M. 1995. *Canadian family policies: Cross–national comparisons.* Toronto: University of Toronto Press.
Barrett, M., and M. McIntosh. 1985. Ethnocentrism and socialist feminist theory. *Feminist Review* 20: 23–47.
Basow, S. 1992. *Gender stereotypes.* Scarborough, Canada: Nelson Canada.
Baxandall, R., and L. Gordon 1995. *America's working women: A documentary history, 1600 to the present.* New York: Norton.
Betteridge, A. 1980. The controversial vows of urban Muslim women in Iran. In *Unspoken worlds: Women's religious lives in non-Western cultures,* edited by N. Falk and R. Gross. San Francisco: Harper & Row.
Bird, C. 1999. Gender, household labor, and psychological distress: The impact of the amount and division of housework. *Journal of Health and Social Behavior* 40(1): 32–45.
Bodman, H. L., and N. Tohidi. 1998. *Women in Muslim societies: Diversity within unity.* London: Lynne Rienner Press.
Boserup, E. 1970. *Women's role in economic development.* London: Allen and Unwin.
Creighton, C., and C. K. Omari, eds. 2000. *Gender, family and work in Tanzania.* Burlington, VT: Ashgate.
Davies, M. 1983. *Third World second sex: Women's struggles and national liberation: Third World women speak out.* London: Zed Books
Dickerscheid, J. D. 1990. Profiles of rural Egyptian women: Rules, status and needs. *International Journal of Sociology of the Family* 20(1): 1–20.
Dickinson, T. D., and R. K. Schaeffer. 2001. *Fast forward: Work, gender and protest in a changing world.* Lanham, MD: Rowman and Littlefield.
Dixon, R. 1982. Women in agriculture: Counting the labour force in developing countries. *Population and Development Review* 8(3): 347–72.
Dumont, L. 1992. *Anthropologie totalite et hierarchie.* Paris: Edition de Centre Pompidou, Philosophie et Anthropologie.
Esfandiari, H. 1997. *Reconstructed lives: Women and Iran's Islamic revolution.* Washington, D.C.: Woodrow Wilson Center Press.
Esposito, J. 1982. *Women in Muslim family law.* Syracuse, NY: Syracuse University Press.
Flora, P. 1986. *Growth to limits: The Western European welfare state since World War II.* Vol. 1. Berlin: Walter de Gruyter.
Friedl, E. 1989. *Women of Deh Koh: Lives in an Iranian village.* Washington, D.C.: Smithsonian Institution Press.
Gannagé, C. 1986. *Double day, double bind: Women garment workers.* Toronto: Women's Press.
Ghorayshi, P. 1993. Gender disparity in education: A challenge for development. *International Journal of Contemporary Sociology* 30(2): 199–215.
Ghorayshi, P. 1994. *Women and work in developing countries: A critical annotated bibliography.* New York: Greenwood Press.
Ghorayshi, P. 1996. Women, paid work and the family in the Islamic Republic of Iran. *Journal of Comparative Family Studies* 27(3): 453–66.
Ghorayshi, P. 1997. Women and social change: Towards understanding gender relations in rural Iran. *Canadian Journal of Development Studies* 18(1): 71–92.
Ghorayshi, P. 1998. Rural women face capitalism: Women's response as guardians of the household. In *Transgressing borders: Critical perspectives on gender, household and culture,* edited by S. Ilcan and L. Phillips. Westport, CT: Bergin and Garvey.

Ghorayshi, P. 2001. Dans la mouvance: Les femmes rurales iraniennes transforment leur vie. *Anthropologies et Sociétés* 25(1): 23–41.

Haeri, S. 1989. *The law of desire: Temporary marriage in Shi'i Iran.* London: I. B. Tauris.

Haeri, S. 1994. Temporary marriage: An Islamic discourse on female sexuality in Iran. In *Women in postrevolutionary Iran,* edited by M. Afkhami and E. Friedl. London: I. B. Tauris.

Hirschberg, S., and T. Hirschberg. 2001. *One world, many cultures.* Boston: Allyn and Bacon.

hooks, b. 1989. *Talking back: Thinking feminist, thinking black.* Toronto: Between the Lines.

Hopkins, N. S. 1992. Women, work and wage in two Arab villages. *Eastern Anthropologist* 44(2): 103–23.

Jackson, C., and R. Palmer-Jones 1998. *Work intensity, gender and well-being.* Geneva: United Nations Research Institute for Social Development.

Joekes, S., ed. 1987. *Women in the world economy: An International Research and Training Institute for the Advancement of Women (INSTRAW) study.* Toronto: Oxford University Press.

Kabeer, N. 1992. Organizing landless women in Bangladesh. *Community Development Journal* 20(3): 203–12.

Kandiyoti, D. 1988. Bargaining with patriarchy. *Gender and Society* 2(3): 274–89.

Keddie, N. 2000. Women in Iran since 1979. *Social Research* 67(2): 405–34.

Kousha, M., and N. Mohseni. 1997. Predictors of life satisfaction among urban Iranian women: An exploratory analysis. *Social Indicators Research* 40: 329–57.

Labrecque, M. F. 1996. The study of gender and generational hierarchies in the context of development: Methodological aspects. In *Women, work and gender relations in developing countries: A global perspective,* edited by P. Ghorayshi and C. Belanger. Westport, CT: Greenwood Press.

Leacock, E., and H. Safa. 1986. *Women's work: Development and division of labor by gender.* South Hadley, MA: Bergin and Garvey.

Lee, C. K. 1998. *Gender and the South China miracle: Two worlds of factory women.* Berkeley, CA: University of California Press.

Long, B., and S. Kahn. 1993. *Women, work and coping.* Montreal: McGill-Queen's University Press.

Loutfi, M. 1985. *Rural women: Unequal partners in development.* Geneva: International Labor Organization.

Mahdavi, S. 1983. Women and the Shii Ulama in Iran. *Middle Eastern Studies* 19(1): 17–27.

McCall, L. 2001. *Complex inequality: Gender, class, and race in the new economy.* New York: Routledge.

Mernissi, F. 1991. *The veil and the male elite: A feminist interpretation of women's rights in Islam.* New York: Addison-Wesley.

Mies, M. 1986. *Patriarchy and accumulation on a world scale: Women in the international division of labour.* London: Zed Books.

Millett, K. 1986. *Going to Iran.* New York: Coward, McCann and Geoghegan.

Moghadam, F. 2000. Ideology, economic restructuring, and women's work in Iran (1976–1996). In *Earnings inequality, unemployment, and poverty in the Middle East and North Africa,* edited by W. Shahin and G. Dibeh. Westport, CT: Greenwood Press.

Moghadam, V. 1988. Women, work and ideology in the Islamic Republic. *International Journal of Middle Eastern Studies* 20: 221–43.

Moghadam, V. 1991. The reproduction of gender inequality in Muslim societies: A case study of Iran in the 1980s. *World Development* 19(10): 1335–49.

Moghadam, V. 1993. *Modernizing women: Gender and social change in the Middle East.* Boulder, CO: Lynne Rienner.

Moghadam, V. 1995. Women's employment issues in contemporary Iran: Problems and perspectives in the 1990s. *Iranian Studies* 28(3–4): 175–202.

Mojab, S. 1987. The Islamic government's policy on women's access to higher education and its impact on the socio-economic status of women. Working paper no. 156. East Lansing, MI: Michigan State University.

Motiee, N., and F. Sarhaddi. 1994. (1373). *Moghaye-seh fa'ali-yat-ha-i tawli-di zanan-i roosta-i dar seh mantagh-i motefavet as yek eghlim* (A comparison of rural women's work in production in three different places in one country). Tehran: Faslnameh-i Oloom-i Ejtemai.

MOW (Meaning of Work International Research Team). 1987. *The meaning of work.* Orlando, FL: Academic Press.

Nafisi, A. 1994. Images of women in classical Persian literature and the contemporary Iranian novel. In *In the eye of the storm: Women in postrevolutionary Iran,* edited by M. Afkhami and E. Friedl. Syracuse, NY: Syracuse University Press.

Naylor, T., W. Willimon, and R. Osterberg 1996. *The search for meaning in the workplace.* Nashville, TN: Abingdon Press.

Neshat, G 1980. Women in the Islamic Republic of Iran. *Iranian Studies* 13(1–4): 165–94.

Nippert-Eng, C. 1996. *Home and work: Negotiating boundaries through everyday life.* Chicago: University of Chicago Press.

O'Connor, J., A. S. Orloff , and S. Shaver. 1999. *States, markets, families: Gender, liberalism and social policy in Australia, Canada, Great Britain and the United States.* Cambridge, UK: Cambridge University Press

Paidar, P. 1995. *Women and political process in twentieth century Iran.* Cambridge, UK: Cambridge University Press.

Parpart, J. L., and K. A. Staudt, eds. 1988. *Women and the state in Africa.* Boulder, CO: Lynne Rienner.

Peterson, S. V., ed. 1992. *Gendered states: Feminist (re)visions of international relations theory.* Boulder, CO: Lynne Rienner.

Phillips, L. 1989. Gender dynamics and rural household strategies. *Canadian Review of Sociology and Anthropology* 26(2): 294–310.

Poya, M. 1999. *Women, work and Islamism: Ideology and resistance in Iran.* London: Zed Books.

Radcliffe, S. A. 1990. Between hearth and labor market: The recruitment of peasant women in the Andes. *International Migration Review* 24(2): 229–49.

Ramazani, N. 1993. Women in Iran: The revolutionary ebb and flow. *Middle East Journal* 47(3): 409–28.

Recchini de Lattes, Z., and C. Wainerman. 1986. Unreliable account of women's work: Evidence from Latin American statistics. *Signs* 11(4): 740–50.

Redclift, N., and T. Sinclair. 1991. *Working women: International perspectives on labour and gender ideology.* London: Routledge.

Reeves, J. 1986. Work and family roles: Contemporary women in Indonesia. *Sociological Spectrum* 7(6): 223–42.

Roos, P. 1985. *Gender and work: A comparative analysis of industrial societies.* Albany, NY: State University of New York Press.

Safilios-Rothschild, C. 1985. The resistance of women's invisibility in agriculture: Theoretical and policy lessons from Lesotho and Sierra Leone. *Economic Development and Cultural Change* 33(2): 299–317.

Salehi-Isfahani, D. 2000. Demographic factors in Iran's economic development. *Social Research* 67(2): 599–620.

Sanasarian, E. 1982. *The women's rights movement in Iran.* New York: Praeger.

Sarhaddi, F. 1992. (1371). *Bar-rasi-i ejtema'i eqtesadi-i naghsh zanan roosta-i dar glim bafi* (A study of the socioeconomic role of rural women in the production of Glim). Tehran: Economic and Agricultural Research and Planning Center.

Sarhaddi, F., A. Nikzat, Z. Sarami, N. Motiee, and M. Khojastefar. 1989 (1369). *Bar-rasi Ejtema'i, eqtesadi dar roosta-i-ahandan* (A socioeconomic study of the village of Ahandan). Tehran: Centre for Rural and Agricultural Research, Ministry of Agriculture.

Seager, J. 1997. *The state of women in the world atlas: Women's status around the globe: Work, health, education and personal freedom.* London: Penguin Books.

Shahidian, H. 1991. The education of women in the Islamic Republic of Iran. *Journal of Women's History* 2(3): 6–38.

Sharifi, Z. 1990. (1369). *Moshkelat-e Mas-oolin va keshavarzan-e zan dar vezarat-e keshavarzi* (Women managers and women farmers' problems in the Ministry of Agriculture). Tehran: Ministry of Agriculture.

Sherkat, L. 2000a. (1379). Goft va gou ba Fatemeh Tarighat Monfared (An interview with Fatemeh Tarighat Monfared). *Zanan* 68: 2–8.

Sherkat, L. 2000b. (1379). Inja zanan kalameh miforoushand (Here women sell words). *Zanan* 71: 16–23.

Smith, D. 1987. *The everyday world as problematic: A feminist sociology.* Boston: North Western Press.

Stacey, J. 1987. Sexism by a subtler name: Post-industrial conditions and post-feminist consciousness. *Socialist Review* 17(6): 7–30.

Stanley, L. 1987. Essays on women's work and leisure and "hidden" work. *Studies in Sexual Politics* 18: 1–16.

Stark-Adamec, C., and J. Andrew. 1995. *Women, work and stress: Developing mechanisms for change by bridging the gap between research and policy.* Ottawa: Social Science Federation of Canada.

Statistical Centre of Iran 1996. (1375). *Census of population and housing.* Tehran: Statistical Centre.

Statistical Centre of Iran. 1998. (1377). *Statistical yearbook.* Tehran: Statistical Centre.

Suda, C. 1989. Differential participation of men and women in production and reproduction in Kakamega District. *Journal of Developing Societies* 5(2): 234–44.

Sydie, R. 1987. *Natural women, cultured men: A feminist perspective on sociological theory.* Toronto: Methuen.

Tabari, A., and N. Yeganeh, eds. 1982. *In the shadow of Islam: The women's movement in Iran.* London: Zed Books.

Tohidi, N. 1991. Gender and Islamic fundamentalism: Feminist politics in Iran. In *Third world women and the politics of feminism,* edited by C. Mohanty, A. Russo, and L. Torres. Bloomington, IN: Indiana University Press.

United Nations. 1980. *Sex-based stereotypes, sex biases and national data systems (ST/ESA, STAT/99).* New York: UN.

United Nations. 1991. *The World's women, 1970–1990: Trends and statistics.* New York: UN.

United Nations. 2000. *The world of women, 2000: Trends and statistics.* New York: UN.

Waring, M. 1999. *Counting for nothing: What men value and what women are worth.* 2nd ed. Toronto: University of Toronto Press.

Yadgar Azadi, M. 1992. (1371). Qezavate zan (Women and judjment). *Zanan* 4: 20–26.

Part IV

Globalization of the Economy: The Risks and Opportunities It Creates for Health

10

Work and Health in Export Industries at National Borders

CATALINA A. DENMAN, LEONOR CEDILLO, AND SIOBÁN D. HARLOW

The *maquiladora* industries are a quintessential example of an export-led development strategy that followed the successful examples of Hong Kong and Korea and is comparable to similar programs in Latin America, in the Caribbean, and increasingly in Asia. Like many of these countries, Mexico defined a specific geographic zone—the area along its northern border, a region that was specifically attractive since products could be assembled closer to markets in the United States—in which special tax regulations applied and goods would be taxed only on the value added to the product before reexportation. These zones created new hubs of industrial activity in regions where there were none, and at their initiation attracted a predominantly female labor force. The *maquiladora* industries and the export processing zones (EPZs) more generally have played a key role in the globalization of the economy and in the creation of the global assembly line.

The *maquiladora* industries have been operating in Mexico since 1965. The word *maquiladora*, of Spanish origin, refers to the practice of contracting for another's mill to grind one's grain, and the term now conveys the idea of working for another, usually in a subordinate or asymmetric relationship.

The Border Industrialization Program, launched in 1965, created the *maquiladora* export industry. Since then, this industry has been a major factor in Mexico's social and economic transformation, spurring large-scale migration to the northern cities, creating an enormous new employment opportunity for women, and stimulating a restructuring of family dynamics. However, it has not become a more integral part of the domestic economy by purchasing raw materials and services locally. Only 3 (Malaysia, Mauritius, and Singapore) of over 70 countries with EPZs (ILO, 1998a) have shown such successful linkages to their national economies; and numerous authors question the impact *maquiladora* industries actually have on sustainable development in Mexico (Gereffi, 1990; Kopinak, 1996; Sklair, 1993).

Maquiladoras are related to and intersect with EPZs. The EPZs have emerged as a popular neoliberal economic liberalization policy initiative intended to enhance developing countries' position in the world market by promoting private and international investment, decreasing government participation and regulation, and promoting exports. In the past four decades, more than 840 EPZs like the *maquiladoras* of Mexico have been created in over 70 countries in Latin America, Asia, and the Caribbean, with a labor force of 27 million workers (ILO, 1998a). Generally, these zones have been established where products can be easily exported and where there is an available labor force to be recruited, sometimes (but not always) on international borders. The exact nature of EPZs varies by region, time period, and type of foreign investment. While the distribution of products exported changes over time, in most regions the products assembled or manufactured are electronic goods, textile goods, televisions, and auto parts, goods that are characterized as being labor-intensive to assemble and produce. However, the most successful EPZ programs, such as those in Malaysia and Singapore, have involved high-tech industries that have increased the number of high-skill, high-quality jobs with better wages and working conditions and linkages to the domestic labor market (ILO, 1998a).

Many multinational corporations have been lured to EPZs by tax benefits and access to a low-wage labor force. In 2000, foreign direct investment reached $1.3 trillion worldwide. Although 75% of this investment remains concentrated in the developed countries, 25% is directed to developing countries such as Mexico, where it is invested primarily in manufacturing and banking, with much of the manufacturing focused on export industries in EPZs (UNCTAD, 2001, xii–xiv). The labor force in the *maquiladora* industries in Mexico (over 1.3 million workers) represents the next to largest work force in EPZs in the world, second only to that of China, making Mexico's experience in export processing one of the oldest and largest in global production strategies (ILO, 1998b).

These global production strategies have specific implications for health, among other issues, and generate a series of questions that need to be carefully framed if we are to evaluate sustainable development on a global level. As companies based in one country are increasingly investing in and locating factories in other countries, bringing their own workplace standards, regulations, and norms concerning the nature and quality of the workplace environment, both the factory-generating and factory-hosting countries are facing a series of questions surrounding health and safety standards in foreign-owned plants: Should workplace standards match those in other industries or plants within the host country or should they match those in the sending country? What are the economic consequences, in terms of costs to the factory and possible job loss, of raising the standards to those in the sending country?[1] How should the health benefits be weighed against the potential economic costs and vice versa? What are the long-term repercussions on health for local populations? What are the implications in terms of reducing or increasing other gender, health, and environmental inequalities? In a globalizing economy, raising and resolving these questions have critical health implications.

In this chapter, we begin to grapple with these issues by examining the nature of working conditions in the mostly foreign-owned export industries. Mexico currently is the developing country with the largest body of literature published in international health journals regarding occupational impacts on workers' health in factories that produce for export.

In this chapter, we summarize the currently available quantitative knowledge of Mexican *maquiladora* workers' health status while illustrating the gaps in knowledge that remain. We conclude by highlighting critical public health concerns that are relevant to other countries that depend on export production as a cornerstone of their development strategies, and discuss policy recommendations for reducing *maquiladora* workers' health risks.

Growth and Importance of the *Maquiladora* Export Industry

Currently, the *maquiladora* export industry is Mexico's fastest-growing national manufacturing industry, and it is the primary industry that both the state and federal governments depend on for job creation and generation of foreign exchange. By 2000, *maquiladora* employment constituted 30% of the total employment in manufacturing industries. Table 10–1 illustrates the increase in *maquiladoras* and in the total number of jobs this type of industrialization has created. By the end of 2000, there were more than 3655 plants and more than 1,338,970 jobs registered under the *maquiladora* industry regime (INEGI, 2001a).

Maquiladoras and the Employment of Women

Maquiladoras play an important role in the Mexican economy because of their contribution to Mexico´s exports and foreign exchange. Of the total net exports, which amounted to $58.7 billion in 1999, petroleum accounted for 17%, *maquiladoras* for 23%, and all other manufacturing for 52%, as illustrated in Figure 10–1.[2] Since the inception of the *maquiladora* export industry, one of its defining characteristics has been the high proportion of female employees—a pattern that has held true globally in EPZs. In some *maquiladora* plants, particularly in the textile industry, the entire labor force was long composed of women (de la O, 1995). While the proportion of female employees in the *maquiladora* export industry has been decreasing since 1975 (Table 10–2), data for 1990 shows that the proportion of jobs in the *maquiladoras* occupied by women, 61% (INEGI, 1994), is significantly higher than the proportion of jobs held by female workers in manufacturing industries nationally—20% (INEGI, 1997)—or in industry in the United States—32% in 2001 (U.S. Bureau of Labor Statis-

Table 10–1. Number of Companies and Jobs in the *Maquiladora* Export Industry in Mexico, 1974–1999

Year	Number of establishments	Employed personnel
1974	455	75,974
1980	620	119,546
1985	760	211,968
1990	1703	446,436
1995	2130	648,263
1999	3297	1,140,528

Source: INEGI (2001a).

tics, 2001). The *maquiladora* industries represent the most important job alternative to working in agriculture, where 12% of women worked in 1990, or the service sector, where 68% of women worked. Although female employment has been dominant in the *maquiladora* industries, few of these industries have policies to accommodate women's occupational and reproductive health needs. On the contrary, *maquiladoras* have often discriminated against pregnant women, prompting international campaigns to modify these practices (Hertel, 2002), and the availability of child-care facilities is severely limited (Saint-Germain, Zapién, and Denman, 1993, 80). Mexican labor law guarantees maternity leave for 45 days previous to childbirth and 45 days after childbirth, and our studies (Denman, 2001) indicate that this law is generally respected by the factories when pregnant women are hired and not fired. Although opportunities for breast-feeding during the work day are guaranteed in theory, in practice they are limited to the few larger factories where child-care facilities are available. (See Chapter 5 by Yimyam and Morrow.)

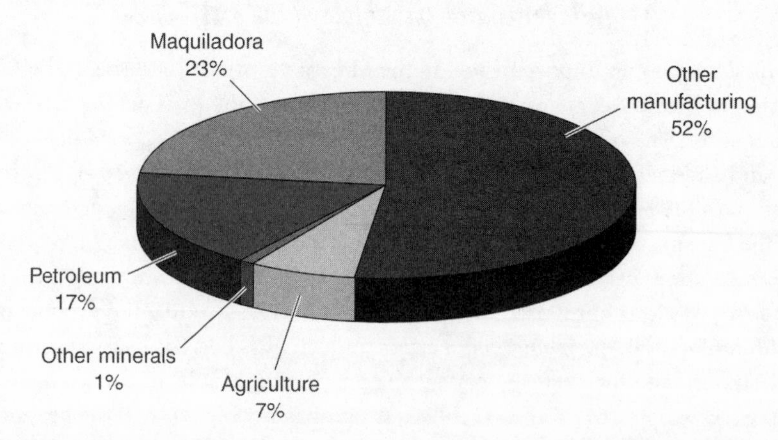

Figure 10–1. Total net exports for Mexico, 1999 (millions of dollars). Source: Data from H. Vázquez Tercero, 2000. Medición del flujo de divisas de la balanza comercial de México. *Comercio Exterior* 50(10): 890–94.

Table 10–2. Direct Labor Personnel* in the *Maquiladora* Export Industry in Mexico, by Sex, 1975–1999

	Women		Men		
	Number	Percentage	Number	Percentage	Total
1975	45,275	78.3	12,575	21.7	57,850
1980	78,880	77.3	23,140	22.7	102,020
1985	120,042	69.0	53,832	31.0	173,874
1990	219,439	60.9	140,919	39.1	360,358
1995	314,172	59.0	217,557	40.9	531,729
1999	515,164	55.9	406,458	44.1	921,622

*This does not include technical and administrative jobs.

Source: INEGI (2001a).

Comparisons of Employment in the Maquiladoras and in Other Industries

Understanding employment in the *maquiladoras* in the Mexican and global context is challenging for a number of reasons. Comparisons of work in *maquiladoras* and other industries in Mexico require recent data collected at the factory level, which are not widely available. Comparisons of employment in the same companies in their home countries and foreign-owned factories pose similar challenges. However, there are data on wages from both *maquiladoras* and other manufacturing industries showing that in addition to differences in tariff regimes and the importation and reexportation of components, one important difference between *maquiladoras* and other Mexican industries (such as manufacturing of goods not intended for export) is that salaries are lower in the *maquiladoras*, although they have risen in the past decade. In 1986, salaries in the border auto-parts *maquiladoras* were $0.36[3] an hour, while workers in the same skill category in non-*maquiladora* auto-parts plants in central Mexico received $1.40 (Carrillo, 1992, 56). The source and consequences of these disparities—as well as wage differences across countries and by gender, documented subsequently—is a topic for another paper. Our discussion of them here serves to highlight the fact that *maquiladoras* raise important questions regarding working conditions in factories located in the home countries compared to those in the foreign-owned plants.

Maquiladora wages have also been considerably lower than those paid for similar jobs in the same industrial sector in the United States and in Asian countries. In 1986, for example, automobile workers performing a similar job averaged $0.60 per hour in Mexico, $1.55 in Korea, $1.87 in Hong Kong, and $13.09 in the United States (Carrillo, 1991). One of the major reasons for the high job turnover in the *maquiladora* industry has been low salaries (Carrillo and Santibáñez, 1993), and it explains why 66% of *maquiladora* workers surveyed by Kopinak (1996, 163–64) responded that better wages, benefits, and bonuses would give them greater job satisfaction.

Within the *maquiladora* industry, salaries for female workers have also been consistently lower than salaries for male workers. In Nogales in 1985, the average monthly salary of female *maquiladora* workers, $87.30, was 83% of that for male workers, $104.89 (Denman, 1991, 45). A study in the state of Sonora, based on the 1980–1995 state employment survey, showed that, by economic sector and employment level, women in each group had, on average, higher levels of schooling and yet received lower wages than did men (Grijalva, 1996). Employment and differential salary policies, which usually are not permitted by collective bargaining agreements in automobile plants, have become common in auto-parts *maquiladora* plants on the northern border through promotion practices that favor men (Zúñiga, 1998). According to Carrillo (1992), this difference has been most apparent in the promotion and hiring policies for better-paid positions.

In addition to providing monetary income for working women, employment can confer status. Here, too, work in the *maquiladoras* differs from work in other industries in Mexico. The prestige of working in the *maquiladoras* has varied by social class, migrant status, and time. For women from rural areas, remunerated work with a set salary, often found in the *maquiladoras*, has been preferred to unemployment in the countryside (which increases dependency on other relatives) or employment as a domestic worker. However, for women from urban areas, jobs in public service or commerce have generally been perceived as preferable to work in the *maquiladoras* (Denman, 2001). In this and other ways, *maquiladoras* raise important questions regarding the effect of globalization and urbanization on local economic conditions, of which this chapter will address one.

Research on Working Conditions and Health in the *Maquiladoras*

Focused research on working conditions and health consequences of employment in the *maquiladora* industries is essential to understanding what, if any, health hazards are associated with work in these emergent industries and to evaluate whether the benefits of employment are potentially eroded or compromised by hazardous working conditions. Although work in *maquiladoras* is obviously less hazardous than some forms of employment (e.g., mining), prudent development policies require health monitoring tailored to evaluate potential risks of new industries to ensure that adverse health changes in the population do not emerge as a consequence of the new forms of employment.

The first published research on *maquiladora* workers' living and working conditions in various border cities appeared during the 1980s (Arenal, 1986; Carrillo and Hernández, 1985; Fernández-Kelly, 1983; Gambrill, 1981; Iglesias, 1985). These anthropological and sociological studies included participant observation, sociodemographic surveys, and ethnographic approaches, including in-depth interviews.

The researchers who conducted those studies pioneered the investigation of health and safety in the *maquiladoras* specifically and in EPZs more generally, and their results were the first to shed light on the potential job hazards in this economic sector. For example, Carrillo and Hernández (1985, 137) described the "poor working conditions in the *maquiladoras* such as lack of ventilation and insufficient light, use of soldering, microscopes and toxic substances" in Ciudad Juarez. Iglesias (1985, 53) catalogued the symptoms women attributed to their work in the *maquiladoras*, including "dizziness, headaches, fatigue, sneezing, coughing; eye inflammation, pain and irritation; skin dryness, irritation, itching, and breakouts; trouble breathing; menstrual irregularities, irritability and insomnia, among others." Similarly, both Fernández-Kelly (1983) and Iglesias (1985) described *maquiladora* workers' poor living conditions—such as inadequate housing and the lack of services such as drinking water, sewage, and transportation—and conflictive family dynamics, including domestic violence, alcoholism, substance abuse, and unequal distribution of the domestic workload in, respectively, Ciudad Juarez and Tijuana.

In the mid-1980s, the first descriptive studies appeared that were specifically designed to catalogue health and safety conditions in the *maquiladoras*. This research (Carlesso and Rodríguez-García, 1985; Carrillo, 1984; Carrillo and Jasis, 1983; Márquez and Romero, 1988; Torres Muñoz et al., 1991) from the northern Mexican cities of Tijuana, Matamoros, and Chihuahua resulted in a copious inventory of self-reported and medical records health problems among *maquiladora* workers, including such illnesses as lumbago and peptic acid syndrome, reproductive health problems such as menstrual cycle disturbances and menstrual pain, and various symptoms and injuries such as bruises and lacerations. Carlesso and Rodríguez-García (1985) and Márquez and Romero (1988) also began to explore the potential connection between these health problems and the working conditions in the factories. However, no quantitative assessments were made of the associations between specific exposures and health outcomes. Thus, the studies of the early 1980s were limited, from a public health perspective, because the data did not clearly quantify the extent of exposure, the level and trends in specific health problems, or the strength of the association between exposures and adverse health outcomes. Nonetheless, these early studies clearly defined a public health research agenda, identifying health conditions that were of concern to workers.

Routinely reported surveillance statistics such as reported occupational accidents and illnesses are also inadequate measures of the potential adverse effects of employment in the *maquiladoras*. Of 5520 reported illnesses, 2793 cases involved hearing impairment and 2243 cases involved respiratory effects. Included among the other cases were: contact dermatitis, traumatic amputation of wrist and hand, sinovitis, and tenosinovitis (IMSS, 2001). The unrealistically small number of illnesses reported highlights the extent of underreporting of occupational illness in Mexico generally. Occupational musculoskeletal disorders are notably absent from the list, although cumulative trauma disorders are a known occupational risk in production assembly, and a higher frequency of problems such as lumbalgia, carpal tunnel syndrome, tendonitis, and tendosinovitis would be expected nationally, as well as within the *maquiladoras* specifically. These are illnesses related to jobs that involve repetitive motion and short work cycles, as in the *maquiladoras.* It is difficult to disaggregate *maquiladora* data from national statistics in Mexico, because all *maquiladoras* are grouped under general manufacturing. The absence of reported musculoskeletal diseases in Mexico is not credible, particularly by comparison with the number of cases in other countries, for example the United States, where the number of repeated trauma cases increased dramatically, from 23,800 in 1972 to 332,000 in 1994 (O'Neill, 1999).

The Mexican Institute of Social Security (IMSS) is the institution responsible for providing medical care and pension programs to private sector employees, diagnosing and treating their occupational diseases and injuries, and maintaining the registry of these diseases and injuries. In 2001 IMSS theoretically covered 56% of the country's population, which includes all private sector workers, their families, and pensionees, as well as 16 million persons living in rural areas. For the year 2001 IMSS had registered 12,234,231 workers, 31% of the economically active population (IMSS, 2001; INEGI, 2001b), while other workers were either covered by government programs or were without care. Data on diagnoses by physicians attending sick workers from non-*maquiladora* industries at an IMSS center in Mexico City show a rate of 93.2 visits per 100 workers per year for illnesses not considered to be occupational (Villegas et al., 1997). When Márquez and Romero (1988) analyzed the same rate at the IMSS center in Matamoros for two *maquiladora* electronics companies, they found morbidity rates of 246.3 and 247.4 visits per 100 workers per year, more than double the rate of workers in Mexico City. However, these data do not permit us to draw conclusions about potential reasons for this apparent increase in morbidity among *maquiladora* workers.

Research on health and safety in the *maquiladoras* has increased since the 1990s, and the broader range of topics investigated in recent years has increased researchers' and policy makers' awareness of how working conditions in the *maquiladora* industries may be linked to workers' health. Nevertheless, the body of literature remains limited, as noted earlier, and the dearth of longitudinal research still prohibits an evaluation of temporal trends in *maquiladora* workers' health risks. In the following section, we review and analyze the findings of 13 studies that have been published in since the 1990s. In four of these studies (Cedillo et al., 1997; GAO, 1993; González Arroyo et al., 1996; Moure-Eraso et al., 1994), researchers evaluated working conditions, occupational hazards, and worker health and safety programs. In seven other studies (Cedillo et al., 1997, González Arroyo et al., 1996, González Block, 2001; Guendelman and Jasis, 1993; Hovell et al., 1988; Jasis and Guendelman, 1993; Moure-Eraso et al., 1997), researchers evaluated general health status and health symptoms, including two studies that involved measures of psychological distress. In four studies (Denman, 1990, 1991; Eskenazi et al., 1993, González Block, 2001), researchers examined infant birth weight and other reproductive outcomes; in another (Balcázar, Denman, and

Lara, 1995), accidents; and in five others (Cedillo et al., 1997; GAO, 1993; Harlow et al., 1999; Meservy et al., 1997; Moure-Eraso et al., 1997), ergonomic risks and musculoskeletal complaints.

Working Conditions, Occupational Hazards, and Safety and Training Programs

The first and most extensive evaluations of working conditions in *maquiladora* plants were commissioned by the U.S. General Accounting Office in 1993. As the North American Free Trade Agreement (NAFTA) was being implemented, the General Accounting Office contracted with the University of California–Los Angeles to assess the occupational safety and health work environment in the Mexican auto-parts industry in response to congressional concerns that disparities in health and safety regulations between the United States and Mexico might lead to job loss in the United States. Of the 104 auto-parts plants, 2 plants from each of six border states were selected for study, based on the objective of including large and small plants and a variety of production processes. Permission to conduct the evaluation was obtained from 8 of the 12 plants, which employed about 13% of all Mexican auto-parts workers. A 2-day survey at each plant included reviews of the written documentation on health and safety programs, discussions with plant managers and with safety and health staff, walk-through industrial hygiene evaluations of each plant, and ergonomic evaluations of specific workstations. The presence of ergonomic, safety, physical, and chemical hazards was assessed on the basis of U.S. Occupational Safety and Health Administration standards (29 C.F.R. 1900) and professional judgments of the researchers, with the consultants focusing on eight specific areas: ergonomics, fire protection, personal protective equipment, hearing conservation, respiratory protection, hazard communication, hazardous energy control, and lead exposure. This study is one of only two studies to date that have involved actual in-plant assessments. [The other one (Cedillo, 1999) related only to psychosocial factors.]

This study clearly documented limitations in the occupational safety and health programs of the individual auto-parts plants, but the focus on only one sector of the *maquiladora* industry limits the generalizability of the results. Nevertheless, ergonomic, safety, physical, and chemical hazards common to many types of light manufacturing and assembly were observed. Some limitations were serious enough to have caused permanent or prolonged damage to workers, but none was considered an "imminent danger" to workers' lives or health—a classification in industrial hygiene evaluations that refers to, for example, atmospheres without oxygen or concentrations of toxins in the environment that require special equipment. The most frequently observed ergonomic hazards involved exposure to processes and technologies that could provoke repetitive motion injuries. Consultants reported ergonomic hazards in all eight plants included in the study. Through interviews with 175 workers in one of those plants, it was determined that 42% of the interviewed workers reported pain in the upper limbs;

37% reported hand-wrist pain; 30% pain in the lower limbs; 25% pain in the neck and shoulders; and 14% pain in the lower back. Most workers in all of the plants were observed to be exposed to such hazards. The most frequently observed safety hazard was machines without safety shields or guards; consequently, the most common injuries reported by the plants were contusions, lacerations, and hand injuries, which were treated in the plants' medical facilities. Noise was the most frequently observed physical hazard, with noise levels measured by direct reading instruments exceeding 90 decibels in six of the plants. Although workers were provided with earplugs, they were often observed not to be using them or not wearing them properly. The use of chemicals was limited, but in those instances where chemicals were employed, the opportunity for skin contact and inhalation was noted during the factory walk-through visits.

Seven of the eight *maquiladoras* had established health and safety programs, yet the programs in all of the plants were either lacking or inadequate in 6 of the 10 areas deemed necessary. For example, none of the plants had ergonomic safety or training programs, although two were in the process of developing them. Most of the plants did not have adequate programs to address hazard communication ($n = 7$), hearing conservation ($n = 7$), and safe machine operations ($n = 5$). In the six plants where material safety data sheets were reviewed, only one had translated all the forms into Spanish. The U.S. parent companies were found to have given health and safety guidance, as well as limited technical support, but the evaluations and audits commonly used in the U.S. plants were not found to have been employed in the Mexican plants.

In 1996, González Arroyo and colleagues (1996)[4] interviewed 177 workers from two cities about their working conditions, health and safety programs at their workplaces, and health symptoms they had experienced in the preceding 6 months. Participants were identified by convenience sampling at the factory entrances of 72 plants and were asked about machine operations, use of chemicals, noise exposure, ergonomic hazards, hazard communication, health and safety training, and availability and use of personal protective equipment. Fifty-four percent of the participants were female. The mean age of workers was 27 years, and the mean length of job tenure was 22 months. Forty-seven percent of the participants worked in electronics, 11% in furniture and woodworking, and 9% in medical supplies processes, with the remainder distributed in a variety of other plants, such as garment, plastics, and metalworking plants.

Chemical exposures were reported by 42% of the participants. Fifty-three percent of these individuals had not received material safety data sheets for the chemicals they handled. Half of the workers reported that they operated machinery, and 26% of this group reported that the machines had no safety-guard features. Forty percent of the workers said they had not received any training regarding hazards associated with their jobs. Thirty-eight percent reported noise as a problem; it was so loud that they had to shout to be heard. González Arroyo and colleagues (1996) simultaneously conducted an in-depth interview with a line supervisor at one electronics *maquiladora*. This respondent noted additional hazards such as the inadequate environmental control of pollutants, including a lack of exhaust ventilation in the soldering area. He also described the lack of health and safety training, of material safety data sheets, and of an emergency plan for chemical spills.

Using the workers' reports, González Arroyo and colleagues (1996) also endeavored to assess qualitatively the *maquiladora* industries' general level of compliance with Mexican regulations requiring employers to provide warning labels and material safety data sheets in Spanish, to provide training, to monitor airborne substances and noise and to maintain them below designated limits, and to provide personal protective equipment. The researchers concluded, on the basis of the workers' reports, that plants may not have been complying with the regulations, particularly regarding hazard communication, workplace monitoring, and safety training. This study clearly documented workers' perceptions of workplace hazards. However, the use of convenience samples limits the generalizability of the findings even to the 72 factories studied. Although multiple industries were represented, except for electronics each sector was represented by only a handful of individuals, thus making cross-industry comparisons impossible. Another limitation was the researchers' reliance on the workers' self-reports, without independent evaluations of the adequacy of personal protective equipment or use of quantitative exposures assessments. Self-reported data at best provide a qualitative assessment of potential risk and presuppose that workers are knowledgeable about potential hazards.

Maquiladora working conditions and health and safety programs were also assessed by Moure-Eraso and colleagues (1997), who conducted a community-based cross-sectional study of 267 *maquiladora* workers in Matamoros and Reynosa. To identify a sample, the researchers employed snowball sampling and obtained key informants through randomly selected households and through church-sponsored community organizations. Structured interviews were conducted with 267 of the 270 workers identified. Ninety-four percent of the participants engaged in production activities, predominantly in electronics plants. Women accounted for 81% of the sample and men for 19%. The mean age of the respondents was 25 years, and 50% had only a primary school education. The average duration of employment was 28 months among the Reynosa respondents and 62 months among the Matamoros ones.

Forty-five percent of the respondents reported exposure to gas or vapors, 43% reported exposure to manufacturing dust during at least part of their shifts, and 41% reported skin contact with chemicals. Physical hazards included noise, which was reported by two-thirds of the participants, and heat and vibration, which were reported by more than half of the workers. More than half of the workers reported that their jobs required high visual demands. Reported exposures to ergonomic risks included repetitive movements (76%), manual labor requiring strength (44%), and heavy physical work (26%). Also, 43% reported having to perform their duties in difficult positions during at least part of the workday. Approximately half of the workers had received health and safety training, and 94% of that group considered their training adequate. However, of eight areas of training asked about in the questionnaire, less than half of those who received any training had received training in all eight. About 50% reported regularly using personal protective equipment.

Women's *maquiladora* working conditions, occupational hazards, and safety and training programs. Various researchers have focused on women's experiences as *maquiladora* workers, since women have composed the majority of the labor force since the inception of the industry. In 1993, Cedillo and colleagues (1997) conducted a cross-sectional pilot study designed to estimate the prevalence of potentially hazardous exposures and of health complaints, and to evaluate the contribution of working conditions to job transitions among women working in Tijuana's *maquiladoras.* A systematic age-stratified (aged 18 to 24 and 25 to 50) sample of 40 women—10 from each of four occupational groups (electronics *maquiladora* workers, other *maquiladora* workers, other workers, nonemployed individuals)—was obtained in each of 12 neighborhoods over a 3-month period. A house-to-house survey was conducted by female community health workers to obtain the desired sample, and 479 women were interviewed. The analysis of working conditions was limited to the 365 women who had worked within the preceding 2½ years and thus could provide detailed information about working conditions in their then-current or most recent job.

Thirty-six percent of the interviewed women were single, and 13% were heads of their households. The respondents' overall educational level was low, with one-third having completed only elementary school. Of the 365 working women, 30% were then employed or had most recently been employed in an electronics *maquila*; 34%, in another type of *maquiladora*; and 36%, in another, non-*maquiladora* job such as retail (15%) or office work (15%). The participants reported having held from one to five jobs, with half of them having had two or more jobs. Among the women who had held more than one job, rotation into and out of some type of *maquiladora* industry and rotation among sectors within the *maquiladora* industries were common. The average duration of employment per job was less than 1 year.

The prevalence of occupational exposures was assessed among the 230 women who worked or had recently worked in a *maquila.* The exposures were many and frequent. Among physical factors, noise was the most prevalent exposure, with 72% and 75% of the women in electronics and other *maquiladora* plants, respectively, reporting that they were frequently or always exposed to noise. Exposures to heat (34%), vibrations (22% and 34%, respectively), and poor ventilation (33% and 35%, respectively) were also commonly reported. Radiation exposure was infrequent, but it was sufficient to have been captured even in this relatively small sample (6% and 8%, respectively). A total of 36% and 39% of the electronics and other *maquiladora* workers, respectively, reported having had at least some chemical exposure. Alcohols and other solvents were used most frequently, followed by chlorinated hydrocarbons in the electronics sector and glues in the other *maquiladora* group. Approximately 20% of the women faced exposure to soldering fumes. Eighty-three percent of women working in a nonelectronic *maquiladora* and 90% of those women working in an electronic factory reported that they worked or had worked on production lines, and 45% to 60%, respectively, reported having dealt with quotas or having received incentives. Experiences with awkward postures were also gauged, and more than 60% of the women reported having worked in such positions.

This study also documented deficiencies in occupational health and safety programs. Although most women who used chemicals reported having received some safety training, more than 90% had had inadequate training. Slightly more than half indicated that their plants had at least minimal safety infrastructures and engineering controls. The women were also asked why they had most recently left a job. Although the primary reasons that *maquiladora* workers cited were personal or family ones [48% (for instance, to stay home and take care of their child)], 16% to 20% had left because of working conditions or health problems they attributed to work. In comparison, 70% of the women who had held non-*maquiladora* jobs had resigned for personal or family reasons, whereas only 4% had left because of working conditions.

This study employed a community-based, random-sampling strategy; used standardized approaches to the assessment of occupational hazards; quantified the prevalence of perceived exposure to occupational hazards among women working in the *maquila*, and provided preliminary data to facilitate the design of more rigorous studies. However, the data were self-reported and thus reflected only perceived hazards. No information was available on levels or durations of exposures. As stated above, self-reported measures can at best provide qualitative assessments of possible hazards. For example, most women who soldered on their job did not appear to consider the fumes a chemical exposure. Cedillo and colleagues (1997) also noted that high turnover rates, rotation between occupational categories, and job turnover related to working conditions and migration status posed methodological challenges for future studies because of the potential difficulty of following workers in longitudinal studies, defining appropriate comparison groups and potential selection for healthy workers in factory-based samples.

In summary, all of the studies described in this section suggest that safety, physical, and ergonomic hazards exist in the *maquiladora* industries. Lack of adequate protection—including machine guards, ventilation, and noise reduction—and the lack of adequate safety and training programs have been reported consistently. Although chemical exposures have been a major concern since the *maquiladora* plants began to dot the northern border area of Mexico, in many plants the use of chemicals has, in fact, been limited. Nonetheless, the evidence suggests that when chemicals have been present, workers have been exposed improperly and have lacked information about the potential toxicity of these exposures. Ergonomic risks were noted in all studies, and these risks remain of particular concern because of the potential for long-term disabling injuries to young workers. In only one of the five studies did researchers focus on a single sector and, within that, provide an in-depth analysis based on in-plant observations. Comparable studies in other sectors are clearly needed.

Studies of Health Status and Health Risks

Quantitative epidemiological studies of health risks generally employ health surveys, medical examinations, or a combination of the two in a representative sample of workers. In order to determine whether the risks among the workers of interest are higher or lower than the risks among workers in other industries or economic sectors or the general population, a comparison population is needed. Studies may be cross-sectional (studies that measure current exposures and current health status) or longitudinal (studies that follow a group of healthy workers to observe the onset of new diseases or health conditions). Since workers tend to be healthier than the general population (the healthy worker effect), comparisons with other working populations are often preferred.

Cross-sectional studies provide information on prevalence and on associations, but because measurement of exposure does not occur before observation of the onset of the disease, causal relationships cannot be assumed. Cohort studies permit the observation of incident cases and enable assessment of the temporal relationships between exposure and disease, but they are generally more time-consuming and can be costly.

General Health Status, Physical Symptoms, and Psychological Distress among Maquiladora Workers

One of the earliest quantitative studies of *maquiladora* workers' health status was conducted by Hovell and colleagues (1988). This community-based study involved a systematic sample of 108 women recruited from seven working-class neighborhoods. After randomly selecting households among those households located at the edge of each neighborhood, the researchers approached every tenth household and interviewed all women aged 15 to 35 years in each household they contacted. Of the women interviewed, 38 worked in a *maquila*, 29 worked in non-*maquiladora* jobs, and 41 were not employed outside the home. The questionnaire was based on a previously validated instrument, the Health Status Index (Kaplan, Bush, and Berry, 1976). The mean scores for mental health indicators in the previous month, gastrointestinal or urinary symptoms in the previous month, and respiratory and musculoskeletal symptoms in the previous year were then compared across occupational groups.

Scores on the health index indicated that female *maquiladora* workers were less likely to report musculoskeletal symptoms or difficulty breathing, and they were less likely to report falls in the previous year than were women in the other occupational groups. Homemakers received the worst scores for six out of nine measured outcomes. However, none of the morbidity indicators differed significantly, once adjusted for age, income, and education. Although *maquiladora* workers did not present more morbidity than other women or seem to be less healthy, this study was limited by the small sample size, its cross-sectional nature, and the failure to consider the possibility of a healthy worker effect.

Guendelman and Jasis (1993) conducted a community-based cross-sectional study of 480 women in Tijuana that was designed to evaluate the health impacts of working in the *maquiladoras*. This study involved a convenience sample of nonpregnant working women aged 16 to 28 years who were stratified by occupation (garment *maquila*, electronics *maquila*, service sector, and homemakers; $n = 120$ per group) and duration of employment (<6, 6–24, >24 months). The average age of the respondents was 21 years. More than 70% of the working women were single compared to 40% of the homemakers. Sixty-seven percent of the participants were originally from Tijuana or had lived there for more than 10 years. Women working in the *maquiladoras* had less formal education, worked longer hours, and earned less than women in the comparison groups. Four measures of health status were examined. *Functional impediments* were defined as "having at least one of fifteen physical symptoms in the previous thirty days that impeded performance." Symptoms ranged from backaches to stomachaches to ear problems. *Depressed mood* was measured by the Center for Epidemiologic Studies' Depression Scale (Radloff, 1977). *Nervousness* in the previous 30 days was measured by the question "In the past 30 days how often have you felt nervous or tense?", and *sense of control* was measured by Cohen's Perceived Stress Scale (Cohen and Williamson, 1988). Health status was compared across occupational groups. In addition, psychosocial risk was measured by Karasek's (1997) Job Content Questionnaire, which assesses the level of job demand relative to job control, as well as levels of social support, job satisfaction, and promotion opportunities. Household strains such as not having enough money to make ends meet and family tension were also assessed.

The prevalence of functional impediments (ranging from 18% to 27%) and of depressed mood (mean score ranging from 15 to –18) did not differ significantly by occupational group, although women working in the electronics *maquiladoras* reported the lowest prevalence and scores. After adjustment for confounding factors, electronics workers had half the risk of functional impairments that service workers faced. Nervousness was reported most often by women working in the service sector and least often by women working in the *maquiladoras*. Level of perceived stress also did not differ significantly by occupational group. When occupational and household stressors were examined, lack of financial resources proved to be an important risk factor for each of the four health outcomes. Guendelman and Jasis concluded that the health of *maquiladora* workers was no worse than that of other working women.

This study was considerably larger than earlier studies, and it included a comparison group of working and nonworking women. However, the study had limitations. The functional impediments measure was a poorly constructed outcomes indicator, as it lumped together multiple symptoms likely to have had distinct etiologies. Since no information was available about the participants' prior work history, the healthy worker effect may also have biased the results. Thus, the primary contribution of this study was the data it provided on psychosocial risks, as opposed to general health status or specific morbidities.

The study by González Arroyo and colleagues (1996) discussed above also included a symptom checklist on which workers were asked to indicate whether they had experienced any of 45 symptoms in the previous 6 months. Workers were also asked whether they had any symptoms caused by their work and whether they had been injured on the job. Symptoms such as fatigue (45%), back pain (41%), headache (33%), upper airway irritation (23%), wrist pain (24%), and upper extremity pain (20%) were common. Twenty-one percent of the 177 respondents reported having symptoms caused by workplace exposures, and 19% reported having suffered a job-related injury. The participants were not asked, however, which specific symptoms or injuries they considered work-related, and the most prevalent symptoms may have been related to ergonomic and irritant exposures. The use of a convenience sample and the lack of a comparison population make it difficult to assess not only the extent to which the reported symptoms were work related but also the prevalence of symptoms in comparison to those among other working populations.

Another study warranting discussion is the large cross-sectional one conducted by González Block (1996). This study used a cluster sample approach to recruit a representative sample of 1278 women working in Tijuana's *maquiladoras*. Although no internal comparison group was included, the results of the survey were compared to data from the Second National Health Survey, as well as to state surveillance data and clinical surveys. Of the 1278 workers identified, 1228 were employed on production lines or as supervisors and participated in this survey; of those, 928 (76%) completed the survey. The study thus included 2.5% of Tijuana's total *maquiladora* worker population as of 1995. The average age of the participants was 26.5 years. Forty-six percent were married or living as married, and 54% were not married. Eighty-two percent were immigrants, and 18% were from Tijuana. On average, the *maquiladora* workers interviewed had more formal education than the female population in Tijuana, with 43% having completed primary school. A total of 160 women (17%) had been pregnant in the 2 years prior to the study. Most of the women (73%) had had more than one job, with 44% reporting between three and eight jobs. Half of the jobs had lasted for 1 year or less.

Information on morbidity was obtained by questionnaire, and no measurements were taken. Unlike previous studies that had focused on health symptoms, González Block's study evaluated the frequency of specific morbidities. Compared with the Second National Health Survey[5] results, the prevalence of hypertension, deafness, and asthma was higher among *maquiladora* workers than among industrial workers nationally. For example, the prevalence of hypertension was 3.8-fold higher in the survey of *maquiladora* workers than among responsents classified as industrial workers in the National Health Survey. Notably, female *maquiladora* workers were less likely to smoke (16.6%) than were Mexican urban women as a whole (18.6%).

In contrast to the study of Guendelman and Jasis (1993), also conducted in Tijuana, this study focused on specific morbidities and recruited a large, representative sample.

González Block's findings suggest that the health status of *maquiladora* workers (particularly with regard to hypertension and asthma) may well be compromised when compared with the health status of industrial workers and pregnant women nationally. However, this study included no information on specific physical, chemical, or psychosocial hazards.

Moure-Eraso and colleagues (1997), employing a symptom checklist (in the study described earlier), were the first researchers to obtain information on chemical and airborne exposures simultaneously and to evaluate associations between reported symptoms and chemical exposures. More than half of the women and men reported having experienced headache (56%), unusual fatigue (53%), and depression (51%). In addition, over a third of the workers reported having experienced forgetfulness (41%), chest pressure (41%), stomach pain (37%), dizziness (36%), and numbness or tingling in the extremities (33%). Reported instances of nausea, stomach pain, urinary problems, and breathing problems were significantly associated with the reported frequency of exposure to airborne contaminants, while reported instances of eye and nose secretions and breathing problems were associated with the reported frequency of exposure to dust. Reported exposures to airborne organics (including solvents, glues, and gasoline) were associated with reported instances of fatigue, chest pressure, and tingling in the extremities. Although this study was limited by its cross-sectional nature, lack of clear time frames for reported symptoms, and lack of information on levels of exposure, it represents a critical first attempt to assess the link between workplace exposures and health status, and it provides suggestive evidence for this link.

Adverse Reproductive Outcomes

Three intriguing studies have suggested that women working in the *maquiladoras* may be more likely than other women to give birth to low-birth-weight babies. One of the earliest studies of the health consequences of working in the *maquiladoras* was a study of medical records conducted by Denman (1990) in Nogales. Infant records over a 2-year period (between 1985 and 1986) were randomly selected at the IMSS hospital in Nogales. Of the 300 records reviewed, the mothers of 169 of the infants worked in a *maquiladora* and the mothers of 131 others in service or retail positions. The frequency of low birth weight was 2.8 times higher among *maquila*-employed mothers compared to other working women (14% and 5%, respectively). In addition, whereas 52% of the low-birth-weight infants of *maquila*-employed mothers had been born prematurely, that was true of only 33% of the infants of other workers.

In a follow-up study, Denman (1991) interviewed all women who had given birth in the IMSS hospital in Nogales during a 6-month period in 1989. Of the 406 participants, 143 worked in the *maquiladoras*, 38 worked in service or retail jobs, and 225 were homemakers. This study reported a slightly lower frequency of low birth weight in both employed groups: 9% for infants of *maquiladora* workers and 3% for those of other workers. The frequency of low birth weight among the homemakers' infants was comparable to that among *maquiladora* workers' infants (10%). Eighty-five percent of the *maquiladora* workers reported laboring more than 9 hours a day (excluding overtime), whereas 37% of the service and retail workers reported laboring for a similar number of hours. The reported overtime hours worked per week were 11.4 among the *maquiladora* workers and none among the other employed women. When asked about potential toxic exposures, 67% of the women who worked in the *maquiladoras* compared to none of the service sector employees reported having been exposed to solvents, paints, degreasers, solder fumes, and other hazards. The *maquiladora* workers identified difficult postures required during most of their shifts as the greatest problem. Although this study showed a difference in the frequency of low birth weight, the sample size of other workers was small. No difference was observed between *maquila*-employed women and homemakers. The study did not adjust for potential confounders such as parity.

Following up on Denman's results, Eskenazi and associates (1993) conducted a secondary analysis of data obtained by Guendelman and Jasis (1993). This analysis included information from the 61 women who had been pregnant and who had worked at the same job during their most recent pregnancy (24 in electronic *maquiladoras*, 15 in garment *maquiladoras*, and 22 in services). Infants' birth weights were compared by their mothers' occupational groups. The garment workers' infants had an average weight of 2987 grams; the electronics workers', 3266 grams; and the service sector workers', 3578 grams. The birth weight difference between the infants of garment industry workers and those of service workers (591 grams) was statistically significant. After adjustment for the mothers' age, parity, education, and smoking status by multiple linear regression, garment workers were found to have had babies who were 653 grams lighter than service workers' infants ($p < .01$) and 316 grams lighter than electronics workers' infants ($p = .11$). Electronics workers' babies weighed 337 grams less than service workers' infants ($p = .06$). In this analysis, occupation proved a better predictor of birth weight than other well-known risk factors such as parity and smoking. Although the sample size was small, this was the first study of pregnancy outcomes that included a comparison between different sectors of the *maquiladora* industry, and it was the first to include adjustments for potential confounders.

A major focus of González Block's (1996) study was also on the reproductive health status of the *maquiladora* population. Among women who had recently been pregnant, 12% reported having given birth more than 2 weeks early, but only 4% reported having had a low-birth-weight (< 2500 grams) infant. This low-birth-weight frequency is considerably lower than that reported in the previously cited studies by Denman (1990, 1991) or in a study of workers in Mexico City (Cerón-Mireles, Harlow, and Sanchez-Carrillo, 1996), all of which involved birth weight information obtained from medical records. However, the reported frequency of preterm delivery was higher in González Block's study than in the one other study of this outcome among Mexican working women (Cerón-Mireles, Harlow, and Sanchez-Carrillo, 1996). In this study, interviews were conducted in 1992 of 2663 workers who had given birth in Mexico

City Hospitals, and the association between low birth weight and working conditions was evaluated with regression models, identifying risk factors for low birth weight as having a work week longer than 50 hours (OR = 1.6; 95% CI = 1.17, 2.28), as well as lacking tangible social support (OR = 1.7; 95% CI = 1.20, 2.33) (Cerón-Mireles, Harlow, and Sanchez-Carrillo, 1996).

In the study of *maquiladora* workers in Tijuana, González-Block also identified the frequency of self-reported gynecological conditions of pregnant women. Twenty-nine percent of the women were found to have had signs of vaginal, urethral, or cervical infection, higher than that reported by national health institutions (IMSS) for the same year for prenatal care among non-*maquiladora* women. Despite higher rates of health problems, workers in *maquiladoras* who had had health problems during pregnancy were less likely to have left their jobs before receiving paid maternity leave than were workers in Mexico City (18% and 42%, respectively) (González-Block, 1996). One explanation for these findings is that women in the *maquiladoras* need to maintain their jobs and their earned income more than other workers in Mexico City.

Although provocative, these findings require follow-up in more methodologically rigorous studies. In future studies, researchers should tease out the precise etiology of the low-birth-weight births. In particular, Denman's (1991) finding of an increased proportion of premature babies among low-birth-weight infants suggests that more studies should focus on gestational age and premature birth. Two possible avenues of research are suggested by González Block's finding that pregnant women working in the *maquiladoras* had an increased frequency of reproductive tract infections, and by recent reports of an association between occupational strain and risk of preeclampsia (Landsbergis and Hatch, 1996; Marcoux et al., 1999).

Accidents

Only one study (Balcázar, Denman, and Lara, 1995) focused specifically on accidents in the *maquiladoras*. Also a cross-sectional study, this investigation included 497 *maquiladora* workers living in Nogales who were identified while attending clinics at the Medical Services of Sonora, an agency that provides health certificates to workers. Seventy-five percent of the workers who had been employed at a *maquiladora* within the previous 6 months and who were seeking a certificate were recruited. The mean age of the participants was 22 years. Fifty percent of the participants were female and 50% were male; 56% were single and 44% were not; 50% had received more than a primary education and 50% had not; and 74% were migrants and 26% were not. The average number of hours worked per week was 51.

Thirteen percent of the workers reported having had an accident while working in the *maquiladoras* within the previous 6 months, and 18% had had a work-related illness. More than 40% of the accidents had required at least 1 disability day. The parts of the body most commonly affected were the hands and the fingers. The accidents most frequently reported were injuries caused by machine operation and tool manipulation, as well as burns and eye damage related to toxic substance exposures. The presence of a doctor or a nurse at any given plant was associated with a reduced risk of accidents. The incidence of accidents was two times greater than the incidence reported by the IMSS in Nogales in 1989 based on the authors' review of data at the mentioned health institution, suggesting that about half of the accidents reported during the interviews had not been registered by the IMSS.

The only other study to provide quantitative information on the prevalence of accidents (González Block, 1996) indicated a lower incidence. In that study, 5.3% of the workers suffered at least one accident per year, with half of those accidents occurring in the *maquiladoras*. Of the 39% of respondents who had received no accident-prevention information, 9% had had at least one accident compared with 3% of those who had received such training.

Musculoskeletal Complaints and Injuries

A major area of concern about the health status of *maquiladora* workers has been the potential for musculoskeletal injuries, given the known ergonomic hazards of assembly line production (Armstrong, 1986; Armstrong et al., 1993). The earliest sociological and ethnographic studies suggested that women who worked in the *maquiladora* industry were experiencing neuromuscular problems (Denman, 1991; Fernández-Kelly, 1983; Iglesias, 1985). The U.S. Government Accounting Office evaluation of occupational hazards in auto-parts plants, discussed earlier, included interviews with 175 workers in one of the larger plants, 42% of whom reported pain in their upper extremities; 37% in their hands and wrists; 30% in their lower limbs; 25% in their neck and shoulders; and 14% in their lower back. However, the study did not provide comparative data or evaluate the association between specific ergonomic risks and reports of pain.

Participants in the study of Moure-Eraso and associates (1997) reported somewhat lower frequencies of musculoskeletal complaints, which were assessed through a standardized questionnaire. Specifically, 21% reported having experienced pain or numbness in their hands within the previous year, 12% reported elbow or forearm pain, and 14% reported shoulder pain. The fact that over half of those experiencing pain reported that it diminished after they had been away from work for at least a week strongly suggests that the pain was caused by their work. In addition, these authors evaluated the association between the experience of pain and exposure to specific ergonomic risks. Shoulder pain and hand/wrist pain were about twice as frequent among respondents who worked all day in uncomfortable postures and whose work involved repetitive movements and forceful manual labor compared to workers with no exposure to these risks. Significantly, level of exposure to specific ergonomic risks was considered in this study; however, adjustments were not made for potential confounding factors other than sex.

Harlow and colleagues (1999), in a further analysis of data from the study of Cedillo and associates (1997), estimated the prevalence of musculoskeletal complaints among the 466 study participants and evaluated differences in the odds of their having a complaint, by occupation and duration of employment, after adjusting for sociodemographic confounders. The frequency of aches or pain in the lower back during the previous 12 months was 30%; in the upper back, 38%; in the neck or shoulder, 26%; and in the hand or wrist, 18%. In general, working outside the home increased a person's risk of having a musculoskeletal complaint. Specifically, *maquiladora* workers had a 40% to 90% increased risk, depending on the body site, compared with women who had not worked in the previous 2½ years. Compared to women who had other types of paid jobs, *maquiladora* workers had a 20% increased risk of self-reported pain in the lower back, the upper back, and the shoulder or neck. Although these researchers did not evaluate exposure to specific ergonomic risks, they did consider the role of the women's living circumstances. Notably, the risk of having a musculoskeletal complaint was found to be associated with women's sociodemographic characteristics and living conditions.

The most comprehensive evaluation of ergonomic risks and musculoskeletal disorders among *maquila*-employed women was conducted by Meservy and colleagues (1997). In this study, 145 of 166 production workers at one medical device assembly plant were interviewed. A modified version of a U.S. National Institute for Occupational Safety and Health questionnaire was used to evaluate the presence of cumulative trauma disorders. Workers were also examined by a physician to identify tendonitis, ganglia, and carpal tunnel syndrome. In addition, workers were videotaped to identify ergonomic risk factors including positions producing postural strain and cycle time (time allotted to complete a required sequence of tasks), as well as the frequency, force, and duration of work-related movements. The mean age of the workers was 25 years, and the mean duration of employment was 3.5 years.

The 12-month prevalence of upper-extremity cumulative trauma disorders was 46% in women and 12% in men, while the prevalence at the time of the interview was 24% and 8%, respectively. Tendonitis was diagnosed in 12% and carpal tunnel syndrome in 4% of the workers examined. Highly repetitive movements, pinch grips, and awkward postures of the wrists were identified as important risk factors for the presence of cumulative trauma disorders. A major strength of this study is that it attempted to evaluate actual disorders rather than symptoms or complaints; however, it did not include a comparison group. The prevalence of ergonomic risk factors and musculoskeletal problems that Meservy and associates found was consistent with the prevalence of those reported in the few other studies available on Mexico (Serratos-Pérez and Mendiola-Anda, 1993).

Discussion and Conclusions

One critical aspect of the globalized and more interdependent nature of the world's economy is the growing use of foreign direct investment, EPZs, and other policies to increase the number of foreign-funded mass production facilities in developing nations. The local specificities of global production are diverse, as Gereffi (1990) points out in his comparison of Southeast Asia and the cases of Brazil and Mexico. The Mexican *maquiladoras* are just one example among many of this trend. The growth of foreign-owned factories has had many repercussions—social, political, and economic. In this chapter, we have focused on the potential health implications of this trend. The difficult questions facing Mexico are the same questions all other countries receiving foreign direct investment will struggle with: What should health and safety standards be in foreign-owned assembly plants? Should they be the same as those in the investing country? Will the health benefits outweigh the potential job losses if standards are set higher than the receiving country's norms? What is the relationship between health and safety standards and the health status of workers?

Most countries do not yet have an answer to these pressing questions. Some are ethical questions involving societal or governmental values, but others can be answered empirically with the appropriate data. The studies reviewed in this chapter, however, point out the lack of critical comparative data and the methodological flaws in the research to date that have limited researchers' ability to assess accurately the nature and level of problems inherent in the *maquiladora* industries. Limited data exist that compare the risks faced by *maquiladora* workers with those faced by workers in other Mexican industries, by workers in EPZs in other developing countries, or by workers in the same industry in the parent country. Standard government reports from the IMSS, the institution responsible for maintaining the registry of occupational diseases and injuries, for example, aggregate the *maquiladora* industry within manufacturing and thus cannot provide statistics on occupational accident and illness cases that originate in the *maquiladora* industries.

While a lack of data on valid comparison groups renders impossible an assessment of the relative danger that workers in *maquiladoras* face, the review provides a good model for the first step in the process of evaluating what standards are needed: namely, documenting not only the absolute percentage of workers who are facing hazards known to be linked with debilitating illnesses and injury, but also the extent of serious health problems. *Maquiladora* workers appear to be at high risk in both cases. They were found to be exposed to solvents, paints, degreasers, and solder fumes. Frequently, they were exposed to noise, heat, vibrations, and poor ventilation. Ergonomic risks were noted in all studies and are of particular concern because of the potential for causing long-term disabling injuries to young workers. Adequate protection against these hazards was also lacking. The studies reviewed also showed that adequate protection (machine guards, ventilation, noise reduction, and so on) and safety and training programs were frequently lacking. Workers also lacked information about the potential toxicity of chemical exposures.

Symptoms of diseases, illnesses, and injuries among *maquiladora* workers—even without adequate comparison groups—appeared to be frequent, as the following examples show. In one study (González Arroyo et al., 1996), nearly one in five workers had been injured on the job in the previous 6 months. A number of studies revealed that female *maquiladora* workers may have been more likely than other women to give birth to low-birth-weight babies and to be at high risk of musculoskeletal disorders, including upper-extremity cumulative trauma disorders.

Research Implications

While the data reviewed are valuable and suggest that workplace conditions in *maquiladoras* may harm workers' health, a number of reasonable hypotheses for poor health among *maquiladora* workers can be posited: rapid industrialization without concomitant services and infrastructures; transnational corporations' double standards with respect to safety precautions, plus chemical and other exposures; the transformative effects on the families of *maquiladora*-factory workers and low wages that do not guarantee adequate living conditions; and the limited possibilities for labor organization to address these problems. The degree to which health and safety standards in *maquiladoras* are responsible for health problems among the workers cannot be determined until researchers acquire critical comparative data such as the following: the extent of health hazards that *maquiladora* workers faced in earlier time periods, as well as the extent of health hazards that workers face in other formal sector Mexican jobs, in other informal sector Mexican jobs, and, in positions with the same companies but in the companies' home countries.

In order to gather these data, researchers need to conduct large-scale, nationally representative, longitudinal surveys on the prevalence of occupational illnesses and injuries across industries. Longitudinal studies are necessary to estimate the burden of disease related to occupational factors, not only in the *maquiladoras* but also in other manufacturing sectors to provide a comparison group. Most of the studies in the *maquiladora* industries to date have had small sample sizes and inadequate controls, and have failed to consider the potential healthy worker effect. The lack of epidemiological studies in other industrial sectors also makes it difficult to draw conclusions about potential adverse effects of working in the *maquiladora* sector. Clearly, substantive efforts by researchers are needed to evaluate health issues of *maquiladora* workers, to support such comprehensive research approaches, and to build international collaborative research and training programs that can generate the needed information. Important social actors in this arena are policy makers who can make occupational health research a priority on the global scientific research agenda; corporate and labor organizations, which have a great deal to contribute as participants in and supporters of the research process; and international agencies with expertise in this area and nongovernmental organizations that can promote and facilitate communication and exchange between groups of researchers in a variety of countries.

Given the high percentage of women in the *maquiladora* workforce, further efforts are needed to increase our understanding of the joint impact of exposures in the domestic space and the workplace. The first studies on the health status of *maquiladora* workers considered the domestic setting only in very general terms, discussing material housing deficiencies, generalized poverty, and, occasionally, issues of family conflict. Only recently has the importance of analyzing the domestic setting, particularly family relationships, as a key determinant of workers' health been considered. Cedillo (1999), focusing on a sample of female workers in electronics *maquiladora* plants in Sonora, suggested that the level of stress-provoking family conflict among female *maquiladora* workers may have been significant, and the author concluded that the impact of stress in the workplace on these workers' health could not be understood in isolation from the levels of stress outside the workplace. Denman's (1990) finding, noted earlier, that homemakers' infants had low birth weights in proportions similar to, and often greater than, those of female *maquiladora* workers' infants also suggests the need to consider relationships between women's domestic and occupational environments more explicitly. (See Denman, 2001, as well as Chapters 5, 7, and 8 in this volume.) Few theoretical models or methodological approaches have been developed to study these joint exposures, thus making risk measurement more difficult and effect analysis more complex in the *maquiladora* population.

More innovative questions about the broader impact of *maquiladora*-type production on cultural changes that may influence health are also warranted. Although many researchers have discussed the transformative impact of the *maquiladora* export industry on family relationships, few have sought to characterize the positive and negative health consequences of this impact. Similarly, the characteristics of work organization—using production lines, having workers comply with standards and production bonuses, allowing workers few breaks (typically, two 15-minute breaks plus one 30-minute lunch break), and assuming high turnover among employees in a plant—promote isolation more than socialization. As women spend less and less time at home because of the demands of work and transportation, there is less chance of their socializing with neighbors or fellow workers. Thus, the often-touted Mexican social support structures, fundamentally the extensive family and social networks, may well be at risk, with important health ramifications. This is the argument put forth by González de la Rocha (2000), who posits that the social support networks in Mexico have been weakened by too many years of hardship and are not endless resources (González de la Rocha, 2000, 34).

Despite the importance of understanding the particular constellations of individual workers' lives, researchers need to develop a framework for understanding the health status of the communities in which *maquiladora* workers live that does not overemphasize individual responsibility. An important unresolved problem is how to focus public health attention on the particular context of *maquiladora* employment while not ignoring either community-level factors (other social and physical factors outside the workplace) or the corporate and governmental sectors' responsibilities in providing necessary infrastructure and general environmental services. Thus, macrolevel studies are also needed that focus on the broad question of health inequalities, such as what proportion of corporate taxes is directed to urban infrastructure and living conditions in the country of origin versus in the country of destination. Given the immense diversity of global patterns of production, it will be necessary to promote cross-country comparisons to understand each region's specific health issues, the differing roles of government and other agencies, and the variety of responses developed by workers.

The contributions of qualitative studies to increase our understanding while identifying the distinct meanings of health for workers and their families cannot be underestimated. Qualitative study designs can delve where quantitative research cannot. One such proposal would be a study of "closest siblings" that would compare health outcomes and practices for individuals with similar family cultural and biological backgrounds who have different work and living conditions. A research project using this design could, for example, identify and compare health outcomes over a period of years of two women from the same family: one who remains in her rural home town and one who migrates to work in the *maquiladoras.*

Policies to Reduce Maquiladora Workers' Risks

Mexican occupational health and safety regulation follows procedures defined by the Mexican standard for all regulations (Ley Federal de Metrología y Normalización), with the Ministry of Labor being the government agency responsible for both regulation and monitoring compliance. In addition, the Ministry of Health has a mandate to address health issues related to workers' exposure to hazardous materials and work environment pollutants. As noted previously, this institution is also responsible for medical care of workers and their families and also for certifying occupational accidents and illnesses. Although a regulatory and health-care infrastructure exists, the capacity for surveillance of occupational illness is very limited, and the professional infrastructure capable of evaluating the health and safety of the work environment is significantly underresourced (IMSS, 2002).

In general, IMSS data on occupational accidents and illnesses reflect crude incident reports, and few or no public reviews or analyses of these data are conducted in the border region or for the *maquiladora* industries. These data have additional limitations. For example, a worker must file a claim for the event to be recorded in the institute's medical-legal database. Also, data specific to the institute cannot be disaggregated by industry. Many companies have medical services to handle minor accidents that are not reported to the IMSS, and since employers' contribution rates are based on the companies' risk-group classifications, there are clear disincentives to reporting such cases. In Mexico, by law, all plants with more than 100 workers should have a physician on the premises. More specifically, a large proportion of *maquiladora* plants have on-site medical services. Ninety percent of the workers interviewed by Moure-Eraso and colleagues (1997), for example, said that their workplaces had medical services. Minor accidents and many illnesses are usually treated in the plant's medical services and consequently are not reported to the IMSS. Many occupational illnesses are thus never recognized as work-related illnesses.

Many incongruities also exist between local, state, and national reports, and the reports lack detailed information on the economic sector in which cases originate. For example, the *maquiladora* industry is aggregated within manufacturing, so standard reporting systems cannot provide statistics on occupational accident and illness cases that originate in the *maquiladoras.* The Ministry of Health, besides handling regulatory responsibilities, provides primary, secondary, and tertiary care to the country's general population. Because these services are directed to the general population for general health problems (not occupational ones), the Secretary of Health does not register occupational illnesses or related accidents.

Mexico has a serious shortage of trained professionals who can evaluate the health and safety of the work environment. This is especially true with regard to ergonomics, industrial hygiene, safety at work, and occupational medicine (Cedillo, 1994). The majority of occupational health professionals are physicians, but no doctoral program in occupational medicine exists. However, there are 14 (Cedillo, 1994) nascent master's degree programs, including an occupational medicine residency for physicians trained by and for the IMSS. If Mexico is to achieve the expertise needed to monitor and audit workplace safety and health, to train workers and supervisors in safe work techniques, and to prevent and attend to occupational illnesses and accidents, these professional training programs must be intensified and developed throughout the country.

Mexico has experimented with voluntary programs for maintaining healthy working conditions and establishing good practices related to environmental pollutant management. To date, voluntary programs such as the "clean industry" program managed by the Ministry of Environment have had a good response only in the non-*maquiladora* industries, such as large chemical plants and other manufacturing plants located in the traditional industrial zones surrounding Mexico City. These programs have promoted financial incentives, introduced technological modifications, improved negotiations between government and industry, and offered low-interest loans for improving environmental controls in industry. (See the examples for Mexico City in Molina and Molina, 2002.)

However, since *maquiladora* plants are engaged in global manufacturing and since global market interest in obtaining International Organization of Standards (ISO) certification is growing,[6] global social pressure and regulation of commerce may play a key role in improving production practices and working conditions in this type of industry in the future. Generating relevant data and subsequently developing health interventions through research are parts of only one strategy for monitoring and improving the health status of the communities in which the Mexican *maquiladora* workers live. National and international pressures are necessary to ensure that transnational companies comply with domestic laws and regulations, international agreements, and corporate policies as strictly as they do in plants in their countries of origin. (See Chapter 11 by Pursey, Baichoo, and Takala.) There is a clear need to develop strategies to monitor corporate policies and how they are carried out in *maquiladoras* (Moure-Eraso et al., 1997). For those transnational corporations that have been certified by ISO or other regulatory systems,[7] it would be useful to assess whether the actual practices of those corporations and their *maquiladora* factories differ from those of uncertified companies. Current efforts to conduct this type of monitoring are in an initial stage.[8] Wider public participation in the discussion and development of labor policy is needed in Mexico, as well as in other countries in the developed and developing worlds. To promote more participation, perhaps it would be useful to build on efforts in the apparel licensing arena—that is, to develop systems that would allow consumers to evaluate production conditions from the point at which a product is initially created to the point of purchase. (See also the discussion in Chapter 12 by Elliott and Freeman.)

To help workers minimize their exposure to workplace hazards, companies, labor organizations, and unions can jointly implement and intensify information sharing, training, and capacity-building programs. In all such programs and in campaigns for just wages, those living and working in the affected countries and other relevant actors need to be incorporated more effectively in the ongoing dialogues.

The role played by international organizations can be critical. For example, in 2001 the World Bank recommended that Mexico decrease many of the workers' benefits currently mandated by Mexican federal labor law.[9] Because the influence of the World Bank and other multilateral agencies on national legislation and policies is substantial, a dialogue needs to be started with agencies on their potential for promoting, rather than worsening, workers' safety and health. A series of concrete actions should include the following: the development of codes of conduct, audits of workplace conditions as well as of the surrounding communities, and verification of health and safety conditions by independent organizations. In order to take these steps, training at all levels—both for workers and for supervisors—is necessary, as well as for medical personnel, transport personnel, community social service and health agencies, in government, and for independent auditors.

ACKNOWLEDGMENT

We are grateful for the research assistance, translation, and editing provided by Blanca Lara, Elsa Cornejo, and Verónica Larios.

Notes

1. Recent studies contracted by the U.S. Trade Deficit Review Commission with Cornell University analyzed the relationship between capital mobility and union organizing, and "conclusively demonstrate(s) that capital mobility and the threat of capital mobility have had a profound impact on the ability of the American workers to exercise their rights to freedom of association and collective bargaining" (Bronfenbrenner, 2000, v).

2. It should be noted that the $6.28 billion that Mexican migrants sent from the United States to their Mexican families is not included here.

3. All dollar amounts in this chapter are in U.S. dollars.

4. Some of this material has been published by Takaro et al. (1999).

5. The Second National Health Survey (NHS-II) was conducted in 1994. Data were collected on 61,524 individuals in 12,615 households at a national level in five geographic regions.

6. This refers to a series of standards developed by the ISO, which was founded in 1947 to facilitate the international exchange of goods and services. *ISO* comes from the Greek *iso*, which means "equal."

7. Less than 1% of Mexican firms fulfill international quality standards, according to the Mexican Institute of Norms and Certification (*La Jornada*, June 6, 2001).

8. See http://www.cepaa.org for more information.

9. They argued that labor reform was sorely needed to promote investment, to make Mexico more competitive in the world market, and to avoid increasing the growth of the informal labor market.

References

Arenal, S. 1986. *Sangre joven: Las maquiladoras por dentro.* México, DF: Editorial Nuestro Tiempo.

Armstrong, T. J. 1986. Ergonomics and cumulative trauma disorders. *Hand Clinics* 2: 553–65.

Armstrong, T. J., P. Buckle, J. H. Fine, M. Hagberg, B. Jonsson, A. Kilbom, I. A. A. Kuorinka, B. A. Silverstein, G. Sjogaard, and E. R. A. Vilkari-Juntura, 1993. A conceptual model for work-related neck and upper limb musculoskeletal disorders. *Scandinavian Journal of Environmental Health* 19: 73–84.

Balcázar, H., C. A. Denman, and F. Lara. 1995. Factors associated with work-related accidents and sickness among maquiladora workers: The case of Nogales, Sonora, Mexico. *International Journal of Health Services* 25(3): 489–502.

Bronfenbrenner, K. 2000. *Uneasy terrain: The impact of capital mobility on workers, wages, and union organizing.* Report submitted to the U.S. Trade Deficit Review Commission. New York: Cornell University. Available from http://www.ustdrc.gov/research/bronfenbrenner.pdf

Carlesso, E. M., and J. C. Rodríguez-García. 1985. *Proceso laboral y desgaste obrero. Caso maquila de procesamiento de mariscos en Matamoros.* Master's thesis. México, D.F.: Universidad Autónoma de México–Xochimilco.

Carrillo, J. V. 1984. Maquiladoras: Industrialización fronteriza y riesgos de trabajo. El caso de Baja California. *Economía: Teoría y Práctica* 6: 97–132.

Carrillo, J. V. 1991. *Mujeres en la industria automotriz.* Cuadernos de COLEF No. 1 [COLEF Working Papers No. 1]. Tijuana, México: El Colegio de la Frontera Norte (COLEF).

Carrillo, J. V. 1992. *Mujeres en la industria automotriz,* Cuaderno de COLEF No. 1 [COLEF Working Papers No. 1]. Tijuana, México: El Colegio de la Frontera Norte.

Carrillo, J. V., and A. Hernández. 1985. *Mujeres fronterizas en la industria maquiladora.* México, DF: Secretaría de Educación Pública (SEP) and Centro de Estudios Fronterizos del Noroeste de México (CEFNOMEX).

Carrillo, J. V., and M. Jasis. 1983. *La salud y la mujer obrera en las plantas maquiladoras: El caso de Tijuana.* Tijuana, México: CEFNOMEX.

Carrillo, J. V., and R. J. Santibáñez. 1993. *Rotación de personal en las maquiladoras de exportación en Tijuana.* Tijuana, México: Secretaría del Trabajo y Previsión Social, and El Colegio de la Frontera Norte.

Cedillo, L. 1994. *Documento de sustento para la propuesta de la Maestría en Ciencias, Concentración en Higiene Ocupacional.* México, DF: Escuela de Salud Pública de México.

Cedillo, L.1999. Psychosocial risk factors among women workers in the maquiladora industry in Mexico. Ph.D. dissertation. Lowell, MA: University of Massachusetts.

Cedillo, L., S. D. Harlow, R. Sánchez, and D. Sánchez. 1997. Establishing priorities for occupational health research among women working in the maquiladora industry. *International Journal of Occupational and Environmental Health* 3: 221–30.

Cerón–Mireles, P., S. D. Harlow, and C. I. Sanchez-Carrillo. 1996. The risk of prematurity and small-for-gestational-age birth in Mexico City: The effects of working conditions and antenatal leave. *American Journal of Public Health* 86(6): 825–31.

Cohen, S., and G. Williamson. 1988. Perceived stress in a probability sample of the United States. In *The social psychology of health*, edited by S. Spacapan and S. Oskamp. Beverly Hills, CA: Sage.

De la O, M. E. 1995. Maquila, mujer y cambios productivos: Estudio de caso en la industria maquiladora de Ciudad Juárez. In *Mujeres, migración y maquila en la frontera norte*, compiled by S. González, O. Ruiz, L. Velasco, and O. Woo. México, D.F.: El Colegio de México and El Colegio de la Frontera Norte.

Denman, C. A. 1990. *Industrialización y maternidad en el noroeste de México.* Cuadernos de Trabajo No. 2 [Working Papers No. 2]. Hermosillo, México: El Colegio de Sonora.

Denman, C. A. 1991. *Las repercusiones de la industria maquiladora de exportación en la salud: El peso al nacer de hijos de obreras en Nogales.* Hermosillo, México: El Colegio de Sonora.

Denman, C. A. 2001. Prácticas de atención al embarazo de madres-trabajadoras de una maquiladora en Nogales, Sonora, México. Ph.D. dissertation. Zamora, México: El Colegio de Michoacán.

Eskenazi, B., S. Guendelman, E. P. Elkin, and M. Jasis. 1993. A preliminary study of reproductive outcomes of female maquiladora workers in Tijuana, Mexico. *American Journal of Industrial Medicine* 24: 667–76.

Fernández-Kelly, M. P. 1983. *For we are sold, I and my people.* Albany, NY: State University of New York Press.

Gambrill, M. C. 1981. *La fuerza de trabajo en las maquiladoras. Resultados de una encuesta y algunas hipótesis interpretativas: Maquiladoras.* México, D.F.: Centro de Estudios Económicos y Sociales del Tercer Mundo.

Gereffi, G. 1990. Paths of industrialization: An overview. In *Manufacturing miracles: Paths of industrialization in Latin America and East Asia,* edited by G. Gereffi and D. L. Wyman. Princeton, NJ: Princeton University Press.

González Arroyo, M., G. Brown, S. Brumis, E. Knight, and T. Takaro. 1996. *The CAFOR survey of maquiladora workers on occupational health and safety in Tijuana and Tecate, Mexico.* Berkeley, CA: Maquiladora Health and Safety Support Network, Comité de Apoyo Fronterizo Obrero Regional (CAFOR), Support Committee for Maquiladora Workers (San Diego), and Labor Occupational Health Program (University of California, Berkeley).

González Block, M. A. 1996. *La salud reproductiva de las trabajadoras de la maquiladora de exportación en Tijuana, Baja California. Diagnóstico para las políticas de salud.* Research report presented to the Instituto Nacional de Salud Pública, El Colegio de la Frontera Norte, and Fundación Mexicana para la Salud.

González Block, M. A. 2001. Salud reproductiva de las trabajadoras de la maquila de exportación en Tijuana: Diagnóstico y retos para las políticas de salud. In *Encuentros y desencuentros en la salud reproductiva. Políticas públicas, marcos normativos y actores sociales*, coordinated by J. G. Figueroa and C. Stern. México, D.F.: El Colegio de México.

González de la Rocha, M. 2000. *Private adjustments: Household responses to the erosion of work.* New York: United Nations Development Programme, Bureau for Development Policy, Social Development and Poverty Elimination Division.

Government Accounting Office. (GAO). 1993. *U.S.–México trade: The work environment at eight U.S.-owned maquiladora auto parts plants.* Report to the Chairman, Committee on Commerce, Science, and Transportation, U.S. Senate. Washington, D.C.: Government Printing Office.

Grijalva, G. 1996. *Empleo femenino: Análisis de la Encuesta Estatal de Empleo en Sonora, 1995.* Hermosillo, México: El Colegio de Sonora. Draft.

Guendelman, S., and M. Jasis. 1993. The health consequences of maquiladora work: Women on the U.S.–Mexican border. *American Journal of Public Health* 83: 37–44.

Harlow, S. D., L. Cedillo, J. N. Scholten, D. Sánchez, and R. Sánchez. 1999. The prevalence of musculoskeletal complaints among women in Tijuana: Demographic and occupational risk factors. Ann Arbor, MI: University of Michigan. Draft.

Hertel, S. 2002. Campaigns to protect human rights in Mexico's maquiladoras: Current research findings. *Columbia University, Institute of Latin American Studies Newsletter* 1: 6–9.

Hovell, M., C. Sepan, R. Hofstetter, B. DuBois, A. Krefft, J. Conway, and H. Jasis. 1988. Occupational health risks for Mexican women: The case of the maquiladora along the Mexican–United States border. *International Journal of Health Services* 18: 617–27.

Iglesias, N. 1985. *La flor más bella de la maquiladora.* México: SEP-CEFNOMEX.

Instituto Mexicano del Seguro Social (IMSS). 2001. *Memoria estadística, 2001. Salud en el trabajo.* México, D.F.: IMSS.

Instituto Mexicano del Seguro Social (IMSS). 2002. *Informe al Ejecutivo Federal y al Congreso de la Unión sobre la situación financiera y los riesgos del IMSS.* June 28, 2002. México, D.F.: IMSS.

Instituto Nacional de Geografía, Estadística e Informática (INEGI). 1994. *Estadísticas históricas de México.* Tomo I [Volume I]. Aguascalientes, México: INEGI.

Instituto Nacional de Geografía, Estadística e Informática (INEGI). 1997. *Encuesta nacional de empleo urbano 1995.* Aguascalientes, México: INEGI.

Instituto Nacional de Geografía, Estadística e Informática (INEGI). 2001a. *Estadísticas de la industria maquiladora de exportación.* Aguascalientes, México: INEGI.

Instituto Nacional de Geografía, Estadística e Informática (INEGI). 2001b. *Encuesta nacional de empleo y seguridad social 2000.* Aguascalientes, México: INEGI.

International Labor Office (ILO). 1998a. Export processing zones: Steady growth provides major source of new jobs. *World of Work* 27: 18–20. Available from: http://www.ilo.org / public/english/bureau/inf/magazine/27/news.htm

International Labor Office (ILO). 1998b. *Labour and social issues relating to export processing zones.* Available from http://www.ilo.org/public/english/dialogue/govlab/legrel/tc/epz/reports/epzrepor_w61/index.htm

Jasis, M., and S. Guendelman. 1993. Maquiladoras y mujeres fronterizas. Beneficio o daño a la salud obrera. *Salud Publica Mex* 35: 620–29.

Kaplan, F. M., J. W. Bush, and C. C. Berry. 1976. Health status: Types of validity and the index of well being. *Health Services Research* 2: 478–507.

Karasek, R. A. 1997. *Job content questionnaire and user's guide.* Lowell, MA: Job Content Questionnaire Center, University of Massachusetts–Lowell.

Kopinak, K. 1996. *Desert capitalism: Maquiladoras in North America's western industrial corridor.* Tucson, AZ: University of Arizona Press.

Landsbergis, P. A., and M. C. Hatch. 1996. Psychosocial work stress and pregnancy-induced hypertension. *Epidemiology* 7(4): 346–51.

Marcoux, S., S. Bérubé, C. Brisson, and M. Mondor. 1999. Job strain and pregnancy-induced hypertension. *Epidemiology* 10(4): 376 –82.

Márquez, M., and J. Romero. 1988. El desgaste de las obreras de la maquila eléctrico-electrónica. *Salud Problema* 14: 9–24.

Meservy, D., A. J. Suruda, D. Bloskwich, J. Lee, and M. Dumas. 1997. Ergonomic risk exposure and upper-extremity cumulative trauma disorders in a maquiladora medical devices manufacturing plant. *Journal of Occupational and Environmental Medicine* 39(8): 767–73.

Molina, L. T., and M. J. Molina (eds.). 2002. *Air quality in the Mexico megacity: An integrated assessment.* Dordrecht, the Netherlands: Kluwer Academic.

Moure-Eraso, R., M. Wilcox, L. Punnett, L. MacDonald, and C. Levenstein. 1994. Back to the future: Sweatshop conditions on the Mexico–U.S. border. Part 1: Community health impact of maquiladora activity. *American Journal of Industrial Medicine* 25: 311–24.

Moure-Eraso, R., M. Wilcox, L. Punnett, L. MacDonald, and C. Levenstein. 1997. Back to the future: Sweatshop conditions on the Mexico–U.S. border. Part 2: Occupational health impact of maquiladora industrial activity. *American Journal of Industrial Medicine* 31: 587–99.

O'Neill, R. 1999. *Europe under strain. A report on trade union initiatives to combat workplace musculoskeletal disorders.* Brussels: European Trade Union Technical Bureau for Health and Safety.

Radloff, L. S. 1977. The CES-D scale: A self report depression scale for research in the general population. *Applied Psychological Measurement* 1: 385–401.

Saint-Germain, M., J. de Zapién, and C. Denman. 1993. Estrategias de atención a hijos de obreras de las plantas ensambladoras de la frontera. *Revista de El Colegio de Sonora* 5: 77–93.

Serratos-Pérez, J. N., and C. Mendiola-Anda. 1993. Musculoskeletal disorders among male sewing machine operators in shoemaking. *Ergonomics* 36: 793–800.

Sklair, L. 1993. *Assembling for development,* 2nd ed. La Jolla, CA: Center for U.S.–Mexican Studies, University of California, San Diego.

Takaro, T. K., M. González Arroyo, G. D. Brown, S. G. Brumis, and E. B. Knight. 1999. Community based survey of maquiladora workers in Tijuana and Tecate, Mexico. *International Journal of Occupational and Environmental Health* 5: 313–15.

Torres Muñoz, M., P. C. Morales, C. M. Sías, and R. G. Villarreal. 1991. *Proceso de trabajo y salud en la industria maquiladora: El caso de una maquiladora textil.* Chihuahua, México: Universidad Autónoma de Chihuahua, Facultad de Enfermería, Programa de Salud en el Trabajo.

United Nations Conference on Trade and Development (UNCTAD). 2001. *World investment report 2001. Promoting linkages.* New York and Geneva: UNCTAD.

U.S. Bureau of Labor Statistics. 2001. *Current population survey.* Available from http://www.bls.gov/cps/cpsaat18.pdf

Villegas, J., M. Noriega, S. Martínez, and S. Martínez. 1997. Trabajo y salud en la industria maquiladora mexicana: Una tendencia dominante en el neoliberalismo dominado. *Cuadernos de Salud Pública* 13: 123–34.

Zúñiga, M. M. 1998. *Cambio tecnológico y nuevas configuraciones del trabajo de las mujeres. Un estudio de caso en una empresa de arneses.* Hermosillo, México: El Colegio de Sonora.

11

Opportunities for Improving Working Conditions through International Agreements

STEPHEN PURSEY, PAVAN BAICHOO,
AND JUKKA TAKALA

Work-related health problems are a significant factor affecting both individual workers and, through their families and friends, the overall health of the community. It is also likely that unsafe workplaces are sources of health-damaging emissions and wastes into the wider environment, but this topic is beyond our scope here. Workers in low-income or low-skill occupations characterized by precarious employment, informality, and small enterprise size are more likely to suffer from the effects of work-related health accidents and diseases. In general, work-related problems are associated with high-risk industries, as well those with low wages, long hours, temporary work arrangements, and high labor turnover. Countries with relatively unequal wage dispersions and labor markets divided sharply between skilled and unskilled occupations tend to have a high incidence of work-related health problems.[1]

Businesses—and, by extension, countries—face a threshold as they move away from low wages, low skills, low productivity, and low occupational safety and health protection onto the "high road" to competitiveness. One of the effects of globalization, or international economic integration, may be to raise this threshold, further exacerbating dualism in the labor market and social inequality.

Public policy can help create an institutional framework that enables businesses, especially micro- and small enterprises, to shift from low-road survival to high-road competitiveness. As a result of globalization, increased international policy coherence is needed to support public policy interventions to this end, especially in lower-income countries.

At its 1999 conference the International Labour Organization (ILO) focused its mission on the goal of Decent Work for All. This overarching objective is defined as "the promotion of opportunities for women and men to obtain decent and productive work, in conditions of freedom, equity, security and human dignity" (ILO, 1999, 3). The strategic objectives of the ILO have been aligned in a Decent Work agenda that aims to ensure that issues related to the world of work are more coherently articulated and pursued, and thus achieve a higher profile in discussions of international economic and social policy integration. One key component of the agenda is the In-Focus Programme on Safety and Health at Work and the Environment, or SafeWork (ILO, 1999). Various mechanisms are available to take the Decent Work agenda forward. These include

- Setting, supervising, and promoting of standards
- Technical assistance
- Research
- Information dissemination
- Voluntary private initiatives
- Partnerships with other agencies

The setting, supervising, and promoting of standards are often linked to technical assistance and research and are the traditional mechanisms for ILO action. But as a result of the ever-increasing pace of worldwide liberalization of trade and economies, as well as technological progress, the world of work has become increasingly competitive and now has to face the rapid changes in working conditions and the environment, as well as in processes and work organization, that are necessary for sustainable development. The traditional command-control approach provided by legislation and binding standards (such as ILO conventions, which are discussed extensively later in this chapter) cannot address these changes fully or cannot be elaborated rapidly enough to cover new hazards and risks arising from these changes. Hence, holistic, coherent, flexible, and sound approaches integral to a company's business cycle and structure at all levels are becoming an increasingly important part of management strategies and can provide the incentives necessary for continual identification, evaluation, and control of hazards and risks in constantly evolving workplaces. For example, the International Council of Chemical Associations (ICCA), a worldwide body representing the chemical industry, has adopted a Responsible Care strategy (ICCA, 2000) and has programs with its members in 46 countries. Occupational safety and health management systems and voluntary private initiatives (such as company codes of conduct and partnerships with other agencies) are innovative approaches that can stimulate a comprehensive and systematic method for ensuring continual improvement in occupational safety and health performance at the company level. Both have considerable potential but pose new and difficult challenges.

The intensity of competition faced by businesses has a mixed impact on occupational safety and health. On the one hand, businesses in the most competitive industrialized countries are generally conscious of the costs of poor occupational safety and health performance. Consequently, they invest in plant, equipment, and occupational safety and health management systems to reduce accidents and health risks (ILO, 2001c, 108). This is probably due to the stricter occupational safety and health regulations in place in the industrialized countries, as well as more resources available for labor inspectorates (such as more and better-equipped inspectors) to ensure compliance. This may apply to many of the larger, often international companies investing in developing countries, which also tend to have access to sources of finance for these investments. In general, laws and regulations concerning safety and health are more extensive in industrial countries; however, the relative weakness of public and private systems for monitoring and remedying hazards in developing countries is an important factor. As highlighted in an ILO report, "Decent Work and the Informal Economy" (2002b), health hazards in micro- and small businesses in many developing countries are widespread partly because these companies are rarely visited by understaffed labor inspectorates but also owing to lack of knowledge of simple, low-cost, productivity- and safety-enhancing techniques for improving work organization (ILO, 2000a). On the other hand, the struggle to survive tempts low-productivity businesses to forgo investments in better occupational safety and health measures or to relocate to countries that demand lower levels of protection and export back to their main market.

The Global Picture on Health

In general, the health situation in the world is improving, and life expectancy has increased over the past 50 years. However, occupational diseases and injuries still force millions of people out of work for shorter or longer periods, some of them forever (Takala, 2000):

- Every year 1.2 million men and women die in occupational accidents and from work-related diseases. By conservative estimates, workers suffer 250 million occupational accidents and 160 million episodes of occupational diseases each year—that is, on average, up to 14% of the labor force suffer some form of work-related loss of earning capacity each year (Annan, 1997).
- This social and economic burden is not evenly distributed geographically. Fatality rates in some European countries are twice as high as in others, and in parts of the Middle East and Asia, fatality rates soar to four times those in the industrialized countries with the best records. Certain clearly hazardous jobs can be 10 to 100 times riskier in poorer than in richer countries.
- Deaths and injuries take a particularly heavy toll in those developing countries where large numbers of workers are concentrated in primary and extractive activities such as agriculture, logging, fishing, and mining—some of the world's most hazardous industries. Children are also likely to be badly affected in these sectors.

- Recent national calculations for European Union (EU) member states show that occupational accidents and diseases lead to an annual cost for the whole society ranging from 2.6% to 3.8% of gross national product (GNP). The ILO's estimate for the whole world is 4% of GNP. A detailed picture of how these costs are divided—as estimated from industrialized countries' data—appears in Figure 11–1. The major single cause of lost output in this context is musculoskeletal problems, usually due to physical work wrongly carried out.

Differences in health status generally dramatically illustrate the divide between the rich and the poor in today's world. The inhabitants of poorer countries suffer disproportionately from communicable diseases (Dorman, 2000).

- In 1998 communicable diseases were responsible for about 34% of all disease worldwide but were nearly twice that—64%—among the fifth of the global population living in the poorest countries. Most of these diseases can be prevented or easily cured with available vaccines and drugs, but poor countries and poor people cannot afford them.
- Human immunodeficiency versus (HIV) prevalence rates of 10% to 15%, which are no longer uncommon, can translate into a reduction in the growth rate of per capita gross domestic product (GDP) of up to 1% per year. Tuberculosis, which is made worse by HIV, takes an economic toll equivalent to $12 billion

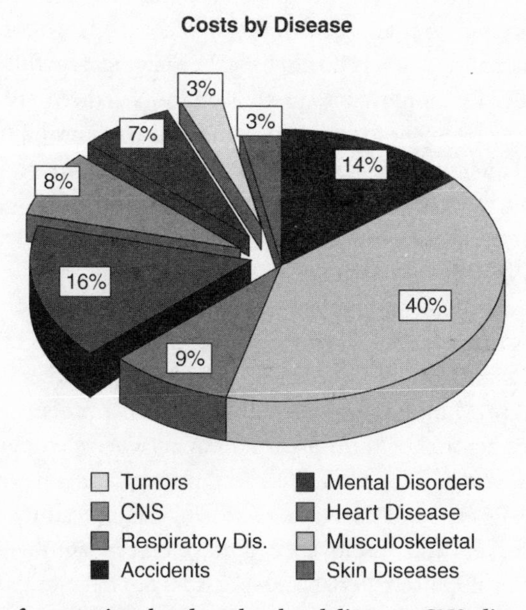

Figure 11–1. Cost of occupational and work-related diseases. CNS: disorders of the central nervous system. *Source*: Takala (2000).

(the annual income of a medium-sized African country) from the incomes of poor communities. The mortality rate of women is rising steeply.
- Africa's GDP might be about $100 billion (or nearly one-third) more by now if programs to eradicate malaria, often a work-related disease in agriculture, had been introduced when effective control measures became available 30 years ago.

Inequalities in Safety and Health Protection

It is generally true that the most dangerous jobs are the ones lowest in the economic hierarchy: precarious employment, informal employment, work in small and medium-sized enterprises, and work performed by groups subject to discrimination and marginalization.

Precarious Employment

Over the past 20 years there has been a steady expansion of work that does not conform to the traditional model of a permanent, full-time relationship between the worker and the employing enterprise. *Nonstandard* work, or *precarious employment*, consists of various alternatives, individually and in combination: temporary employment, leased employment, part-time employment, and multiple employments. Various factors explain this trend. In some countries, new laws have encouraged employers to hire people on short-term contracts to avoid statutory conditions concerning redundancy and dismissal that apply to workers on contracts without specified time limits. In others, part-time workers do not have the same rights as full-time employees, creating an incentive for employers to use this option. Furthermore, part-time work is sometimes more convenient for workers with family responsibilities, and employers have organized their work rosters to attract them. Furthermore, the introduction of new technologies, especially in the information and communication field, has made it easier for businesses to subcontract parts of their operations (Bertola, Boeri, and Cazes, 1999; ILO, 2002b).

Outsourcing can lead to employment relationships that are essentially nonstandard in the sense just noted, even when the worker and the subcontractor have a formally standard relationship. In some cases of outsourcing, a worker may be nominally self-employed but to all intents and purposes may be dependent on and under the direction of a contractor. The term *precarious* or *contingent* employment has been applied to nonstandard work that has the effect of attenuating the employment relationship: reducing its expected duration, increasing its uncertainty, or undermining the claims that workers and employers can make on one another by virtue of the employment relationship itself. Part-time work does not fall into this category, but it can have similar effects insofar as it reduces the degree of commitment entailed in employment.

Information on status in employment,[2] which is available for some 112 countries, provides an indication of trends. A high proportion of self-employed workers could be taken as an indication of low job growth in the formal economy and a high rate of job creation in the informal economy. A large proportion of workers in unpaid family work is typical in largely rural developing economies. Using this indicator, there are important differences between developed and developing countries. Within developed countries, the proportion of wage and salaried workers is as high as 80% or even 90% of the total employed; the self-employed typically account for 10% to 15%, although this share increased in most countries in the 1990s; and unpaid family workers account for as low as 0% to 4%. Within formal employment, part-time work and temporary work have grown faster than full-time employment. Transition economies have similarly high proportions of wage and salaried workers, although since 1995 there has been a declining trend. Self-employment has been increasing, sometimes as a secondary activity. Among some of the more developed Asian economies, the proportions of self-employed workers and unpaid family workers are very low. But in poor countries such as Bangladesh and Pakistan, these proportions are around 70% of total employment. In Latin American countries, where the major share of new jobs has been in the informal economy, self-employment accounts for 25% to 40% of total employment. Men are more likely than women to be self-employed in all regions of the world, but women clearly outrank men as contributing family members. Downsizing of larger firms has led to a separation of *noncore* workers, whose work can be put out to subcontractors or undertaken by a transient workforce on short-term contracts, from *core* employees the business needs to retain because their knowledge and skills are essential to its operations. Women also predominate in noncore paid employment situations as home workers and casual employees, while men predominate in the core regular employee status. Although an imperfect measure, status in employment data show that, globally, formal employment has increased markedly less than other forms of employment (see Chapter 1 of the ILO *World Employment Report 2001*, 2001d).

How these trends are related to globalization is a matter of continuing debate, beyond the scope of this discussion, but proposed causes include changes in technology, increased international competition, and new patterns of consumer demand, as well as regulations, laws, and other aspects of government policy (for a more extensive discussion, see ILO, 2001d). It is important, however, that increased informality and precariousness in employment, and the social and economic policy challenges these trends pose, are occurring at the same time that markets are opening up to international trade and investment. However, little attention has yet been given to the implications of changing employment patterns for safety and health at work.

Over the past 10 years, evidence has been accumulating that work that is precarious in employment terms is likely to be physically precarious as well. Every form of precarious employment has been linked to increased risk, and studies have often shown the specific mechanisms involved (Quinlan, 1999). Outsourced and contract workers more often than not receive less training and have less awareness of their rights; in some instances, they do not even know who their employer actually is. Pressures to maximize output and minimize time often lead the workers involved to cut corners and take greater risks—a fact that makes precarious workers attractive to some employers (Salminen, 1995). Accident rates are systematically higher for such groups, including the self-employed. Moreover, safety and health problems often go unrecognized in the case of leased and outsourced workers because accident data are not categorized by the industry or establishment in which the accidents actually occur. Results from the U.S. National Academy of Sciences and the National Research Council survey (1998) showed that temporary workers—along with racial and ethnic minorities, migrants, and workers with less education—are at greater risk than comparable "regular" workers (Dorman, 2000).

One of the more worrisome characteristics of precarious employment is that these workers have little input and often no control over their work conditions. Nonpermanent workers have less knowledge about their work environment. According to one survey, 30% feel constrained by their status to "refuse work environment deficiencies," while 41% said it was more difficult for their voices to be heard (Aronsson, 1999). Precarious workers are far less likely to be represented on safety and health committees. Among the aspects of work over which precarious workers have less control are the freedom to choose when to take personal leave and the ability to change the temperature, lighting, ventilation, and work location. Taken together, a number of studies have painted a picture of increasing polarization of the labor force, with the bottom tier excluded from many of the workplace protections long taken for granted in industrialized societies.

The safety and health concerns of precarious workers have begun to attract the attention of policy makers. The European Agency for Safety and Health at Work (1999), reporting on its survey of EU member governments, found that five governments had paid particular attention to the situation of atypical workers during the past decade, and seven were intending to do so during the coming 3 to 5 years. The corresponding numbers for governments' attention to self-employed workers' situations were three and eight.

Informal Employment

Informal employment, or work that is not recognized or protected under legal and regulatory frameworks, encompasses a wide range of income-generating activities. For the most part, this type of work is concentrated in developing countries, although there are signs of a reemergence of an informal economy in the industrialized world. In all probability, workers in the informal economy are at high risk relative to their industry and occupation. This is due to the small scale of the enterprise; the intensely competitive nature of both labor and product markets; and the general absence of public occupational safety and health monitoring, enforcement, or supportive services. It is also attributable to the widespread poverty among informal workers themselves, since other risk factors include poor nutrition, infectious diseases, unsanitary living conditions (which are also often working conditions), and the weakness of representative organizations such as trade unions, farmers, and small business associations in giving voice to these workers' grievances (Forastieri, 1999). It would be valuable to have more information on occupational injury and illness rates, but credible numbers are virtually nonexistent. One intriguing recent study from China, however, has cast some light on this critical issue (Yu et al., 1999). Five years of occupational accident data (from 1989 to 1993) were presented for a sample of town and village enterprises in Shunde City, a rapidly growing industrial region. Town and village enterprises vary enormously, from joint ventures with multinational corporations to essentially informal enterprises financed off the books and organized through family or other personal connections. The legal status of town and village enterprises is unclear, particularly during the period under investigation, as the Chinese authorities have gradually changed their attitude toward private business activities over the past 15 years of gradual market reforms. In particular, there is no occupational safety and health legislation governing the town and village enterprise sector in China. Overall data on Shunde City's work-related injury and fatality rates are presented in Table 11–1.

A *major injury* was defined in this study as one that resulted in at least 105 lost workdays in a year. Given the virtual absence of social insurance available to injured workers, these would indeed be major impairments. If these injury and fatality rates remained constant over time, and if we assume that these accidents are randomly distributed (that is, each year's distribution is independent), any given worker, over the course of his or her 30-year work career, would face a more than 1-in-12 chance of such an event. An even graver picture emerges regarding the statistics for construction workers. Construction is of particular interest because it is one of the most hazardous sectors of economic activity, even in the most developed countries. From 1989 to 1993, construction accounted for 4.8% of the employment in this sample; its major injury and fatality rates per 100,000 workers were, respectively, 904 and 274. They indicate that the 30-year combined risk is just under one in three. The cumula-

Table 11–1. Major Injury and Fatalities in Shunde City, China

Year	Major injury	Fatalities
1989	56	29
1990	51	25
1991	175	18
1992	258	26
1993	266	39

Note: Sample of 392 enterprises; employment = 116,577.

Source: Yu et al. (1999).

tive fatality rate alone is slightly under 8%. In light of this information, a majority of small (fewer than 100 employees) enterprises in the Shunde sample indicated that they had no formal system in place for managing occupational safety and health.

Workers in Small and Medium-Sized Enterprises

One would expect a higher incidence of occupational safety and health problems at small and medium-sized enterprises for several reasons. First, many occupational safety and health interventions have a substantial overhead cost, and the smaller the firm, the smaller the revenue base over which these costs can be distributed. Second, the level of expertise is frequently lower at small and medium-sized enterprises. Third, the environment in such enterprises is generally more competitive and finance is more difficult to obtain, leading to shorter time horizons (lower investment in general) and fewer expenditures on what may be perceived as nonessential items such as guards on machines or effective ventilation and lighting. Fourth, smaller firms tend to receive less frequent inspections, either because they fall below a threshold stipulated by law or because inspection services are overstretched. The often harsh reality is that even where, in theory, safety and health regulations apply to smaller enterprises, in practice inspections are infrequent and follow-up visits to check whether recommendations for change have been implemented are even more rare because of the small number of inspectors and the vast numbers of small-scale operators.

Factors Associated with Precarious Employment

It should be borne in mind that not all workers have an equal likelihood of ending up in the employment categories surveyed thus far. Both women and children are, for different reasons, disproportionately represented in precarious employment and in small and medium-sized enterprises in particular. In the case of women, currently little is known about their comparative health status, primarily because of the lack of gender-disaggregated data. The information deficit may also be a result of more research being devoted to injuries and fatalities, which are more prevalent in male-dominated sectors, rather than to diseases and pain, which often affect workers in occupations with a high proportion of women. Concerning children, the U.S. National Academy of Sciences and the National Research Council conducted a major study (1998) and found that while children are not generally more susceptible to risk physiologically, social and psychological pressures make it less likely that children will refuse or question hazardous work. The consequences of a major accident or illness early in life, of course, can be especially devastating. Considering the restrictions on the employment of minors in the United States, measured rates of occupational injury are high and fatalities are a problem, particularly in agriculture. One of the reasons cited for the occupational safety and health problems of young workers is their concentration in precarious, part-time, and small-establishment employment.

Overall, it seems that all groups with lower socioeconomic status have, on average, more dangerous working conditions. Workers with low levels of educational attainment and skill qualifications are often able to find employment only in enterprises that are on the margins of the economy (Forasteri, 1999). Thus, based on the U.S. experience, racial and ethnic minorities have higher accident rates, as do immigrants and workers with less formal education. Indeed, the ultimate test of this relationship is probably income itself, and here the evidence suggests that low income is associated with higher risk, even, for most workers, when other factors affecting wages are controlled for (Dorman and Hagstrom, 1998). Taken together, studies point to profound equity problems in the distribution of risk: those who suffer the most from poor working conditions are also the most likely to bear other social and economic costs.

This portrait of groups at risk is cast in general social terms, but it has a particular salience for economics. Certain forms of employment appear to be more dangerous, and certain groups are congregated in them. The kinds of jobs created and the distribution of those jobs are both economic phenomena; and they stem from the choices, rational or otherwise, that enterprises, workers, and governments make in their pursuit of economic goals. In particular, the global trend toward more informal or precarious employment suggests that fundamental economic forces are at work. Although we have barely begun the enormous effort to identify—and, hopefully, counteract—these forces, it would seem that the competitive pressures on employers have led to a search for ways to reduce labor costs through various forms of outsourcing designed to downsize regular employment. For now, it is enough to note that these forms of employment present an obstacle to the improvement of occupational safety and health conditions and exacerbate the unequal exposure to those conditions within society. These effects should be taken into consideration when employment policies are weighed.

The Impact of Competition on Investment in Workplace Safety and Health

Adopting high standards of safety and health is both a benefit and a cost to an employer. On a narrow economic rationale, where the benefits are higher than the costs, firms will usually act to reduce hazards. Of course, firms are not entirely economic, or bottom line, in their motivation. Owners and managers may act to reduce hazards out of a sense of morality or social duty, or out of a need to comply with occupational safety and health legislation. However, the scope of such noneconomic behavior is limited if the costs eventually force them out of business because competitors have less social conscience or have not faced the same legal obligations, or if customers are not prepared to pay a premium for buying "clean" products.

In trying to assess the extent to which any given firm will act voluntarily to prevent safety and health hazards, one has to examine the factors affecting the cost–benefit balance to the firm and its impact on the firm's competitive position in the market.

(When regulations and requirements exist, the pressure of legal mandates, rather than of the cost–benefit balance, becomes the impetus for a firm's attention to safety and health hazards.) One of the key factors of such an analysis is where the burden of costs and the acquisition of benefits fall between the firm as a separate economic unit, workers, and society at large. Study of this issue requires an examination of the impact of laws concerning occupational health and safety on firm behavior. Where all firms in a particular market observe the same standards, the costs are passed to consumers. However, if the standards are unevenly applied, or if firms choose to adhere to higher standards than those legally required, their competitive position may be adversely affected.

The calculus involves factors such as the cost to the firm of compensating workers or their dependents for loss of earning power and medical expenses as a result of death, injury, or ill health. The loss of production as a result of an accident, including damage to equipment, is a further factor. Workers' knowledge that a colleague has been killed or has suffered a work-related injury or disease tends to reduce productivity, whereas their confidence that safety measures are in place is a positive stimulus to work performance. Indeed, it would appear that some firms carry a certain amount of extra capacity to absorb lost production caused by accidents, but this too has a price.

One of the problems, of course, is that many firms do not account for these costs accurately and may be unaware of how damaging unsafe work is to their productivity and profitability. But assuming that these costs and benefits are understood and that they point to a case for action to reduce hazards, firms still need to offset the investment needed to reduce or eliminate dangers to safety and health at work. Some hazard-reducing investments are relatively cheap or may simply involve good housekeeping measures such as cleaning and tidying work areas. Others, however, may be more costly, requiring new machinery or alternative materials. In either case, the basic principles of investment apply. The rate of return is compared with the cost of the capital required over the lifetime of the investment. In many cases, such analysis comes out strongly in favor of investing in safety and can give an employer a competitive advantage in the marketplace. In others, however, the analysis can be negative, especially if competitors do not take similar action or the benefits accrue over a long period of time while the costs are more immediate, increasing the risk that a firm will not recoup its outlays.

An additional factor in a wider social cost–benefit calculus is that not all costs of hazards are paid by the firm, since some also fall on the worker and the community. The systems used to compensate for loss of earnings and medical expenses may not be entirely funded by employers—for example, by requiring firms with poor safety records to pay higher insurance premiums. Medical expenses may be subsidized by the state, and the firm may not compensate loss of earnings by other household members who are caring for sick or injured workers. And last but not least, the polluter may not pay the environmental contamination costs resulting from unsafe working practices.

Differing National Approaches to Cost–Benefit Analyses

The extent to which a complete accounting of the internal and external costs of unsafe working practices is undertaken varies within and between countries. In general terms, a system that clearly identifies and allocates costs to the firms responsible for hazards requires a relatively sophisticated institutional framework, plus well-crafted and well-applied laws and regulations. For example, well-funded but inappropriately designed public insurance schemes for health care and workers' accident compensation may inadvertently end up subsidizing unsafe work or act as a disincentive to investment in safe work.

Firms with a strong market position that are not threatened by competitors may choose to invest in safe work—using internally generated capital rather than external finance—and either pass the costs on through price increases to customers or absorb them gradually as productivity improves. At a time of low unemployment, firms with a reputation for dangerous workplaces may not be able to attract new employees and thus may be obliged to improve standards. Conversely, high unemployment may force workers to take a risk in accepting jobs in hazardous workplaces because no alternatives are available. As competition for global markets intensifies, governments also face a dilemma in formulating strategies to improve safety and health at work. Strengthening the national regulatory system is an important way of preventing competition from inhibiting needed safety improvements. But where firms are competing internationally, this may lead to loss of markets to competitors from other countries not applying comparable standards unless the benefits from safer conditions yield quick results in terms of increased productivity.

Firm-level decisions on investing in safe work are thus importantly influenced by competition in both product and labor markets and by the legal obligations applying in different locations. Although it is possible to achieve and retain a high degree of competitiveness through safe working practices, market conditions can make it easier or more difficult to follow this path.

Safe work creates no obstacles to being competitive and successful. In fact, no country—and no company, in the long run—has been able to jump to a high level of productivity without making sure that the work environment is safe. Figure 11–2 shows the broad relation between national competitiveness (IMD, 2000) and the rate of fatal accidents (ILO, 2000b). Although quality products are generally associated with quality production processes and command a premium in the marketplace, the underlying question remains: How can public policy interact with firms to create a path toward competition based on ensuring safe work and protecting communities—and especially their most disadvantaged members—from the costs of ill health? This is an issue with which the ILO and its constituents have considerable experience. However, this knowledge now needs to be reassessed in the light of the quickening pace of international integration, or what has come to be known as *globalization.*

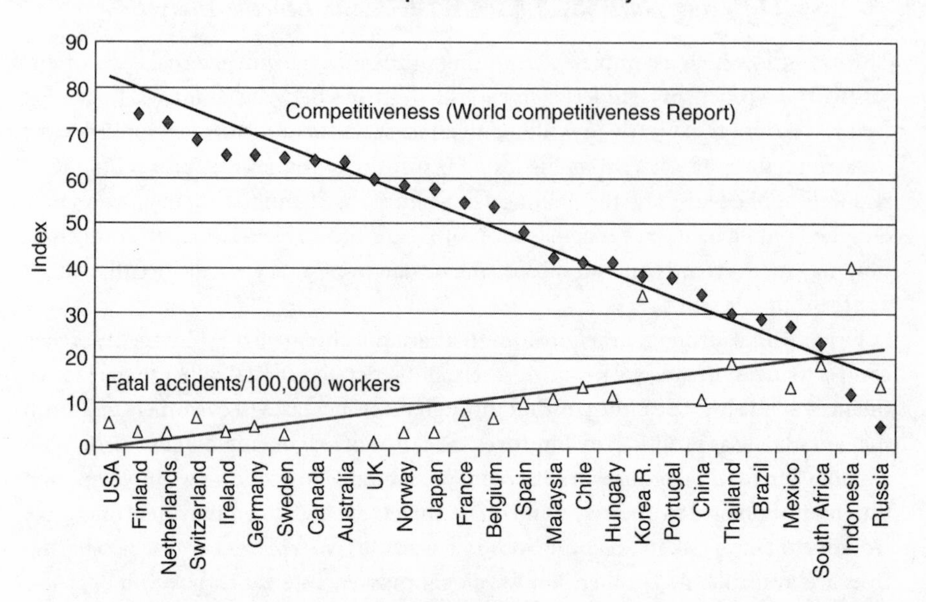

Figure 11–2. National competitiveness. Sources: International Institute for Management Development (2000); International Labor Office, 1999.

The Internationalization of Public Policy in Response to Globalization

Public policy on occupational safety and health has evolved over a long period, but its modern history began in the nineteenth century and quickly acquired an international dimension. Much of the ILO's standard setting in the early 1920s concerned occupational safety and health. However, a large part of the current legal and institutional framework was constructed in the post-1945 period. The greatest progress was made in the industrialized countries in the era of what might be termed *national welfare capitalism.* From an economic point of view, the key characteristic of this period was that the territorial boundaries of markets largely coincided with the jurisdiction of states. One feature of this period was that laws and regulations about safety and health at work and systems of social protection included most firms selling and producing in national markets. Products produced in other countries had only a limited share of such predominantly national markets and in any case came mostly from other industrial countries with similar social systems (Standing, 1999).

Tariff and quota protection of markets and controls on capital flows gradually fell in the period up to the 1980s, but barriers to international commerce were substantially dismantled only in the last two decades of the twentieth century. The term *globalization* came into common parlance in the 1990s when the effects of the information and communication revolution, along with the spread of democratic forms of governance, added to the trend toward internal and external liberalization (Standing, 1999). Although it is premature to talk of a single global market, the twenty-first century has opened with states facing the problem that the territorial boundaries of markets are no longer the same as those within which their laws and institutions operate. Governments are thus increasingly conscious not only of the potential effect that enterprises' competitive positions may have on global markets but also of the degree to which their countries appear attractive to foreign direct investors. The EU, in building a single market (reducing and eliminating barriers to trade, capital flows, and labor mobility between EU member states), has recognized the importance of developing an EU-wide system of safety and health protection that ensures that all member states will move ahead more or less synchronously in improving standards, even as they face competition in both home and foreign markets from producers with lower standards.

It would seem that most enterprises are facing increasingly fierce competition for market share not only from established companies but also from new and potential entrants to the market, although it would be hard to measure such trends statistically. Firms that have captured the productivity advantages of high standards of safety and health protection are not likely to reduce levels of protection. However, others—particularly small and medium-sized enterprises or those using various forms of precarious employment or subcontracting—may face, or perceive, a higher threshold in breaking through to a virtuous spiral of high safety and health standards and high productivity. If, as is quite likely, for many small enterprises the threshold is in fact considerably lower than they believe, public agencies must actively intervene to spread the understanding that the costs of improving safety can be negligible, certainly by comparison with the benefits. By comparison with the past, international coordination and cooperation are of greater significance in assisting such firms to move to a strategy of improving safety and health as part of efforts to improve their competitiveness.

Perspectives for the ILO in an Integrated Multilateral System

The ILO has recently become a focus of attention in the debates about how to shape the processes of globalization to ensure that its potential benefits are spread more evenly and its costs shared among and within countries. In attempting to assess whether the institution can meet this challenge, it is important to know what the ILO does and how it is able to influence international and national policies.

The ILO's Traditional Forms of Action

The ILO's primary means of action to promote cooperation and coordination in and around the labor market, including issues related to occupational safety and health, are standard setting, technical assistance, and research. The ILO has a number of occupational safety and health *conventions* that, when ratified, commit the member state to render effective the provisions engendered in the convention within its national legal system and to provide information to relevant ILO supervisory mechanisms for this purpose.

Conventions are usually accompanied by *recommendations*, which supplement conventions with more detailed provisions that enable the underlying principles of the convention to be set out and stated more precisely, and that serve as a guide to national policies. Recommendations, however, do not have the binding force of conventions. Further guidance, especially in the occupational safety and health field, is provided by *codes of practice*, which are technical standards providing the basic requirements for implementation of the principles contained in conventions and recommendations. A new type of "soft standard" that directly targets enterprises is the newly published guidelines on occupational safety and health management systems (ILO, 2001a). This standard follows the principles outlined in ILO conventions, but it follows the form of other systems-based standards, namely, those on quality and environmental management (International Standards Organization 9000 and 14000, respectively). Taken together, these standards constitute a comprehensive and influential guide for governments, employers, unions, and all others responsible for protecting workers' health against hazards.[3]

Action on these standards is, however, a matter for competent national authorities. In the case of ratified conventions, regular reports are required and are scrutinized by experts and an international tripartite committee, which can draw attention to problems and make recommendations where observance is found wanting. The conventions also provide for a complaints procedure. The act of ratification of a convention thus demonstrates and reinforces the political decision to incorporate the principles it contains into national law and practice and accept international oversight of their observance. Critics of the ILO say that this form of voluntary acceptance of international peer review is effective only where a government is already prepared to adopt policies that conform to international standards. Others that tolerate weak safety and health practices and do not ratify conventions escape scrutiny. Some go further and argue that international standards are, of necessity, too general to have a decisive impact and often appear inappropriate to the specific problems of often very different countries' circumstances.

Side by side with the guidance offered in international labor standards, the ILO offers technical assistance as a further support for countries that are ready to commit to the observance of international standards but lack the capacity to do so. It offers advice and training to government enforcement agencies, employers, and trade unions in drafting legislation and regulations pertinent to the establishment of public agencies. Technical assistance is usually funded by extra contributions to the ILO from industrial countries' aid budgets. It is thus a means of overcoming the social divides that characterize the disparities in occupational safety and health performance internationally.[4] The ILO's advocacy role is backed up by research demonstrating the advantages, particularly to small and medium-sized enterprises, of improved occupational safety and health performance. Well-informed employers and trade unions are often the most effective conduits for efforts to improve safety and health at work. If, as we are suggesting, economic analysis of the costs and benefits of improving safety and health is increasingly important, given competitive pressures in global markets, such research becomes an increasingly vital means of both developing firm-level strategies and supporting public policies.[5]

Cooperation with Business, Trade Unions, and Nongovernmental Organizations

In addition to these traditional forms of action, two new areas of activity have opened up for the ILO in recent years. With the emergence of global supply chains often driven by large, well-known multinational companies such as Nike, General Motors, and TESCO, the general public is increasingly aware of differences in labor standards. Although wage levels and labor costs generally are linked to national levels of per capita income, the public sees owners of global supply chains as being in a position to transfer, within their own operations and those of subcontractors, improved employment and environmental practices. Even in 1977, the ILO Tripartite Declaration of Principles on Multinational Enterprises and Social Policy (ILO, 1977, paragraph 38) urged companies to maintain the highest standards of safety and health, in conformity with national requirements, bearing in mind their relevant experience within the enterprise as a whole, including any knowledge of special hazards. They should also make available to the representatives of the workers in the enterprise and, upon request, to the competent authorities and the workers' and employers' organizations in all countries in which they operate, information on the safety and health standards relevant to their local operations, which they observe in other countries. In particular, they should make known to those concerned any special hazards and related protective measures associated with new products and processes. They, like comparable domestic enterprises, should be expected to play a leading role in the examination of causes of industrial safety and health hazards and in the application of resulting improvements within the enterprise as a whole.

The ILO is working with businesses, trade unions, and nongovernmental organizations as part of the United Nations Secretary General's Global Compact initiative, which encourages corporations to commit themselves to action to promote basic human and labor rights and environmental principles. This initiative includes efforts to improve the safety and health performance of subsidiaries and subcontractors, with a view to meeting minimum standards in these areas. In an increasingly competitive world, coordinated action by leading employers can demonstrate intentions in far-reaching ways. Respect for workers' right to organize and represent their concerns to management is particularly important to the development of sound management systems for the avoidance of work hazards and environmental damage.

Action by companies alone, however, is no replacement for national policy. The ILO has argued that the system of multilateral cooperation and coordination built up since 1945 is underperforming in the era of globalization. An increasingly integrated global economy requires from the multilateral system a more integrated policy response.

Decent Work for All and Core Labor Standards

In 1999 the ILO launched an initiative to improve policy coordination under the title of Decent Work for All.[6] The approach encapsulated in this goal is to improve the ILO's own policy integration across the fields of labor standards, employment, social protection, and social dialogue, and to connect its work to that of other multilateral agencies. One vehicle for such policy coherence is the poverty reduction process now underway in many of the poorest developing countries (ILO, 2001b). This will require the ILO to operationalize the concept of decent work, first, through dialogue with governments, employers, trade unions, and international agencies and, second, within national strategies aimed at reducing the incidence of extreme poverty by half by 2015.

One key area now is the creation of more and better jobs by establishing institutional support for small and medium-sized enterprises. This support will encourage the enlargement of employment opportunities and the progressive improvement of working conditions. Work that is not safe cannot be said to be decent. Thus, making work safe is a major component of this approach and will require investment in the capacity of government agencies, employers, and workers' organizations to identify and act on hazards at work.

Integrated policy frameworks will require a much better understanding of how fiscal, financial, and trade policies interact with policies designed to improve the functioning of labor markets. Improved policy integration is particularly important in the fields of occupational safety and health and community health, where the policy and regulatory environment within which firms operate can have a major influence on hazard avoidance and the health of disadvantaged social groups and communities. Analysis of the social and private costs and benefits of occupational hazards and of the mechanisms for their reduction is essential to the design of sound public policy, which in turn needs to develop along internationally coherent lines, given increasing market integration.

One of the most contentious areas is the relationship between international efforts to open markets through trade liberalization and universal observance of core labor standards. Attention has focused on a limited number of Fundamental Principles and Rights at Work, referred to in the 1998 ILO Declaration as "*enabling rights.*"[7] A recent

ILO paper ("Organizing, Bargaining and Dialogue for Development in a Globalizing World": International Labor Organization Working Party, 2000) surveying the available information on the relationship between, on the one hand, the rights to associate freely, organize, and bargain collectively and, on the other hand, trade, investment, and economic performance found no evidence that abuse of these rights enhanced a country's competitive advantage.

An underlying reason for increased attention to the trade-related aspects of policies dealing with such things as the environment and labor is the steady shift in the World Trade Organization (WTO) and the General Agreement on Tariffs and Trade agenda from issues related to commercial transactions across borders to rules affecting competition between foreign and domestically produced goods and services within national jurisdictions. Justifications for particular national standards or subsidies are usually made by reference to goals other than trade. The WTO is thus being pushed or pulled into a number of difficult trade disputes over the allegedly discriminatory and protectionist character of certain national laws. Questions have started to be raised as to whether measures justified on the grounds of public health are interfering with trade, either deliberately or inadvertently. A recent case involving Canada versus France over whether a French law banning the use of asbestos constituted an unfair trade practice raised many controversial issues regarding the capacity of a trade law system to adjudicate on matters that extend to other spheres of competence and expertise. The ILO is still studying the implications of the reasoning used by the WTO to find in favor of France's ban on all asbestos imports. Clearly, trade in hazardous products, and perhaps at some point in products made by hazardous processes, is set to become a major source of friction unless resolved by international agreements that balance the goals of freer trade and better health within a more coherent multilateral system.

With the objective of enhancing policy coherence, the ILO aims to develop dialogue and joint research with other international agencies. The connections between workplace safety and wider social and economic policies are a neglected issue in many countries. At the core of the ILO's approach is the need to respect workers' rights to organize to protect themselves from dangerous working practices and to work with employers in finding safer ways of structuring the production process. Coupled with improved information services to both management and trade union representatives, social dialogue at the workplace and in the design of company policies, laws, and regulations is an effective way of escaping the trap of low productivity and low safety that is at the core of the problem of advancing safe work in an increasingly competitive global economy.

Within the multilateral system, the role of the ILO is to ensure that all countries progressively raise their occupational safety and health performance in their pursuit of decent work for all people. Evaluating the ILO's performance in meeting this challenge is an underresearched area.

Conclusion

The ILO estimates that approximately 2 million workers lose their lives annually due to occupational injuries and illnesses, with accidents causing at least 350,000 deaths a year. For every fatal accident, there are an estimated 1000 nonfatal injuries, many of which result in lost earnings, permanent disability, and poverty. The death toll at work, much of which is attributable to unsafe working practices, is the equivalent of 5000 workers dying each day, 3 persons every minute (ILO, 2002c). Community health and occupational health and safety experts need to increase their collaboration and grasp the opportunities available for more integrated responses to the global toll taken by work-related accidents and illness.

This chapter has argued that action to reduce and eliminate hazards at work is a vital component of policies to reduce inequalities at work and in the community. Such action also needs to form part of a wider strategy to reduce inequality amongst nations.

A second theme in this chapter is an examination of the impact of the international integration of markets on the effectiveness of national policy regimes for safety and health at work. The conclusion is that efforts are needed to avoid undermining measures to reduce and eliminate hazards by improved coordination of policies at the international level. This is an important part of the mandate of the ILO.

While better regulation and enforcement built on common international standards are a good part of the answer, attention also needs to be paid to creating pathways for underperforming enterprises to realize the productivity gains from safe working conditions that can help their businesses to survive and prosper. For firms and workers on the fringes of increasingly global markets, breaking through to safer work, higher productivity, and commercial success can require a significant investment of time or capital. Public policies need to focus more on helping firms move over this threshold. This is particularly important in developing countries, especially the poorest. Increased financial and technical assistance to enable micro- and smaller businesses to improve their safety and health at work should form part of the poverty reduction strategies supported by the international development community.

Notes

1. The authors acknowledge the work of Peter Dorman, especially his working paper for the ILO "The Economics of Safety, Health, and Well-Being at Work: An Overview."

2. The labor force data in the ILO's Key Information on Labour Markets 3 distinguishes three main categories of the total employed: wage and salaried workers or employees; the self-employed (who are sometimes further disaggregated into employers and own-account workers); and contributing family members.

3. Many transition countries have revised their safety and health laws over the past ten years, often using ILO Convention 155 and Recommendation 164 as guides. Recent examples in-

clude Estonia, Latvia, Belarus, Moldova, Bosnia Herzegovina, Croatia, FYR Macedonia, and Yugoslavia.

4. A recent example of this type of activity was a series of ILO workshops in Brazil that helped pave the way for changes in law and practice and the ratification of Convention 174 on the Prevention of Major Industrial Accidents. This convention was itself a response to issues highlighted by research on the causes of the disaster in Bhopal, India, where in 1984 more than 2,500 people were killed and over 200,000 injured due to the leakage of methyl isocyanate from Union Carbide Corporation's pesticide factory.

5. Work Improvements in Small Enterprises (WISE) is an ILO program that has been proven effective in generating simple, low-cost improvements linking productivity and product quality to better and safer workplace conditions.

6. The report proposed that the goals of the ILO should be the promotion of "opportunities for women and men to obtain decent and productive work, in conditions of freedom, equity, security and human dignity."

7. These standards concern (*a*) freedom of association and the effective recognition of the right to collective bargaining; (*b*) the elimination of all forms of forced or compulsory labor; (*c*) the effective abolition of child labor; and (*d*) the elimination of discrimination in employment and occupation.

References

Annan, K. A. 1997. Occupational health and safety: A high priority on the global, international and national agenda. Editorial. *African Newsletter on Occupational Health and Safety* 7: 51.

Aronsson, G. 1999. Contingent workers and health and safety. *Work, Employment and Society* 13(3): 439–59.

Bertola, G., T. Boeri, and S. Cazes. 1999. Employment protection and labour market adjustments in Organization for Economic Co-operation and Development countries. International Labor Organization (ILO) Employment and Training Papers 48. Geneva: ILO.

Dorman, P. 2000. *The economics of safety, health, and well-being at work: An overview.* Geneva: International Labor Organization. Available from http://www.ilo.org/public/english/protection/safework/papers/ecoanal/ecoview.htm

Dorman, P., and P. Hagstrom. 1998. Compensating wage differentials for dangerous work reconsidered. *Industrial and Labour Relations Review* 52: 116–35.

European Agency for Safety and Health at Work. 1999. *Economic impact of occupational safety and health in the member states of the European Union.* Bilbao, Spain: European Agency for Safety and Health at Work. Available from http://agency.osha.eu.int/publications/reports/302/en/EC.IM-EN.pdf

Forastieri, V. 1999. Improvement of working conditions and environment in the informal sector through safety and health measures. Working paper. SafeWork. Geneva: International Labor Organization. Available from http://www.ilo.org/public/english/protection/safework/sectors/informal/inform1.htm

International Council of Chemical Associations (ICCA). 2000. Responsible Care Status Report 2000. Available at: http://www.cefic.org/activities/hse/rc/icca/Report2000.pdf

International Institute for Management Development (IMD). 2000. *Work competitiveness yearbook 2000.* Lausanne, Switzerland: IMD. Available from http://www.imd.ch/wcy

International Labor Organization (ILO). 1977. ILO Tripartite Declaration of Principles on Multinational Enterprises and Social Policy. Geneva: ILO.

International Labor Organization (ILO). 1999. Decent work. Report of the Director-General to the International Labor Conference. Geneva: ILO.

International Labor Organization (ILO). 2000a. Job quality and small enterprise development. Working paper number 4. In Focus Programme on Boosting Employment through small enterprise development (IFP/SED). Geneva: ILO.

International Labor Organization (ILO). 2000b. *Yearbook of labor statistics 2000.* Geneva: ILO.

International Labor Organization (ILO). 2001a. Guidelines on occupational health and safety management Systems. Geneva: ILO.

International Labor Organization (ILO). 2001b. Reducing the decent work deficit. Director-General's report to the June 2001 International Labor Conference, Geneva.

International Labor Organization (ILO). 2001c. Seventh survey on the effect given to the Tripartite Declaration of Principles Concerning Multinational Enerprises and Social Policy Part I. Geneva: ILO.

International Labor Organization (ILO). 2001d. *World employment report 2001.* Geneva: ILO.

International Labor Organization (ILO). 2002a. Occupational safety and health and employment. In *A global agenda for employment.* Geneva: ILO. Available from http://www.ilo.org/public/english/employment/geforum/download/globalagenda.pdf

International Labor Organization (ILO). 2002b. Decent work and the informal economy. International Labor Conference, 90th Session. Geneva: ILO.

International Labor Organization ((ILO). 2002c. Workers' Memorial Day ceremony to focus on emergency workers, firefighters. Press release, April 24. Available from http://www.ilo.org/public/english/bureau/inf/pr/2002/18.htm

International Labor Organization (ILO) Working Party on the Social Dimension of Globalization. 2000. Organizing, bargaining and dialogue for development in a globalizing world. GB.279/WP/SDG/2. Geneva: ILO.

Loewenson, R. 1997. Health impact of occupational risks in the informal sector in Zimbabwe. Geneva: International Labor Organization. Available from http://www.ilo.org/public/english/protection/safework/papers/infzimb/index.htm

National Academy of Sciences and National Research Council. 1998. *Protecting youth at work.* Washington, D.C.: National Academy Press.

Quinlan, M. 1999. The implications of labour market restructuring in industrialised societies for occupational health and safety. *Economic and Industrial Democracy* 20(3): 427–60.

Salminen, S. 1995. Does pressure from the work community increase risk taking? *Psychological Reports* 77: 1247–50.

Standing, Guy. 1999. *Global labour flexibility.* Basingstoke, UK: Macmillan.

Takala, J. S. 2000. Indicators on death, disability and disease at work. *Asian–Pacific Newsletter on Occupational Health and Safety 2000* 7(1). Available from http://www.occuphealth.fi/e/info/asian/ap100/indicators02.htm

Yu, T.-S. I, Y. Liu, J. Zhou, and T. Wong. 1999. Occupational injuries in Shunde City—a county undergoing economic change in southern China. *Accident Analysis and Prevention* 31: 313–17.

12

The Role Global Labor Standards Could Play in Addressing Basic Needs

KIMBERLY ANN ELLIOTT
AND RICHARD B. FREEMAN

The scene could be Seattle in 1999, Prague in 2000, or Genoa in 2001: Dark-suited government functionaries and helmeted police confront weirdly attired young protesters chanting "Hey, hey, ho, ho, globalization has got to go." The functionaries huddle behind closed doors to discuss the need for multilateral trade agreements monitored by international organizations run by fellow functionaries. The protestors outside demand protection for workers and the environment equal to that provided to investors and intellectual property rights owners.

The battle between the proponents of unfettered globalization and the proponents of globalization with standards to protect labor and the environment has replaced the struggle between communism and capitalism over the best way to deliver the benefits of modern production to people around the globe. On the side of expanded globalization, many economists, international organizations, and developing country governments believe that free trade of goods and services and foreign investment promote the growth of less developed countries, and they fear that labor and environmental standards will undermine their competitiveness in global markets. The critics see global standards as a scheme to lower the comparative advantage of poor countries, and they believe that trade sanctions to enforce standards are protectionism in disguise.

Embracing an alternative vision of globalization, many nongovernmental organizations and human rights activists, as well as most trade unions, believe that unencumbered free trade increases income inequality and creates a race to the bottom for workers worldwide. Many of these groups, particularly from developed countries, want trade agreements that include global labor standards and trade sanctions to enforce them. Nongovernmental organizations and unions from developing countries are often in the middle of this debate, favoring higher standards in their own countries but opposing the linking of those standards to trade for fear that their exports, and therefore jobs, will suffer.

Who is right? Which is the road to economic progress in less developed countries: free trade or global labor standards? What practical steps can the world community take to improve labor standards without harming trade with less developed countries?

We argue that the globalization–labor standards debate has posed the problem of standards and trade incorrectly. Free trade and labor standards are complementary, rather than competitive, ways to raise living conditions in less developed countries. They are political complements because neither can advance far without the other. They are policy complements because global integration directs attention to labor conditions in poor countries, and this attention creates consumer demands for global labor standards to improve conditions. This, in turn, gives multinational corporations an incentive to go beyond legally mandated minimum standards in their overseas operations. Furthermore, improved labor standards can increase the benefits of free trade to less developed countries' workers and can expand the constituency for free trade in developed economies. By contrast, ignoring labor standards guarantees continued confrontation between adherents of free trade and adherents of global standards that could block future trade agreements and wider sharing of the benefits of trade. The central problem with standards in less developed countries is not that standards depress trade but that institutional weaknesses make it difficult to enforce or deliver decent working conditions in low-income and nondemocratic or marginally democratic countries.

Our argument proceeds in three parts. The first section of this chapter describes the labor standards at the heart of the debate; the rationale for global rather then local standards; and the conditions under which standards improve or worsen economic well-being in less developed countries. The second section provides evidence on the economic effects of standards and trade and their interconnection. The third section highlights the problem of delivering standards in less developed countries and argues for an increased role for global institutions, as well as a major effort to improve standards in export processing zones (areas of countries designed to produce for the global market, with various tariff and other concessions), to demonstrate the positive effects of globalization on the well-being of workers in less developed countries.

Defining Global Core Labor Standards

The starting point for the debate over labor standards and globalization is often whether there are any standards, other than the prohibition of slavery, that are universally accepted. Those who say no argue that all other labor market regulations must depend on a country's local preferences and level of development—what it can afford (Bhagwati, 1995; Srinivasan, 1994). Those who say yes argue that additional labor standards should be regarded as fundamental because they are basic human rights or because they are essential to a well-functioning labor market. But there are still disagreements as to which particular standards should be in the *core* (Freeman, 1996; OECD, 1995; Portes, 1994).

As a matter of policy priority, the world community has endorsed four standards as core at this time. From 1998, *all* 175 International Labor Organization (ILO) member governments and their labor and employer constituents were committed to promoting four objectives as defined in the "Declaration on Fundamental Principles and Rights at Work":

- Freedom from forced labor
- Nondiscrimination in the workplace
- The "effective abolition" of child labor
- Freedom of association and the right to organize and bargain collectively

No one today questions the *prohibition of slavery and coerced labor*, but it is important to recall that slavery was an accepted practice in the ancient world and in the U.S. South prior to the Civil War.[1] Chattel slavery persists in the world today only in a few isolated pockets, mainly in sub-Saharan Africa. However, the poorest and most vulnerable people continue to be exploited by other forms of coerced labor, particularly in South Asia, and the struggle to eliminate it in practice continues (ILO, 2001).

Nondiscrimination is a recent addition to the menu of labor standards. Not long ago, firms frequently said that they would not hire women or minorities because of their gender or ethnicity. The fact that nondiscrimination has become a core standard about which there is little controversy in principle (save possibly on sexual preference) indicates how rapidly yesterday's radical opinions can become today's norms. Even more than with forced labor, however, translating principle into practice in eliminating discrimination has a long way to go in most countries (World Bank, 2001).

Because *child labor* is overwhelmingly the product of poverty, it is in practice a very nuanced standard. Many families and children in poor countries rely on the labor of children for survival. Recognizing this, ILO members in 1999 approved Convention 182, which calls on countries to take "immediate and effective measures to secure the prohibition and elimination of the *worst forms* [emphasis added] of child labor," including forced labor, labor linked to illicit activities such as prostitution and drug trafficking, and "work which, by its nature or the circumstances in which it is carried out, is likely to harm the health, safety or morals of children" (www.ilo.org). By early 2002, 117 countries had ratified Convention 182, putting it well on its way to the goal of universal ratification by 2003.[2]

The freedom of association and right to collective bargaining standard is the most controversial because it increases the power of workers relative to the state or capital. Unlike most voluntary organizations, trade unions can gain sufficient independent political and economic power to threaten nondemocratic or semidemocratic regimes, to shift the distribution of income, and to alter authority relations at workplaces and in society more broadly.

The core standards relate to the rules that govern labor market transactions broadly and are thus comparable to rules in product markets that allow capitalist economies to function—protection of property rights, freedom of transactions. Core standards also empower workers to negotiate other standards with employers and to arrive at an outcome that best serves their interests.

Many other labor protections and benefits are called *cash standards*, because they mandate particular outcomes that raise labor costs. The division between core and cash standards is, to be sure, a fuzzy one, since all standards have components of cost and moral standing. The core standard of freedom of association, for instance, often raises the cost of labor as unions negotiate higher wages. Cash standards are not, moreover, less important than core standards in human well-being. Occupational health and safety standards that protect life and limb could be more important than nondiscrimination. Better to be alive and healthy and facing some discrimination than to suffer from an awful occupational injury or death. We argue that the differentiation between core and cash issues is especially valuable, however, in assessing standards in a global economy.

Global or Local Labor Standards?

At the global level, we contend that the key difference between core and cash standards is that the core standards can be applied universally, regardless of a country's economic situation or development status. While the principles and specific conventions underlying core standards allow countries latitude in choosing how to implement them in ways that fit with local needs and customs, the goal is universal ratification. Cash standards cannot readily be applied globally because, by definition, they mandate outcomes that typically vary with the ability to pay—by country and often by sector.

On the side of the debate against any core global standards, many proponents of unencumbered globalism argue that diversity in standards is a legitimate source of comparative advantage and that, slavery aside, each country should determine its own standards based on local conditions and preferences. In their view, universally applied standards risk driving up labor costs in less developed countries and undercutting their comparative advantage in labor-intensive commodities. Many believe this is in fact the intention of unions in developed countries that lobby for a "social clause" in trade agreements (Bhagwati, 1995; Brown, Deardorf, and Stern, 1996; Srinivasan, 1994).

If the world consisted solely of democracies, the argument against global labor standards would carry substantially more weight. However, authoritarian regimes rule many countries, a fact that makes their choice of standards problematic at best, particularly when almost all such regimes prevent freedom of association.[3] The workers whom standards are designed to protect have little or no say in their determination. If the world community insisted on specific ways to implement core standards, the diversity argument might again have weight. But the focus of the core standards is on the fundamental *principles* of working, not on the specifics of the regulations. Even the detailed obligations of the ILO conventions allow for a great deal of flexibility in implementation and diversity among countries. The parallel is with rules about protection of property and transactions, which all capitalist countries need in order to function but which vary in numerous ways, depending on legal traditions and national histories.

Finally, to the extent that there are pressures for a "race to the bottom from the bottom" (Chau and Kanbur, 2000), in which some less developed countries find advantages in increased coercion of workers, child labor, and discrimination, global standards place an identifiable floor on that process. Global standards can help less developed countries overcome problems associated with being a "*first mover*" in improving standards and suffering competitive losses due to higher associated costs.

Public Attitudes toward Labor Standards

The vast majority of the public in the United States, the United Kingdom, and, we would surmise, many other countries support global labor standards.[4] Here we review two public opinion polls: (*1*) a 1999 survey of almost 2000 Americans by the University of Maryland's Program on International Policy Attitudes, which asked people their views about labor standards in less developed countries and trade policy, and (*2*) a 1997 Catholic Agency for Overseas Development (CAFOD) survey of consumers in the United Kingdom that asked about the factors that influence purchasing decisions.

In one section of the survey, the Program on International Policy Attitudes presented people with arguments for and against labor standards and asked whether they agreed or disagreed. Seventy-four percent said that they agreed with the argument that "countries who do not maintain minimum standards for working conditions have an unfair advantage because they can exploit workers and produce goods for less." Eighty-three percent agreed that countries should have to meet minimum standards "because it is immoral for workers to be subject to harsh and unsafe conditions in the workplace." By contrast, only 37% accepted the argument that requiring countries to raise their standards would "force some companies to eliminate the jobs of poor people who desperately need the work." And just 41% agreed that "it is up to each country to set its own standards . . . [and] the international community should not intrude by trying to dictate what each country should do within its borders" (University of Maryland, 2000, 22).

These figures show that most respondents found convincing arguments for minimum labor standards, whereas far fewer accepted the arguments against standards. But respondents did not blindly accept all standards, nor were the distinctions they drew entirely in line with the core versus cash standards dichotomy. They recognized the potential problems in global wage standards, with more than 80% realizing that workers in foreign countries could not expect to earn U.S. wages. Opposition to child labor was common, but many more were concerned about safe working conditions than about the right to unionize.

Finally, considering standards and trade, 90% of respondents in the University of Maryland survey said that "free trade is an important goal for the United States, but it should be balanced with other goals, such as protecting workers, the environment, and human rights—even if this may mean slowing the growth of trade and the economy." Even more striking was the near unanimity (93%) that "countries that are part of international trade agreements should be required to maintain minimum standards for working conditions."

The British survey showed a similar pattern. When prompted, 42% of British consumers surveyed said that they would take into account whether people "worked in an environment that did not affect their health" when buying a product from a developing country; and when prompted on wages, 44% felt workers should be "paid enough to live on." Overall, child labor and safe working conditions were second and third behind only quality as issues these consumers reported taking into account when buying products from developing countries, and 92% of the respondents thought British companies should have to abide by minimum agreed-upon labor standards for their workers in developing countries (Tallontire, Rentsendorj, and Blowfield, 2001, 11).

With massive popular support for standards and with 175 countries agreeing on the ILO definition of core standards, one might imagine that the advocates of global labor standards had won the debate. But the business community, most governments of less developed countries and many trade economists remain skeptical about whether globally enforced standards can improve economic well-being in less developed countries or whether they will simply reduce trade and rates of economic growth. Moreover, signing on to core standards does not mean enforcing standards, so that the battle continues in another way: over how much resources and effort to give to enforcement.

Can Standards Improve Economic Well-being?

The argument over whether any nonmarket intervention can improve well-being is a perennial one in economics. Some economists regard markets as nearly perfect and governments or other social institutions as fallible. They argue that labor standards are unnecessary because a perfectly functioning labor market will produce the best of all possible worlds. For example, Martin and Maskus (1999, 7) argue that "in a competitive market in which employers possessed accurate information about worker productivity, it is difficult to envisage how [gender] discrimination could be maintained for long." Economists of this bent usually oppose trade unions for fear that collective bargaining will drive wages above market levels, reducing employment. They stress that in developing countries, unions exacerbate economic inequalities as well, because membership is concentrated in the relatively high-wage modern sector (Srinivasan, 1994).

On the other side, economists who regard markets as fallible and governments and social institutions as agents of democracy argue that standards can improve outcomes. In this framework, unions elected by workers have "*collective voice*" effects—which can improve productivity—and these effects often dominate their monopolistic tendencies—which raise wages (Freeman, 1993; Stiglitz, 2000). These economists also note that standards can resolve market imperfections, particularly when workers suffer from a lack of information about such things as health hazards. They favor unions to improve labor's bargaining power and to give workers a voice in national debates over policy priorities and reforms (Freeman, 1993; Rodrik, 1999; Sen, 1999; Stiglitz, 2000). These economists suggest three tests of how *global* standards affect workers in low-wage countries: (*1*) whether the standards increase spending on less developed countries' products by reassuring consumers that goods are produced under decent conditions (Elliott and Freeman, 2003b), (*2*) whether the standards alter terms of trade in favor of less developed countries' goods (Brown, Deardorff, and Stern, 1996), and (*3*) whether standards help firms and governments in less developed countries avoid a race to the bottom among themselves (Chau and Kanbur, 2000).

Evidence on the Economic Effects of Standards and Globalization

The most telling argument against labor standards is that they undermine developing countries' comparative advantage in world markets, cutting off a major route to economic growth. Alternatively, low labor standards might give a country a competitive edge in a particular low-wage sector, such as apparel, but might not affect its overall comparative advantage or might even discourage movement into higher-skill, "better" sectors. The extent to which standards affect competitiveness depends on the degree to which standards are violated in traded goods sectors *relative* to domestic production, plus the costs of bringing conditions up to standards.

Violations of Labor Standards in Less Developed Countries

Forced labor appears to be rare, particularly in export industries. The International Confederation of Free Trade Unions (ICFTU) reviewed labor practices in 51 countries and found little or no evidence of forced labor in 32 of them. In the countries where the ICFTU found forced labor, moreover, it was typically bonded or child labor in domestic services or rural areas, not in the traded goods sector. The ILO (2001) has similarly concluded that the most common forms are typically not linked to trade. Still, forced labor has been discovered in exporting activities. According to the *New York Times (*March 1, 2001), one recent case involved Chinese exports of binder clips that were assembled by female prison laborers working long hours with no pay. The

ILO report also contained details about forced labor by Haitian migrant workers in the Dominican Republic's sugarcane industry, the output of which is exported largely to the United States.

Child labor is also more common in agriculture and domestic services than in export industries and is also strongly correlated with poverty. Still, there are export sectors where child labor has contributed to production: rugs, soccer balls, and some plantation agriculture, most recently cocoa, have gained the most notoriety. One researcher regressed the proportion of textiles and apparel in total exports on various proxies for labor standards compliance and found that more child labor is associated with higher exports of such labor-intensive goods (Rodrik, 1996). However, a similar analysis by Morici and Schulz (2001) did not reveal a statistically significant link between child labor and textile exports when an indicator of respect for union rights was included.

By contrast, workplace *discrimination* against women or ethnic groups is found in most countries to some degree. Whether discrimination increases or decreases trade depends on whether discrimination is more intense in traded goods than in other sectors. Discrimination in traded goods, for example in an export sector, reduces the effective labor supply to that sector and thus lowers production and exports (Maskus, 1997). In this case, adherence to an antidiscrimination standard would increase exports and trade. By contrast, if discrimination is more intense in the non–traded goods sector, it will increase the relative supply of labor to traded goods and thus increase trade, so that adherence to nondiscrimination would reduce trade.

In many poor countries discrimination discourages female employment, except in the garment industry. For example, in the apparel industry in Bangladesh, young women are overrepresented in sewing jobs and underrepresented in more skilled jobs in apparel factories and in all other sectors of the economy. Manufacturers reportedly prefer to employ women in sewing jobs because they are more docile, less likely to join unions, and more likely to accept lower wages, in part due to discrimination in other sectors (Paul-Majumder and Begum, 2000). The result is an increased supply of female workers in the apparel sector, which tends to lower prices and increase production and exports of clothing relative to what would hold true otherwise. In short, discrimination outside of the export sector benefits consumers of export goods at the expense of discriminated groups.[5]

Finally, many governments and employers seek to prevent workers from unionizing by restricting *freedom of association.* In some cases, the motivation is political; in other cases, it is the fear that unions will raise costs and deter investment. Bangladeshi government officials, employers, and foreign investors have resisted ILO and U.S. pressures to allow unions into their nation's export processing zones by arguing that unions would deter investment and lower exports. Indeed, unionization rates are frequently lower in export processing zones than in the rest of the economy (ILO, 1998; U.S. Department of Labor, 1989–90), due in part to government restrictions that discourage union organizing in export processing zones.[6]

Table 12–1 summarizes empirical evidence on the relationship between labor standards and trade and foreign investment.[7] In a cross section of 45 developing countries, Mah (1997) found negative associations between total exports as a share of gross domestic product (GDP) and dummy variables indicating whether or not core ILO conventions have been ratified, but he failed to control for any other potential explanatory variables. By contrast, Rodrik (1996) included other variables and found no statistically significant relationship between convention ratification and exports of textile and apparel by less developed countries. Ratification, however, is not a particularly good proxy for enforcement of labor standards. In 77 countries, Morici and Schulz (2001) used the Organization for Economic Cooperation and Development (OECD) (2000) qualitative index of respect for union rights and found that union rights are significantly and negatively correlated with higher exports of textiles and apparel. However, the addition of a variable measuring the difference between male and female illiteracy, as a proxy for discrimination, weakens this result substantially, suggesting that it could reflect other factors correlated with unionism.[8]

Going beyond competitiveness, Palley (1999) found a strong positive relationship between improvements in labor standards and subsequent economic growth in 15 developing countries from various regions.[9] Rama (2001), however, found a negative correlation between union density and growth in a sample of Latin American countries. Reviewing the economic effects of unions more broadly, a World Bank study concluded that unions had different effects on the economy, depending on local conditions, including institutional and legal arrangements and the competitive environment (Aidt and Tzannatos, 2002). When product markets are competitive (as is likely with free trade), unions have limited scope for raising wages. When product markets are monopolized and there is little transparency or accountability, unions often behave as firms do in such an environment—by lobbying, pressuring, and fighting to retain a share of the monopoly profits for themselves. But the problem lies not with the union or firm but with the noncompetitive market structure.

More broadly, we find it implausible that unions can make countries noncompetitive or undo their comparative advantage except in very peculiar situations. Unions do not set wages; they bargain with employers and are fully aware of the employment consequences of their bargaining. Adherents to the unfettered globalization point of view also fear, however, that unions might make it politically difficult to undertake the economic reforms that the international financial community believes are necessary for economies to function well. In fact, unions are often in the forefront of protests against International Monetary Fund (IMF) or World Bank stabilization and structural reform programs. But suppressing union activity does not guarantee that reforms will follow or, if enacted, will succeed. It is more likely to guarantee that workers, who typically bear a large share of the adjustment burden, will have no place in political debates over economic reform and thus no stake in their success. Rama and Tabellini (1995) have suggested that reforms should focus on the product market, which will lead to complementary adjustments in labor markets. When reforms

Table 12–1. Empirical Evidence on Labor Standards and Comparative Advantage

Source and sample period	Countries	Dependent variable	Independent variables	Statistically significant variables
Mah (1997)	45 developing countries	Exports/GDP	*Dummy variables indicating ratification of ILO conventions:*	
			Freedom of association (87)	**Negative**
			Organizing, bargaining (98)	**Weakly negative**
			Forced labor (29)	
			Abolition of forced labor (105)	
			Nondiscrimination (111)	**Strongly negative**
			Real interest rate	
Rodrik (1996) 1985–88	All countries reporting data	Labor cost per worker	Per capita income	Strongly positive
			No. of ILO conventions ratified	**Positive**
			No. of core conventions ratified	**Positive**
			Child labor incidence index	**Strongly negative**
			FH democracy indicator (with 1 = strong democracy)	Positive
Rodrik (1996) 1985–88	Same as above	Textile and apparel exports as share of total exports	Population/land	Positive
			Average years of schooling	Negative
			No. of ILO conventions ratified	
			No. of core conventions ratified	
			Child labor incidence index	
			FH democracy indicator	
			Statutory hours worked	**Positive**
			Union density	
			Paid vacation (days)	

Study	Sample	Dependent variable	Explanatory variables	Result
Rodrik (1996) 1985–88	Sample countries with per capita GDP < US$6000, 1985	Same as above	Population/land	Positive
			Average years of schooling	Negative
			Child labor incidence index	**Weakly positive**
			Statutory hours worked	**Positive**
			All others same as above and insignificant	
Rodrik (1996) 1985–88	All countries reporting data	U.S. foreign direct investment/capital stock	Population	Strongly negative
			Black market forex premium	Weakly negative
			Income growth	Strongly positive
			FH democracy indicator	Strongly positive
			Child labor incidence index	**Negative**
			No. of ILO conventions ratified	
			No. of core conventions ratified	
Morici and Schulz (2001) 1990–94	Countries in OECD (2000) sample with consistent data	Labor cost per worker	Value added per worker	Strongly positive
			OECD index of union rights (1 = best to 4 = worst)	**Strongly negative**
			Child labor index (Rodrik)	**Weakly negative**
			Child labor (%)	**Weakly negative**
Morici and Schulz (2001) 1990–94	Same as above	Exports of textiles, apparel to OECD as share of all exports to OECD	Labor cost per worker	Negative
			OECD index of union rights (1 = best to 4 = worst)	**Strongly positive**
			Child labor index (Rodrik)	
			Child labor (%)	
Morici and Schulz (2001) 1990–94	Same as above	US FDI/capital stock	GNP	Strongly positive
			OECD index of union rights	**Weakly negative**
			Child labor index (Rodrik)	
			FH democracy indicator	Weakly positive
			Black market forex premium	

Source: Adapted and updated from Brown (2000).

Variables related to labor standards are in boldface type.

FH = Freedom House

improve the operation of an economy to the detriment of a small group of unionized workers, the governments of less developed countries should mobilize other constituencies that would benefit from the proposed economic reforms (Forteza and Rama, 2000) or try to compensate the affected workers rather than repressing freedom of association.

In sum, empirical studies conducted thus far suggest a negative but not robust correlation between labor standards and labor-intensive exports, and reject the notion that standards impede growth or development more broadly. Moreover, because most studies have measured standards by nominal adherence rather than measured enforcement, and because the analyses have been based on crude cross-country regression models, all of the evidence is weak. Indeed, we doubt the key proposition of these studies—namely, that adherence to core labor standards raises company costs enough to affect exports or growth (Freeman, 1996). When the United States passed its antidiscrimination legislation and developed affirmative action policies in the 1970s, some economists feared that such steps would raise costs and lower efficiency. The evidence, however, has been to the contrary.

Similarly, while child labor and forced labor can lead to lower costs and contribute to increased output (and exports) of low-skill, low-wage goods in the short run, such policies have their own economic problems. Child labor inhibits the accumulation of human capital. And forced labor so violates human rights that producers using it risk loss of markets once consumers find out about its existence. A recent World Bank (2001) study on gender equality suggested that while discrimination may boost labor-intensive exports, it negatively affects well-being and impedes development overall. Many countries, such as the Philippines and the Dominican Republic, are also finding that labor unrest increases when workers have no voice in their working arrangements and that labor force instability, in turn, deters foreign investment and can cause time-sensitive foreign buyers, including apparel firms, to turn elsewhere (ILO, 1998).

Trade, Growth, and Inequality

Proponents of unfettered globalization hold that globalization is an important—some say the most important—contributor to economic growth and that it benefits the bulk of the population (Dollar and Kraay, 2001; Frankel and Romer, 1999; Srinivasan and Bhagwati, 1999). Removing trade barriers leads to a more efficient allocation of resources. The result is a higher level of output but not necessarily a higher rate of growth of output, which is the key to economic development. Trade affects growth *rates* only if it increases the growth rate of labor or human or other capital (physical or financial), or if it spurs technological innovations that increase productivity (Rodrik, 1999; Srinivasan and Bhagwati, 1999).

Many empirical studies have shown that the level of trade is positively related to economic growth but they have not shown that the linkage runs from trade to growth rather than the converse, or that particular trade policies result in faster growth. Some analysts believe trade and growth are causally linked (Bhagwati, 1995; Dollar and Kraay, 2001; Srinivasan, 1994). Others are more skeptical and stress the need for institutions that protect property, support individual and collective activities in the market, and reduce social conflict (Rodriguez and Rodrik, 2001). It is not lack of trade that has made Africa a development disaster but lack of stable democratic governance that protects property and lives (Freeman and Lindauer, 1999).

But even if the proponents of unfettered globalization are correct and trade and particular trade policies improve growth rates, the majority of workers may not gain. In theory, low-paid workers in less developed countries gain from trade, while higher-paid workers lose, thus reducing the inequality. But there is a disturbing body of evidence that trade, and particularly foreign investment, increase rather than decrease inequality. Latin American countries that have reduced their trade barriers have shown increases in income inequality, though trade liberalization was invariably part of a package of economic reforms, making it hard to isolate its distinct impact (Green, Dickerson, and Arbache, 2000 [on Brazil]; Harrison and Hanson, 1999; Revenga, 1995; Robbins, 1994 [on Chile]; Robbins and Gindling, 1999 [on Costa Rica]; Robertson, 2000 [on Mexico]). By contrast, South Korea and some other emerging markets that have grown through trade have seen income inequalities fall. In their analysis, Dollar and Kraay (2001) found that, in general, the poor have gained proportionately from growth and trade, but that two of the most prominent globalizers in recent years, Chile and China, have had large increases in inequality (Dollar and Kraay, 2001; Rodrik, 1999). More broadly, among 23 globalizers identified by Dollar and Kraay, 10 had seen increased inequality, 9 had seen increased equality, and 4 had had little or no change.

In sum, the effects of globalization on the distribution of income vary across countries. One implication is that just as freer trade can reduce the potentially negative effects of unions on the economy, unions and the other core labor standards can ameliorate the potentially negative effects of globalization on income distribution. Trade and standards working together can produce better outcomes than either can singly.

Openness and Standards as Complements

The link between trade and labor standards is not new (Charnovitz, 1987). The ILO, according to the preamble of its constitution, was created after World War I because its founders believed that "universal and lasting peace can be established only if it is based upon social justice" and that "the failure of any nation to adopt humane conditions of labour is an obstacle in the way of other nations which desire to improve the conditions in their own countries." Efforts after World War II to build an international economic system that would promote peace as well as prosperity addressed similar issues.

However, the planned International Trade Organization failed because of strong congressional opposition in the United States and only lukewarm support in the rest of the world. The more limited General Agreement on Tariffs and Trade, which survived because it did not require U.S. Senate ratification, included only a single labor provision, permitting countries to ban goods produced with prison labor. Nevertheless, developed countries have steadily improved their labor standards and social protections. Indeed, Rodrik (1997) argues that an expanding social safety net, thus far mainly in richer countries, has gone hand in hand with increased trade in order to reduce the risks associated with increased openness. And, as a recent OECD (2000) study showed, some poor countries have been better at protecting freedom of association than others at similar income levels. For example, even though they have similar (low) levels of income, Egypt is in the OECD's worst category for freedom of association, and has much higher rates of child labor and female illiteracy than Suriname, which is in the OECD's best category for freedom of association (OECD, 2000, 28). The feared race to the bottom has not inevitably occurred, even as trade has exploded.

We view the historical pattern of trade and labor standards improving together not as an aberration but as supporting the notion that they are indeed complements. Consistent with our view, an OECD study (1996, 109–12) of the interactions between the development of trade and labor standards across countries showed a generally positive relation. The authors looked at trade liberalization in 44 countries from 1980 to 1994 to see whether there had been any pattern in the sequencing of reforms, as well as changes in freedom of association and bargaining rights. They found no clear pattern between trade reform and subsequent changes in labor standards; but they noted that by the mid-1990s, the relatively more open countries had better standards, while the most restrictive trade regimes had been more likely to repress freedom of association. Excluding six countries with insufficient information on labor rights, trade reforms had in no cases been followed by a worsening of labor rights, and in no cases had improved labor rights impeded trade reform. Thus, they concluded that there is a "mutually supportive relationship between successfully sustained trade reforms and improvements in association and bargaining rights" (ibid., 112). In a similar vein, Rodrik (1999; 2000, 1) has argued that lowering trade barriers reduces opportunities for corruption and "creates a new set of stakeholders while disenfranchising the previous ones." Among those new stakeholders are workers in export sectors and the consumers of their products.

Two Successful Trade–Labor Linkages

Proponents of the unfettered globalization view of the world often assume that labor standards will rise more or less automatically with incomes, so that no external intervention is needed (or desirable) to improve standards over time. They hope (believe) that even in authoritarian regimes, economic openness will promote political openness and higher labor standards, so that there is no need for external pressures from the world trading community. However, we find this argument unacceptable. The issue is not whether economic development can facilitate political freedom and rising labor standards in the long run, but whether in the interim decades or century, external pressures linked to trade can accelerate the process or target particularly severe problems. The question that deserves attention is whether advanced countries can use trade as a means to improve standards in the here and now.

Below, we discuss two cases from the 1990s that which show how trade leverage can improve labor conditions in some settings.[10] These two examples involve the United States and other nations; they were chosen as cases we know well. Similar cases exist for Europe and other actors. The first case involves child labor in Bangladesh, where threats of boycotts led to changes that improved the lives of poor children. The second shows how the promise of market access was used to improve conditions in the garment sector of Cambodia.

The Bangladeshi garment sector. In 1993, U.S. Senator Tom Harkin (Democrat, of Iowa) introduced the Child Labor Deterrence Act to bar the importation of manufactured goods from any foreign industry that uses child labor (exclusive of agriculture and other family work). In that same year, a U.S. television show ran a story showing children in a Bangladeshi factory who were sewing clothing destined for Wal-Mart. Fearing that they would lose access to the U.S. market, which accounts for 43% of their total apparel exports, the Bangladesh Garment Manufacturers and Exporters Association entered into negotiations with U.S. nongovernmental organizations, with input from U.S. Ambassador David Merrill, on how to respond.

Pharis Harvey (1995), the executive director of the International Labor Rights Fund (ILRF) and the cochair of the U.S. Child Labor Coalition, has described how the proposed Harkin bill and nongovernmental organizations' threats of a consumer boycott got the Bangladeshi association to address the child labor problem constructively. From Harvey's perspective, the negotiations waxed and waned, depending on the seriousness with which the Bangladesh Garment Manufacturers and Exporters Association viewed the threat of U.S. sanctions. After the Republican Party won control of the U.S. Congress in 1994, the talks stalled. In May 1995, the Bangladeshi association's members rejected a cooperative agreement that had been negotiated and, to avoid potential trade sanctions, agreed to fire all underage workers by the end of October. Shortly afterward, the Child Labor Coalition, which had threatened a consumer boycott of Bangladeshi clothing if an agreement was not reached, mailed a notice of the boycott to its members and to the U.S. and Bangladeshi press. Negotiations resumed 4 days later. At this stage, the ILO and UNICEF (the United Nations Children's Fund) joined the negotiations, and on July 4, those two organizations signed a memorandum of understanding with the Bangladesh Garment Manufacturers and Exporters Association providing that all children working in the sector would be removed, but not until schools were available for them, and that no new children would be hired. The parties also agreed on joint funding and a monitoring plan to be overseen by the

ILO. Since the memorandum of understanding was signed in 1995, 353 schools have been created, and the incidence of child labor in Bangladeshi garment factories has dropped dramatically.

This case underscores the power of trade threats to get the attention of factory owners who use child labor. Equally important, it shows the value of international cooperation to ensure that those children will have a better future. It is important to appreciate that both the nongovernmental organizations and international organizations concerned with child labor issues are acutely aware that children and their families can be made worse off if sanctions are imposed or the children are simply thrown out into the street. Harvey (1995) has also emphasized that the Child Labor Coalition recognized the riskiness of boycotts, in part because they are difficult to remove when conditions improve and in part because they are the last resort in the case of utterly intransigent exporters or governments. Even with the good intentions of the ILRF and the Child Labor Coalition, moreover, the agreement would have been difficult to reach—and virtually impossible to enforce—without the involvement of the ILO and UNICEF and the resources that they could bring to the table.

The U.S.–Cambodia bilateral textiles agreement. In 1998, the United States and Cambodia signed a 3-year bilateral textiles agreement in which U.S. negotiators offered to expand Cambodia's export quota by 14% if "working conditions in the Cambodia textile and apparel sector substantially compl[ied] with" local law and internationally recognized core standards. In their first review in December 1999, U.S. officials concluded that "substantial compliance" had not been achieved but that progress had been made. The United States offered a lesser 5% quota increase, conditioned on Cambodia reaching agreement with the ILO on an independent monitoring program.

Some ILO officials were initially leery of the proposal, fearing that external monitoring would further weaken the existing local capacity. The ILO agreed to the plan only after gaining a commitment from U.S. officials to provide $500,000 for a parallel program to provide technical assistance and training to the Cambodian labor ministry. The United States also provided $1 million of the $1.4 million cost of the 3-year monitoring program, with the Cambodian government and Garment Manufacturers' Association of Cambodia splitting the balance (Office of the U.S. Trade Representative press release, May 18, 2000). U.S. officials granted the initial 5% quota expansion in May 2000 and added another 4% the following September, in recognition of further improvements in workers' rights. The total 9% quota expansion was extended for 2001, but the remaining 5% potential increase was withheld as an incentive for continued improvements (*Inside U.S. Trade*, January 19, 2001).

The Cambodian government viewed the arrangement as a way to gain trade quotas and to improve standards for its workers. Commerce Minister Cham Prasidh told the *Wall Street Journal* (February 28, 2000, 1) that Cambodia was interested in more than just the quota increase and said, "We didn't want foreign factories taking advantage of our workers either." However, other developing countries and U.S. importers discouraged Cambodia from accepting the bargain because they opposed any precedent linking trade and labor standards, even if it made that country and its workers better off. U.S. importers claimed that Cambodia was benefiting little, if at all, from the agreement because the initial quota level was set below that of other comparable exporting countries (*Inside U.S. Trade,* February 5, 1999, 13).[11] After the initial decision not to grant the full quota increase, critics claimed that the United States was not sincere and that U.S. decisions were driven by unions with protectionist motives. When the partial quota increases were granted in 2000 and 2001, however, the Union of Needletrades, Industrial and Textile Employees (UNITE) supported the decision, while the American Textile Manufacturers Institute, representing the industry, opposed it (*Inside U.S. Trade,* January 19, 2001).

The agreement appears to have improved conditions in the Cambodian garment sector. Although hours remain gruelingly long and wages low, and although enforcement of standards is invariably spotty, wages and benefits have improved, and the Cambodian government has stepped up monitoring of factories in the sector, according to the *Wall Street Journal* (February 28, 2000, 1) and the *Financial Times* (April 7, 2000, 5). Perhaps most important, the incentives in the agreement, the resulting ILO presence, and the knowledge gained by the workers regarding their rights have given workers the confidence to stand up for their own rights by forming unions and demanding changes when they feel conditions are not acceptable, as reported in the previous sources and in *Time* ([Asian edition], July 10, 2000). Since 1997, 75 garment factories have been organized by unions, and in July 2000, garment workers successfully pressured the government to establish Cambodia's first minimum wage ($45 per month, according to the *New York Times* [July 12, 2001]). In January 2002, the Bush administration extended the agreement for another 3 years but declined to say whether it would negotiate similar provisions in agreements with other countries, such as Vietnam (www.ustr.gov).

Using International Organizations to Improve Labor Conditions in Less Developed Countries

The continued debate over standards and trade notwithstanding, global labor standards are being adopted throughout the world. In the 1990s more countries signed ILO conventions, which are more detailed and specific than the declaration on fundamental principles, than ever before. Between 1991 and the first half of 2002, the total number of all conventions ratified by countries grew from 5555 to 7013. A campaign to promote ratification of selected core conventions launched in 1994 to mark the 75th anniversary of the ILO's founding increased the number from 800 to nearly 1000.[12] And ratifications of the core convention condemning the worst forms of child labor were coming in at the fastest rate in ILO history.

Poor countries as well as rich ones are ratifying conventions, though there are some notable outliers among rich countries, such as the United States (Fig. 12–1). But ratification does not mean that countries comply with standards (Chau and Kanbur, 2001). Enforcement lags behind ratification for a number of reasons, ranging from corruption to lack of adequate enforcement resources in most countries and political opposition to independent unions by authoritarian regimes in some. It is not enough for the world community to gain agreement to standards. The ILO and the world trade system need mechanisms and resources to help less developed countries overcome barriers to compliance.

Building these mechanisms and resources requires, first of all, improved information about standards and their enforcement. Workers have to know they have rights before they can take action to assert those rights and to improve conditions. Recognizing this, the ILO, the ICFTU, and national trade union organizations recently launched a global campaign to post a list of the core worker rights in every workplace in the world.

Consumers also need information in order to reward "good" firms and punish "bad" ones by their buying decisions and thereby harness market power to raise labor standards globally. As noted earlier, surveys suggest that consumers care about the conditions under which the goods they buy are produced, but they typically lack the information to act on their preferences. Nongovernmental organizations play a crucial intermediary role in gathering such information and presenting it to consumers compellingly. As a result of the growing antisweatshop movement in recent years, a variety of nongovernmental organizations, public–private partnerships, and for-profit organizations have

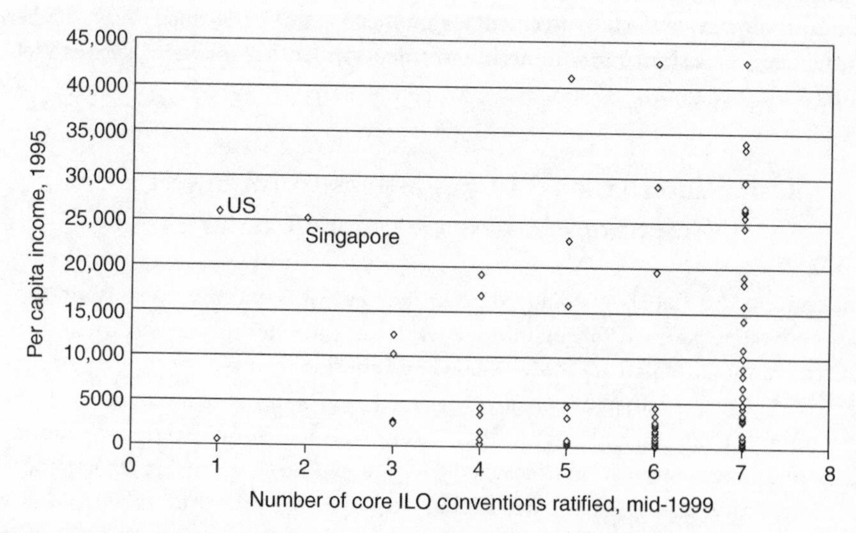

Figure 12–1. Convention Ratification and Income. N = 77. Correlation coefficient = 0.09; excluding US and Singapore = 0.22. Source: OECD (2000)

emerged to provide monitoring and verification services to help consumers find products meeting minimum standards (Elliott and Freeman, 2003b).

Finally, information is essential for governments, the ILO, and other international organizations to bring pressure on recalcitrant governments to improve their compliance with standards. Enforcement of law, standards, and norms relies on publicity, rewards, and penalties, and the use of each of those tools must be based on accurate and compelling information. Both the WTO and the ILO recognize the importance of information. The WTO uses the Trade Policy Review Mechanism, a form of peer review, to catalog and publicize each member's trade barriers in the hope that this information will stimulate pressures for further liberalization from those who bear the costs—both at home and abroad (www.wto.org/english/tratop_e/tpr_e/tpr_e.htm). Traditionally, the ILO has relied largely on publicity, through an extensive supervisory mechanism, and on rewards, in the form of technical assistance, to countries that seek to improve standards. In 1998, the ILO expanded its scrutiny of core labor standards around the world when its members approved the Declaration on Fundamental Principles and Rights at Work.

The ILO: From Paper Tiger to Mighty Mouse?

Despite its constitutional structures for monitoring and review, the ILO for many years was the weak sister of international organizations, with little money or authority. The agency, which was created as part of the League of Nations in 1919 and then incorporated into the United Nations system, was caught for many years between the ongoing struggles of communist countries with capitalist ones, industry with labor, and advanced countries with less developed countries. During the cold war it lost considerable moral authority and suffered from the U.S. withdrawal, from 1977 to 1980, from the agency.

One unanticipated benefit from the trade–labor debate in the 1990s has been increased support for the ILO and progress in strengthening its tools for improving labor standards, including the drafting of international conventions, technical assistance and advice on national laws, and supervision of compliance with international norms (Elliott, 2000, 2001). Proponents of the unfettered globalization view regard a strengthened ILO as less dangerous to free trade than tying standards to trade through the WTO or related agreements. The WTO's Dispute Settlement Understanding is more formalized and binding than the ILO's complaints system, with WTO trade retaliation explicitly serving as the ultimate sanction to enforce the rules. Perhaps at the next world trading conference, the dark-suited functionaries will offer their own "Hey, hey, ho, ho, give more money to the ILO" chants in response to those of the protestors. However, U.S. President George W. Bush proposed cutting funds for the ILO in his first two budgets (ILO, 2002).

For its part, the ILO has raised the profile of its supervision of core labor standards and approved a new convention calling for immediate action against the worst forms of child labor. For the first time in its history, the ILO has moved toward penalizing countries that flagrantly contravene core labor standards. Article 33 of the ILO constitution provides that if satisfactory compliance is not forthcoming, "the Governing Body may recommend to the International Labor Conference such action as it may deem wise and expedient to secure compliance therewith." In 1999, the International Labor Conference, at which ILO members sit in plenary to make administrative and policy decisions, suspended technical assistance to Burma and barred it from most meetings. A year later, the conference recommended that members take action to ensure that their relations with Burma did not in any way support the use of forced labor.

In a major step toward increased transparency, the follow-up mechanism for implementing the "Declaration on Fundamental Principles and Rights at Work," which spelled out the four core labor standards, requires that all governments report on the consistency of their laws and practices with these standards, regardless of whether they have ratified the related conventions (for details, see www.ilo.org/public/english/standards/decl/index.htm). And the ILO director general's "global report" assesses the overall status of each of the core standards (one per year in a 4-year cycle) and highlights specific problems in particular countries. Though criticized for "naming names" when the first report was released in 2000, Director General Juan Somavia insisted that specificity was critical to the credibility of the process. This process may already have borne fruit, as Saudi Arabia, which, along with its Gulf neighbors, was sharply criticized in the global report for barring unions, announced in early 2001 that it would permit the formation of "worker organizations."

Another objective of the follow-up mechanism is to identify priorities for ILO technical assistance, and donor governments have responded. Financial support for ILO technical assistance increased from $76 million in 1999 to $121 million in 2000, with the International Program for Elimination of Child Labor being the major beneficiary. In recent years, the resulting increase in the activities of this program has been evident in various countries through tangible progress in moving children from work to school or rehabilitation programs. Prominent cases include the Bangladeshi garment sector and the Pakistani production of soccer balls and surgical instruments (Elliott and Freeman, 2003b). But to sustain these activities and to expand them into other areas, the ILO will need further funding increases, as well as institutional reforms to make it an activist agency rather than a passive one.

The Somavia administration at the ILO has struggled to energize the organization, but turning around a large bureaucracy is difficult. Even with its renewed activism, ILO supervision of core labor standards compliance relies mainly on self-reporting by governments or on complaints from self-selected constituent monitors. The extent to which the ILO moves from being a paper tiger to a real player will be judged in part on whether its actions on Burma and in naming violators' names become the norm or are aberrations. At the same time, the ILO must balance the need to confront larger and more powerful members that violate labor standards with a pragmatic concern for the limits of ILO leverage and the costs of picking fights it cannot win.

Labor Standards in Trade Agreements

Many adherents to the global standards view of the world insist that the only way to give teeth to standards is to include them in trade agreements and to use trade sanctions to enforce them. In 1984, the U.S. Congress added workers' rights conditions to the U.S. Generalized System of Preferences, which grants preferential trade benefits to developing countries. In the Omnibus Trade and Competitiveness Act of 1988, Congress also added labor rights to the list of U.S. negotiating objectives for the Uruguay Round of multilateral trade negotiations, but to no effect. During the 1992 presidential campaign, candidate Bill Clinton insisted that a side agreement on labor standards (as well as one on environmental issues) was the price of his support for the North American Free Trade Agreement. The resulting North American Agreement on Labor Cooperation relies on "monetary assessments" rather than sanctions and requires only that member countries enforce their own labor laws. It has resulted mainly in studies and consultations between the American and Mexican labor ministries. At this writing, no dispute has been referred to an arbitral panel that could impose penalties for nonenforcement.[13]

At the end of President Clinton's second term, U.S. trade negotiators agreed with Jordan to include labor and environmental issues in the main text of an agreement creating a bilateral free trade area and to make those provisions subject to the same dispute resolution procedures, including the possibility of sanctions, as in all other parts of the agreement. Although the U.S.–Jordan free trade agreement has hortatory language encouraging the parties to strive to comply with core labor standards as identified by the ILO, neither agreement establishes minimum, internationally accepted standards that must be met as part of the deal. Despite the relatively weak language, proponents of labor standards in trade agreements welcomed the Jordanian deal as a precedent, and many Republicans and members of the business community strongly opposed it for the same reason (*Inside U.S. Trade*, October 27, 2000). The agreement, which was motivated primarily by foreign policy concerns, was approved in the wake of the September 11, 2001, attacks on the World Trade Center in New York City and the Pentagon in Washington, D.C.

In the WTO, members from less developed countries have resisted U.S. entreaties even to create a working group on labor issues, much less to consider how labor standards could be incorporated into trade discussions. While unions and some nongovernmental organizations in these countries generally support international efforts to raise labor standards in their countries, they typically share the concerns of their governments about linking enforcement to trade agreements for fear that such authority would be abused for protectionist purposes. The European Union and some individual member states have also criticized the unwillingness of the United States to rule out the use of trade sanctions to enforce labor standards. And the WTO has refused requests to consider trade-related labor standards when conducting trade policy reviews, leading the ICFTU to take up the task in recent years (the reports are available on their website at www.icftu.org).

As the trade agenda moves beyond reciprocal tariff concessions to rule writing, it is not clear how effective its enforcement powers will prove to be in any new areas. The pressures to allow for more flexibility in the implementation of the agreement on intellectual property, particularly with respect to drugs, is only the most prominent example of the problems the WTO is increasingly likely to face as it expands into behind-the-border regulatory areas.

In short, both the ILO and the WTO, by themselves, have problems advancing their agendas, and this fact puts at risk both further globalization and the enforcement of global labor standards. To move the globalization-standards issue to a new and more fruitful plane, these organizations should harness the natural complementarity between globalization and standards. The place to do that, in our view, is in export processing zones.

Making Export Processing Zones a Beacon of Standards

Export processing zones are the most readily identifiable face of globalization. According to the ILO (1998), there were 845 such zones around the world in 1997, more than half in North America (320) and Asia (225) and another 133 in Latin America and the Caribbean. The specific features of export processing zones—whether they are physically isolated, industry specific, or more integrated into the local economy—vary widely from country to country. But they all share the aim of attracting foreign investment and creating jobs by promoting exports, and they use similar incentives, including tax holidays and duty-free imports, dedicated infrastructure, and, in labor-intensive sectors, low labor costs. Given these characteristics, export processing zones are a logical place for the ILO and the WTO to work together to demonstrate that trade and labor standards can raise living standards in poor countries.

A few countries explicitly apply lower labor standards in the zones than in the rest of the economy. The website for Bangladeshi export processing zones, for example, advertises its "production-oriented labour laws," including prohibitions on unions and on strikes within the zones (www.bangladesh-epz.com/p_law.htm). More often, however, governments look the other way or engage in de facto collusion with export processing zone investors to discourage union organizing in the zones, and they make little effort to enforce national labor laws in these areas (ICFTU, 1996; ILO, 1998; Romero, 1995; U.S. Department of Labor, 1989–90). By guaranteeing freedom of association and by helping countries—or pressuring them to—enforce labor codes in these zones, the world trading community and the ILO could restore badly needed credibility to the international trading system.

In addition, some export processing zones are likely to decline in importance when the Multi-Fiber Arrangement is phased out in 2005. Under this agreement, the United States and the European Union restrict imports of textiles and apparel through an elaborate system of country-specific import quotas. This has the effect of creating a comparative advantage for low-productivity countries simply because they have unfilled quotas, while potentially more productive suppliers are quota constrained. Combined with China's entry into the WTO in 2002, the Multi-Fiber Arrangement phaseout could mean that many smaller countries relying on low-wage, low-skill labor to produce apparel will no longer be competitive.

In the new competitive environment for textile and apparel exports, increased productivity and higher quality will be more important, putting a premium on increased worker training and relatively peaceful industrial relations. Thus, a joint WTO–ILO project to make export processing zones a best-practice model in core labor standards compliance, funded by developed countries and the World Bank, could assist poor countries in adapting to the Multi-Fiber Arrangement phaseout and moving up the development ladder.

The starting point for such a project should be a baseline survey of standards in export processing zones, to be done either by the WTO and the ILO or by the ILO itself. Either way, the result should be a website that lists basic facts about export processing zones in various countries—whether labor laws apply equally in and outside zones, unionization rates in zones and the rest of the country, average hours and wages, accident rates, the percentage of women in the labor force, and so forth. While increased human and financial resources would be required, improving the collection and dissemination of such data is already an ILO objective, and this project could be used to give further momentum to that effort. This would provide the world community—from governments to consumers to human rights activists—with the information on which to base decisions.

The next task for such a project would be for the ILO to develop operational criteria for the term *best practice* in labor standards. If the ILO were accorded sufficient resources to do credible monitoring, it could develop a certification system for export processing zones or (given likely country politicking against such an official system) at least provide the information so that nongovernmental organizations and others could provide the appropriate scoring system, much as the Fraser Foundation, the Heritage Foundation, and Freedom House rate countries on their economic and political freedoms. Certification would provide useful information to investors looking for a stable and productive industrial relations environment and to consumers who prefer products made under decent conditions. (For a discussion of the potential obstacles to and limitations of this proposal, see Elliott and Freeman, 2003a, Chapters 2 and 3.)

Finally, as a last resort, export processing zones (or firms within them) with egregious violations of core standards could be subject to trade restrictions. This approach also could be negotiated (in theory, at least) in the ILO and without WTO participation, as has occurred with various multilateral environmental agreements. But the WTO *should* also be involved. After all, its job is to discipline trade distortions. Violations of core labor standards that are meant to attract foreign investment or to promote exports are a trade distortion as much as subsidies or other forms of aid to traded sectors, and the WTO should not ignore them (Elliott and Freeman, 2003a, Chapter 4).

With or without the WTO, however, trade measures to enforce labor standards are unlikely to be a significant part of any global labor standards initiative. The not wholly unfounded fear of developing countries that such measures would be manipulated to discriminate against their exports makes the issue simply too sensitive. Moreover, the benefits of a transparency project such as that just described should not be underestimated. Some countries might be shamed into changing particularly egregious practices, while others might decide to market themselves as reputationally less risky for large brand-name retailers and as having more stable labor relations.

Conclusion

"The impact of economic growth depends much on how the *fruits* of economic growth are used . . . success depends on the growth process being wide-based and economically broad" (Sen, 1999, 43, 46).

The main theme of this chapter is that globalization and labor standards are intrinsically linked. Globalization moves the world production frontier to higher levels. For this reason, opposition to globalization is ultimately harmful to workers in less developed countries. Standards can help transform such an upward shift in production possibilities into enhancement of the well-being of those in greatest need, rather than benefiting, largely or entirely, those who already have relatively good living conditions. For this reason, opposition to improved labor standards in those countries is also harmful to workers.

As a result of globalization, there is a great opportunity to advance growth and to distribute the fruits of growth widely and broadly. What the global economy needs is to put the globalization and standards agendas together into a unified package for raising living standards around the world. Trade policy reform should be part of a broader set of institutional reforms because development requires not only "getting the prices right," as proponents of unfettered globalization believe, but also getting behavior right, as proponents of labor standards believe. Trade and standards are sufficiently linked that they can do much more good together than if they are pushed separately.

ACKNOWLEDGMENT
The authors would like to thank Jody Heymann, an anonymous reviewer, and J. David Richardson for their thoughtful and very helpful comments on this chapter. The opinions herein are those of the authors alone and do not necessarily reflect the views of any of the institutions with which they are affiliated.

Notes

1. Some southern criticisms of abolitionists during the era of slavery resemble arguments made today against labor standards being forced on poor countries: "The pilgrim zealots of

New England, with 'humanity' and 'philanthropy' upon their lips, and jealousy and hatred of the southern labor system stamped upon their hearts, make war upon the constitutional rights of fifteen free, sovereign, and independent States, to gratify their malice and glorify their immaculateness (hypocrisy), *at the expense of others*—invariably in the name, and professedly on the behalf, but always to the irreparable injury and disadvantage of, the negro race" (T. W. MacMahon, *Cause and Contrast: An Essay on the American Crisis* [Richmond, VA.: West and Johnston, 1862], 64).

2. http://www.globalmarch.org/worstformsreport/ratification/182.html. Accessed November 10, 2001.

3. Freedom House (2001) rates China, Burma, and Vietnam as "not free" countries and ranks Singapore, Malaysia, and Turkey as only "partly free," which, relative to the "free" category, means that "the level of oppression increases, especially in the areas of censorship, political terror, and the *prevention of free association.*"

4. We can only surmise that large numbers of consumers in other countries also support global labor standards, because we are not aware of similar polls outside the United States and the United Kingdom. But there is evidence of these concerns, particularly in Europe, where the *fair trade* movement, which seeks to ensure a minimum price and decent working conditions for small farmers and artisans in developing countries, began. There are also numerous efforts in Europe to promote codes of corporate conduct incorporating minimum labor standards, including the Ethical Trade Initiative in the United Kingdom and the Clean Clothes Campaign in the Netherlands, and elsewhere.

5. Dollar and Gatti (2000) and Klasen (2000) provided empirical evidence on the links between gender discrimination and growth, income inequality, and development. The case studies and a summary of the report, *Engendering Development*, are available on the World Bank's website, www.worldbank.org

6. The ILO pointed to wildcat strikes and other instances of labor unrest as evidence that a worker demand for more or better representation exists in the export processing zones. Indeed, if lower unionization in export processing zones were a matter of worker preference, the governments and employers would not have to enact policies that make union organization more difficult than in the rest of the economy.

7. More comprehensive surveys of the effects of core labor standards as they relate to trade may be found in OECD (1996, 2000), Maskus (1997), and Brown (2000).

8. The union rights variable becomes only marginally significant with this specification. For further analysis, see Elliott and Freeman (2003a).

9. Countries in the analysis were Argentina, Brazil, the Dominican Republic, Ecuador, Fiji, Guatemala, Honduras, South Korea, Panama, Peru, the Philippines, Suriname, Thailand, Uruguay, and Venezuela.

10. Another similar case involved soccer balls produced with child labor in Pakistan. That case is not summarized here for reasons of space, but information on it can be found in Elliott (2001) and U.S. Department of Labor (1998).

11. It is difficult to test this claim, but data on quota levels elsewhere in Southeast Asia do not appear to support it. Using per capita textile and apparel exports under the Multi-Fiber Arrangement as a crude measure, the figure for Cambodia was 24 square meters (M2) per person, which compares to 8.2 M2 per person for Association of Southeast Asian Nations as a whole, 9 for Bangladesh, 12.4 for the Philippines, 21.3 for Thailand, and 5 for Indonesia (Department of Commerce, Office of Textiles and Apparel, "Major Shippers Report," March 2001; International Monetary Fund [2001]).

12. The increase from 1989 to 1994 is almost entirely due to accessions by former members of the Soviet Union, the former Yugoslav federation, and other members of the Communist bloc.

13. In the years since the North American Free Trade Agreement was negotiated, Canada has signed bilateral trade agreements with Chile and Costa Rica that include provisions on labor standards similar to those in the North American Free Trade Agreement side agreement and enforceable through the assessment of fines only in the former case (Elliott, 2001). [We are not aware of any other trade agreements that address labor standards.]

References

Aidt, T., and Z. Tzannatos. 2002. *Unions and collective bargaining: Economic effects in a global environment.* Washington, D.C.: World Bank.

Becker, G. S. 1971. *The economics of discrimination.* Chicago: University of Chicago Press.

Bhagwati, J. 1995. Trade liberalisation and "fair trade" demands: Addressing the environmental and labour standards issues. *World Economy* 18(6): 745–59.

Brown, D. 2000. International trade and core labour standards: A survey of the recent literature. Labour Market and Social Policy Occasional Papers No. 43, DEELSA/ELSA/WD (2000) 4, October. Paris: Organization for Economic Cooperation and Development.

Brown, D., A. V. Deardorff, and R. M. Stern. 1996. International labor standards and trade: A theoretical analysis. In *Fair trade and harmonization: Prerequisites for free trade?*, edited by J. N. Bhagwati and R. E. Hudec. Cambridge, MA: MIT Press.

Catholic Agencies for Overseas Development. 1997. *Attitudes towards ethical shopping.* Research study conducted by MORI, London.

Charnovitz, S. 1987. The influence of international labour standards on the world trading system: A historical overview. *International Labour Review* 126(5): 565–84.

Chau, N. C., and R. Kanbur. 2000. The race to the bottom, from the bottom. Ithaca, NY: Cornell University, Department of Applied Economics and Management.

Chau, N. C., and R. Kanbur. 2001. The adoption of international labor standards conventions: Who, when, and why? Conference presentation prepared for the Brookings Trade Forum, Washington, D.C., May.

Dollar, D., and R. Gatti. 2000. Gender inequality, income, and growth: Are good times good for women? Working paper no. 1, Policy Research Report on Gender and Development. Washington, D.C.: World Bank.

Dollar, D., and A. Kraay. 2001. *Trade, growth, and poverty.* Development Research Group. Washington, D.C.: World Bank.

Elliott, K. A. 2000. Getting beyond no: Promoting worker rights and trade. In *The WTO after Seattle,* edited by J. J. Schott. Washington, D.C.: Institute for International Economics.

Elliott, K. A. 2001. The ILO and enforcement of core labor standards. International economics policy brief no. PB00-6 (updated April 2001), Institute for International Economics, Washington, D.C.

Elliott, K. A., and R. B. Freeman. 2003a. *Can labor standards improve under globalization?* Washington, D.C.: Institute for International Economics.

Elliott, K. A., and R. B. Freeman. 2003b. White hats or Don Quixotes: Human rights vigilantes in the global economy. In *Emerging labor market institutions for the 21st century,* edited by R. B. Freeman, J. Hersch, and L. Mishel. Chicago: University of Chicago Press for the National Bureau of Economic Research.

Forteza, A., and M. Rama. 2000. Labor market rigidity and the success of economic reforms across more than 100 countries. Working paper no. 2521. Washington, D.C.: World Bank.

Frankel, J. A., and D. Romer. 1999. Does trade cause growth? *American Economic Review* 89(3): 379–99.

Freedom House. 2001. *Freedom in the world.* Available from www.freedomhouse.org

Freeman, R. B. 1993. Labor market institutions and policies: Help or hindrance to economic development? In *Proceedings of the World Bank annual conference on development economics 1992.* Washington, D.C.: World Bank.

Freeman, R. B. 1996. International labor standards and world trade? Friend or foe? In *The world trading system: Challenges ahead,* edited by J. Schott. Washington, D.C.: Institute for International Economics.

Freeman, R., and D. L. Lindauer. 1999. Why not Africa? Working paper no. 6942. Cambridge, MA: National Bureau of Economic Research.

Green, F., A. Dickerson, and J. Saba Arbache. 2000. A picture of wage inequality and the allocation of labour through a period of trade liberalisation: The case of Brazil. Study 00/13, Department of Economics, University of Kent, Canterbury, UK.

Harrison, A., and G. Hanson. 1999. Who gains from trade reform? Some remaining puzzles. Working paper no. 6915. Cambridge, MA: National Bureau of Economic Research.

Harvey, P. 1995. Historic breakthrough for Bangladesh kids endangered by industry inaction. *Worker Rights News* no. 12 (August): 1.

International Confederation of Free Trade Unions (ICFTU). 1996. *Behind the wire: Anti-union repression in the export processing zones.* Brussels: ICFTU.

International Labor Organization (ILO). 2002. Washington Report: Congress Sets Funding for Child Labor, *ILO Focus,* vol. 15, no. 1, Spring 2002. Available at: http://www.US. ilo.org

International Labor Office, International Labor Organization (ILO). 1998. Labour and social issues relating to export processing zones. Report for discussion at the Tripartite Meeting of Export Processing Zones—Operating Countries (TMEPZ/1998). Geneva: ILO.

International Labor Office, International Labor Organization (ILO). 2001. *Stopping forced labor.* Global report under follow-up to the Declaration on Fundamental Principles and Rights at Work. Presented by the director-general to the International Labor Conference, Geneva, June.

International Monetary Fund. 2001. International Financial Statistics, various issues. Washington, D.C.: IMF.

Klasen, S. 2000. Does gender inequality reduce growth and development? Evidence from cross-country regressions. Working paper no. 7, Policy Research Report on Gender and Development. Washington, D.C.: World Bank.

Mah, J. S. 1997. Core labour standards and export performance in developing countries. *World Economy* 20(6): 773–85.

Martin, W., and K. E. Maskus. 1999. Core labor standards and competitiveness: Implications for global trade policy. October 4. Washington, D.C.: World Bank.

Maskus, K. E. 1997. Should core labor standards be imposed through trade policy? Policy research working paper no. 1817, August. Washington, D.C.: World Bank.

Morici, P., with E. Schulz. 2001. *Labor standards in the global trading system.* Washington, D.C.: Economic Strategy Institute.

Office of the United States Trade Representative, 2000. Press release 00-39, "USTRAnnounces Apparel Quota Increase for Cambodia." Washington, D.C.: Office of the United States Trade Representative, May 18. Available at http://www.ustr.gov

Organization for Economic Cooperation and Development (OECD). 1995. *Trade and labour standards: A review of the issues.* Paris: OECD.

Organization for Economic Cooperation and Development (OECD). 1996. *Trade, employment, and labour standards: A study of core workers' rights and international trade.* Paris: OECD.

Organization for Economic Cooperation and Development (OECD). 2000. *International trade and core labour standards.* Paris: OECD.

Palley, T. I. 1999. The beneficial effect of core labor standards on economic growth. Technical working paper no. T010, Public Policy Department. Washington, D.C.: AFL-CIO.

Paul-Majumder, P., and A. Begum. 2000. The gender imbalances in the export oriented garment industry in Bangladesh. Background paper for the World Bank policy research report *Engendering development.* Washington, D.C.: World Bank.

Portes, A. 1994. By-passing the rules: The dialectics of labour standards and informalization in less developed countries. In *International labour standards and economic interdependence,* edited by W. Sengenberger and D. Campbell. Geneva: International Institute for Labour Studies.

Rama, M. 2001. "Globalization, Inequality and the Labor Market Policies," Development Research Group, June 23. Washington, D.C.: World Bank.

Rama, M., and G. Tabellini. 1995. Endogenous distortions in product and labor markets. Working paper no. 1413. Washington, D.C.: World Bank.

Revenga, A. 1995. Employment and wage effects of trade liberalization: The case of Mexican manufacturing. Working paper no. 1524. Washington, D.C.: World Bank.

Robbins, D. 1994. Worsening relative wage dispersion in Chile during trade liberalisation and its causes: Is supply at fault? Discussion paper no. 484. Cambridge, MA: Harvard Institute for International Development.

Robbins, D., and T. H. Gindling. 1999. Trade liberalisation and the relative wages of more skilled workers in Costa Rica. *Review of Development Economics* 3: 140–54.

Robertson, R. 2000. Trade liberalisation and wage inequality: Lessons from the Mexican experience. *World Development* 23(6): 827–49.

Rodriguez, F., and D. Rodrik. 2001. Trade policy and economic growth: A skeptic's guide to the cross-national evidence. In *NBER macroeconomic annual 2000.* Cambridge, MA: National Bureau for Economic Research.

Rodrik, D. 1996. Labor standards in international trade: Do they matter and what to do about them. In *Emerging agenda for global trade: High stakes for developing countries,* edited by R. Z. Lawrence, D. Rodrik, and J. Whalley. Policy essay no. 20. Washington, D.C.: Overseas Development Council.

Rodrik, D. 1997. *Has globalization gone too far?* Washington, D.C.: Institute for International Economics.

Rodrik, D. 1999. *The new global economy and developing countries: Making openness work.* Policy essay no. 24. Washington, D.C.: Overseas Development Council.

Rodrik, D. 2000. Trade policy reform as institutional reform. Cambridge, MA: Harvard University.

Romero, A. T. 1995. Labour standards and export processing zones: Situation and pressure for change. *Development Policy Review* 13: 247–76.

Sen, A. 1999. *Development as freedom.* New York: Knopf.

Srinivasan, T. N. 1994. International labor standards once again!" In *International labor standards and global economic integration: Proceedings of a symposium.* Washington, D.C.: Bureau of International Labor Affairs.

Srinivasan, T. N., and J. Bhagwati. 1999. Outward-orientation and development: Are revisionists right? Festchrift in honor of Anne Kreuger, September. Available at: http://www.columbia.edu/~jb38/Krueger.pdf

Stiglitz, J. 2000. Democratic development as the fruits of labor. Keynote address, Industrial Relations Research Association, Boston, January 8.

Tallontire, A., E. Rentsendorj, and M. Blowfield. 2001. *Ethical consumers and ethical trade: A review of current literature.* Policy series 12. Chatham, UK: Natural Resources Institute.

University of Maryland, Program on International Policy Attitudes. 2000. *Americans on glob-*

alization: A study of public attitudes. College Park, MD: University of Maryland. Available from www.pipa.org/OnlineReports/Globalization/global_rep.html

U.S. Department of Commerce, Office of Textiles and Apparel, 2001. Major shippers report. March. Washington, D.C.: Department of Commerce.

U.S. Department of Labor, Bureau of International Labor Affairs. 1989–90. *Foreign labor trends: Worker rights in export processing zones.* FLT 90-32. Washington, D.C.: Government Printing Office.

U.S. Department of Labor, Bureau of International Labor Affairs. 1998. *By the sweat and toil of children: Efforts to eliminate child labor,* Vol. 5. Washington, D.C.: U.S. Department of Labor.

World Bank. 2001. *Engendering development through gender equality in rights, resources, and voice.* Research policy report. Washington, D.C.: World Bank.

Index